C. SCHMITT ▮ I. DEISENHOFER ▮ B. ZRENNER ▮ (Eds.)

Catheter Ablation of Cardiac Arrhythmias

C. SCHMITT I. DEISENHOFER B. ZRENNER (Eds.)

Catheter Ablation of Cardiac Arrhythmias

A Practical Approach

WITH 201 FIGURES IN 400 SEPARATE ILLUSTRATIONS, MOST IN COLOR AND 16 TABLES

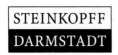

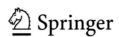

Prof. Dr. med. Claus Schmitt
Dr. med. Isabel Deisenhofer
Dr. med. Bernhard Zrenner
Deutsches Herzzentrum München
Lazarettstraße 36
80636 München
Germany

ISBN 3-7985-1575-1 Steinkopff Verlag Darmstadt

Cataloging-in-Publication Data applied for
A catalog record for this book is available from the Library of Congress.
Bibliographic information published by Die Deutsche Bibliothek.
Die Deutsche Bibliothek lists this publication in the Deutsche Nationalbibliografie;
detailed bibliographic data is available in the Internet at <http://dnb.ddb.de>.

Steinkopff Verlag Darmstadt
a member of Springer Science+Business Media

www.steinkopff.springer.de

© Steinkopff Verlag Darmstadt 2006
  Printed in Germany

Medical Editor: Dr. Annette Gasser   Production: Klemens Schwind
Cover Designer: Erich Kirchner, Heidelberg
Typesetter: K+V Fotosatz GmbH, Beerfelden
Printing and binding: Universitätsdruckerei Stürtz, Würzburg

SPIN 11557340   85/7231-5 4 3 2 1 0 – Printed on acid-free paper

Preface

Catheter ablation has revolutionized the treatment of cardiac arrhythmias. Having started with AV node ablation with direct current for refractory atrial tachyarrhythmias at the beginning of the 1980s, the breakthrough for catheter ablation came with the use of radiofrequency current for ablation of accessory pathways in WPW syndrome. Modification of AV node conduction (instead of AV node ablation) in AV nodal tachycardias and ablation of cavotricuspid isthmus-dependent atrial flutter followed. With the advent of 3D mapping systems, more complex cardiac arrhythmias could be approached such as right and left atrial and ventricular tachycardias. A further milestone was ablation of atrial fibrillation by pulmonary vein isolation in the late 1990s and finally ablation of ventricular fibrillation has come into focus by elimination of potential triggering ventricular ectopies.

This book intends to introduce the fascinating world of invasive clinical electrophysiology. It offers a comprehensive overview as a practical guide for mapping and ablation of the most common arrhythmias. Colored intracardiac tracings together with fluoroscopic and 3D images reflect the situation in the EP lab and will lead you to successful interventional electrophysiological procedures.

Catheter ablation is in most instances a curative treatment and we hope that many ongoing electrophysiologists will share our enthusiasm for this important field in interventional clinical cardiology.

Munich, Germany, April 2006

CLAUS SCHMITT
ISABEL DEISENHOFER
BERNHARD ZRENNER

Table of contents

Table of authors

Dr. med. Isabel Deisenhofer
Deutsches Herzzentrum München
Lazarettstraße 36
80636 München
Germany

Dr. med. Heidi Estner
Deutsches Herzzentrum München
Lazarettstraße 36
80636 München
Germany

PD Dr. med. Gabriele Hessling
Deutsches Herzzentrum München
Lazarettstraße 36
80636 München
Germany

PD Dr. med. Martin Karch
I. Medizinische Klinik
des Klinikums rechts der Isar und
Deutsches Herzzentrum der TU München
Ismaningerstraße 22
81476 München
Germany

Dr. med. Christof Kolb
Deutsches Herzzentrum München
Lazarettstraße 36
80636 München
Germany

Dr. med. Armin Luik
Deutsches Herzzentrum München
Lazarettstraße 36
80636 München
Germany

Prof. Dr. med. Gjin Ndrepepa
Deutsches Herzzentrum München
Lazarettstraße 36
80636 München
Germany

Dr. med. Andreas Pflaumer
Deutsches Herzzentrum München
Lazarettstraße 36
80636 München
Germany

Dr. med. Alexander Pustowoit
Deutsches Herzzentrum München
Lazarettstraße 36
80636 München
Germany

Prof. Dr. med. Claus Schmitt
Deutsches Herzzentrum München
Lazarettstraße 36
80636 München
Germany

PD Dr. med. Michael Schneider
Rhön Klinikum AG
Salzburger Leite 1
97616 Bad Neustadt a. d. Saale
Germany

Dr. med. Jürgen Schreieck
Klinikum der Eberhard-Karls-Universität
Kardiologie
Postfach 2669
72016 Tübingen
Germany

Dr. med. Sonja Weyerbrock
Deutsches Herzzentrum München
Lazarettstraße 36
80636 München
Germany

Dr. med. Bernhard Zrenner
Deutsches Herzzentrum München
Lazarettstraße 36
80636 München
Germany

Abbreviations

A	Atrial
ABP	Atrial premature beat
ACT	Activated clotting time
AF	Atrial fibrillation
AP	Accessory pathway
ART	Antidromic reentrant tachycardia
AT	Atrial tachycardia
AVNRT	AV nodal reentrant tachycardia
AVRT	Atrioventricular reciprocating tachycardia
BBB	Bundle branch block
bpm	Beats per minute
CL	Cycle length
CMP	Cardiomyopathy
CS	Coronary sinus
dis	Distal
FAT	Focal atrial tachycardia
HBE	His bundle electrogram
HRA	High right atrium
ICD	Implantable cardioverter defibrillator
IVC	Inferior vena cava
LA	Left atrium
LAO	Left anterior oblique
LBBB	Left bundle branch block
LV	Left ventricle
LVOT	Left ventricular outflow tract
M	Mahaim
MA	Mitral annulus
MAP	Mapping catheter
MAT	Multifocal atrial tachycardia
ORT	Orthodromic reentrant tachycardia
PES	Programmed electrical stimulation
PJRT	Permanent form of junctional reciprocating tachycardia
prox	Proximal
PV	Pulmonary vein
RA	Right atrium

RAO	Right anterior oblique
RBBB	Right bundle branch block
RF	Radiofrequency
RV	Right ventricle
RVA	Right ventricular apex
RVOT	Right ventricular outflow tract
S	Stimulus
SP	Slow pathway
SR	Sinus rhythm
SVC	Superior vena cava
SVT	Supraventricular tachycardia
TA	Tricuspid annulus
TV-IVC	Tricuspid annulus – inferior vena cava
V	Ventricular
VBP	Ventricular premature beat
VF	Ventricular fibrillation
VT	Ventricular tachycardia

1 Basic principles

Bernhard Zrenner, Christof Kolb, Armin Luik, Gjin Ndrepepa

Over the last four decades, cardiac electrophysiological studies (EP) have gained widespread accceptance for the diagnosis and treatment of cardiac arrhythmias. The spectrum of tachyarrhythmias that can be cured by catheter ablation has increased dramatically and includes most types of supraventricular and ventricular arrhythmias. Transvascular catheterization for the diagnosis and treatment of arrhythmias has become routine in cardiology. In recent times, we have witnessed tremendous developments in the fluoroscopic and nonfluoroscopic mapping techniques, ablation catheters and energy sources used for ablation.

This rapid evolution of cardiac electrophysiology accentuates the need for guidelines and for the education of EP professionals as well as for basic technical standards required in the EP laboratory. Part of these requirements will be addressed in this chapter. The chapter will also offer a basic knowledge regarding cardiac anatomy seen from the viewpoint of the clinical electrophysiologist as well as show basic principles upon which clinical EP studies are based.

▌ Historical aspects

The recording of extracellular electrical signals of the heart was performed in animals at the beginning of 20th century [48] and led to the first bipolar mapping by Lewis in 1914 [43]. Durrer and Wellens were the first who systematically used programmed electrical stimulation of the heart to disclose the mechanism of arrhythmias. The first recording of the His bundle potential in humans was reported by Scherlag et al. [61] in 1969. The recording of a His bundle electrogram was the landmark event with which the era of invasive procedures for diagnosis of arrhythmias began. The technique of His bundle recordings was swiftly standardized and used in conjunction with the programmed stimulation technique by a number of investigators

to study atrioventricular conduction defects, supraventricular and ventricular tachycardias and bradycardias in a short time following its introduction. During the 1970s and 1980s, simultaneous recordings by multiple endocavitary catheters were increasingly used for investigation of various arrhythmias.

In the 1980s, several computerized multichannel systems for endocardial and epicardial mapping became available. Direct current atrioventricular node ablation was the first transvenous therapeutic alternative to medical antiarrhythmic treatment for patients with atrial tachyarrhythmias [23]. In the following years, accessory pathways, focal atrial tachycardia and ventricular tachycardia were successfully treated by direct current (DC) ablation. DC ablation (fulguration) was performed with high-energy shocks and was associated with a significant risk of heart perforation and proarrhythmia. Alternative energy sources were, therefore, investigated and introduced into clinical practice. In the late 1980s, radiofrequency current at 500 kHz became the standard energy source for ablation of tachyarrhythmias [10, 32]. The success achieved with radiofrequency current in patients with atrioventricular nodal reentrant tachycardia, accessory pathways and focal atrial tachycardia transformed catheter ablation into the therapeutic option of choice for these arrhythmias [35]. The development of detailed mapping and stimulation techniques enabled the understanding of atrial flutter and focal atrial tachycardia as a prerequisite for successful invasive treatment. Radiofrequency ablation was also used to treat ventricular tachycardias with acceptably good results. In the 1990s, an exponential increase of electrophysiological procedures occurred and clinical cardiac electrophysiology received the status of a separate unit or department in many countries.

Within the last decade, complex arrhythmias like atypical atrial flutter or intraatrial reentrant tachycardias in patients after surgery for congenital heart disease were also approached by catheter ablation with high success rates. The first attempts of the treatment of atrial fibrillation by catheter ablation were also made within this period of time. It started with efforts to reproduce the surgical Maze procedure by catheter techniques [24, 66], but this was soon suspended due to poor results. Catheter ablation of atrial fibrillation took a new impetus with the work of Haissaguere et al. who targeted arrhythmogenic foci, mostly located within the pulmonary veins, responsible for arrhythmia initiation [25]. The technique evolved rapidly and now consists of the isolation of the pulmonary veins (segmental ostial [26] or circumferential [51] pulmonary vein ablation) with additional linear lesions placed in strategic locations within the left atrium. Despite the encouraging results, effective treatment of atrial fibrillation still remains a "hot topic" in clinical electrophysiology.

The last decade also witnessed the development of a number of high-resolution computer-based nonfluoroscopic three-dimensional mapping systems which enable integrated electroanatomical mapping. New versions of these systems allow the integration of images of cardiac chambers such as those obtained by high-resolution computed tomography or magnet resonance imaging. The most recent technical innovation enables the investigator to steer catheters from a distance (remote navigation) by using magnetic technology rather than moving catheters by hand at the operating table [21]. This technique reflects the need for highly accurate and reproducible catheter placement and navigation. Current experience is rather limited but the results appear promising. Besides these innovations, transcatheter alternative energy sources for ablation like cryothermal energy and special ablation tools like balloon catheters for pulmonary vein ablation have become available and more developments are on the way.

1.1 Cardiac anatomy for the electrophysiologist

The knowledge of the anatomy of the heart is mandatory for daily work in the EP laboratory. The initiation and/or maintenance of arrhyth-

mias like atrial fibrillation, atrial flutter, atrioventricular nodal reentrant tachycardia or tachycardia related to atrioventricular accessory pathways are linked to discrete anatomic structures so that the anatomic information greatly helps in their successful targeting by ablative means. Anatomic information is of crucial importance to avoid complications (i.e., during transseptal puncture) or to titrate the ablation energy in specific regions of the heart to avoid damage of coronary arteries or extracardiac structures in close proximity to the heart (phrenic nerve during ablation in the right atrial free wall, vagal nerves and esophagus during ablation in the posterior wall of the left atrium). For example, to avoid phrenic nerve damage, the course of the nerve may be investigated by high-output stimulation in the right atrial free wall.

In the following, the anatomic features most important for the electrophysiologist and their association with arrhythmias are discussed.

1.1.1 Position of the heart within the chest

The conventional fluoroscopic screen presents the patient's thorax in an upright position, even if the patient is recumbent. The heart is positioned within the mediastinum with one-third of its mass to the right of the midline. Its long axis is directed from the right shoulder towards the left hypochondrium. The short axis corresponds to the plane of the atrioventricular groove and is oriented closer to the vertical than the horizontal plane. There are slight variations to this position from patient to patient which may be accentuated by various diseases. There are also changes related to respiration [4]. Anteriorly, the heart is covered by the sternum and the costal cartilage of the 3rd to 5th ribs. Posteriorly, the heart is in close proximity to the esophagus and the tracheal bifurcation. On the right and left side, the heart is in contact with the respective side of the lungs. Inferiorly, the heart has extensive contact with the diaphragm. The right border of the cardiac silhouette in the conventional fluorogram of the thorax consists of three components: superior vena cava (superior), the right atrium (middle) and the right ventricle (inferior part). The superior vena cava has more or less a vertical position, whereas as the right ventricle extends horizontally along the diaphragm to the apex. The

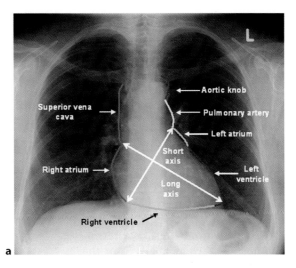

a

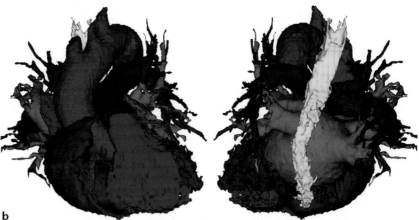

b

Fig. 1.1. a Anteroposterior chest fluorogram. The external contour of the heart and the great vessels is outlined by colored lines. **b** Computed tomography (CT) derived from the segmentation software of the Carto merge 3D electroanatomical mapping system. The image shows the anterior (**b** left) and posterior aspects of the heart (**b** right). Images are derived from the 3D electroanatomical mapping system Car-toMerge. The superior vena cava, the right atrium, the right ventricle and the pulmonary artery are colored in blue, the left atrium with the pulmonary veins. The left atrium with the pulmonary veins, the left ventricle, the aorta with the coronary arteries are coloured in red and the oesophagus is coloured in yellow

left contour has four components (from top to bottom): aortic knob, pulmonary trunk, a small portion of the left atrium and the left ventricle (Figure 1.1).

It is known that the traditional terminology describing the "right-sided" and "left-sided" cardiac structures is not entirely correct. Magnetic resonance imaging and other examinations of the heart have definitely proven that so-called "right-sided" structures are more anterior than right and the so-called "left-sided" structures are more posterior than left [14]. Thus, in the sagital view through the thorax, taken at the midline, the most anterior part of

the heart is the right ventricle and the most posterior part of the heart is the left atrium [4].

1.1.2 Anatomy of the right atrium

The position and the anatomic constituents of the right atrium are crucial for clinical electrophysiology. The sinus node, the atrioventricular node and the His bundle are located in the right atrium. The right atrium harbors the entire reentry circuit for common type atrial flutter which is one of the most common sustainable cardiac arrhythmias. Importantly, the right atrium is the most common access route to the heart during EP studies.

The right atrium has three components: the appendage, the venous part and the vestibule. The interatrial septum is shared with the left atrium and is discussed separately. *The appendage* has the shape of a blunt triangle, is located anterior and laterally and has a wide junction to the venous part across the terminal groove. The appendage also has an extensive junction to the vestibule which represents the smooth-walled right atrial myocardium that inserts into the leaflets of the tricuspid valve. The internal surface of the appendage is lined by pectinate muscles which originate from the crista terminalis. Arising almost at a right angle from the crista terminalis, the pectinate muscles cover the entire interiority of appendage and extend to the lateral and inferior walls of the right atrium. The atrial myocardium between the pectinate muscles is very thin. Whatever the degree of the extension of the pectinate muscles is, they never reach the tricuspid valve always leaving a smooth muscular part surrounding the valvular orifice *(the vestibule)*. *The venous component* receives the superior and the inferior caval veins and extends from the terminal groove (sulcus terminalis) to the interatrial groove [28, 71]. The thickest region in the right atrium is at the top of the terminal groove (5 to 8 mm thick). In general, the right atrial muscle becomes thinner towards the vestibular part with the anterior and posterior vestibular parts being as thin as 2 mm [28]. There is no evidence for the existence of histologically specialized tracts within the right atrium that link the sinus node with the atrioventricular node. Instead, the observed preferential routes of impulse propagation are dictated by atrial geometry [37].

The crista terminalis and the sinus node

One of the most characteristic morphological features of the interior right atrium is the presence of the crista teminalis. The crista terminalis is a well-developed horseshoe-shaped muscular structure (2 to 10 mm thick) that separates the trabeculated part of the right atrium (pectinate muscle) from the posterior, smooth wall (venous component) of the right atrium. Cranially, the crista terminalis originates in the interatrial groove and is always confluent with the Bachmann's bundle, another muscular fascicle that extends to the left atrium [57]. From its

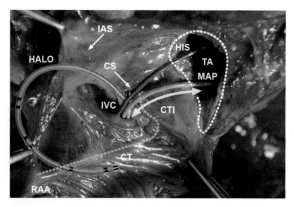

Fig. 1.2. Right atrial cut open view with focus on the atrial flutter isthmus (yellow arrow). The ablation catheter (MAP) is positioned at the ventricular site of the tricuspid ring. A Halo catheter is placed along the trabeculated lateral right atrium. *CS* coronary sinus ostium, *CT* crista terminalis, *CTI* cavotricuspid isthmus; *HIS* quadripolar catheter placed at the HIS bundle, *IAS* interatrial septum, *IVC* inferior vena cava, *MAP* ablation catheter, *RAA* right atrial appendage, *TA* tricuspid annulus

origin the crista terminalis takes a lateral and inferior course turning in beneath the orifice of the inferior vena cava ending in a series of ramifications in the area known as the lateral entry of the cavotricuspid isthmus (Figure 1.2). One of the most important functional characteristics of the crista terminalis is anisotropic conduction with a fast velocity in the longitudinal direction and a slow velocity in the transversal direction (up to 10:1 longitudinal/transversal conduction velocity ratio) due to the higher density of gap junctions at the end-to-end connections [55, 64]. Due to this feature, the crista terminalis serves as a functional block that prevents shortcuts in the impulse propagation in the intercaval region, thus, serving as a lateral stabilizer to the reentry circuit of atrial flutter. In some forms of atypical atrial flutters, the crista terminalis can be crossed in the transversal direction by the activation wavefronts [73]. Apart from the participation in the genesis of common type atrial flutter, the crista terminalis itself serves as an important arrhythmogenic substrate for atrial tachycardias [39] potentially reflecting the presence of cells with pacemaking activity. The crista terminalis corresponds to the terminal groove on the external surface of the right atrium. The structure can be visualized by using intracardiac ultrasound (see Figure 8.10) during EP studies. Experienced operators may feel and localize the crista terminalis by catheter movement in the horizontal direction within the right atrium.

The sinus node is mostly found at the anterior and the superior aspect of the crista terminalis (or terminal groove from outside the atrium) near the ostium of the superior vena cava but it varies in location [58]. The node is a structure (mostly subepicardially located) with a length ranging from 8 to 21.5 mm (mean 13.5 mm and in more than 50% of specimens >16 mm) with the long axis parallel to the terminal groove. The constituent parts of the node consists of the head, the body and the tail. Various shapes such as fusiform, horseshoe or crescent-like have been described [58]. Histologically, nodal cells are packed within the dense connective tissue and are smaller and paler than working atrial myocardial fibers. Nodal cells are not encapsulated by a discrete fibrous border; instead in the majority of cases peripheral nodal regions (85%) constitute specialized nodal cells intermingled with working myocardial cells [58]. This structure may favor local reentry in inappropriate sinus tachycardias.

Apart from serving as pacemaker of the heart, the sinus node region is involved in the arrhythmogenesis (inappropriate sinus tachycardia) and, thus, is subject to modification by ablative therapy.

▌ Cavotricuspid isthmus

This structure is central to the understanding of ablative therapy of atrial flutter. The cavotricuspid isthmus area is defined as the part of the lower right atrial free wall bordered by the eustachian valve/ridge posteriorly, the tricuspid annulus anteriorly and the os of the coronary sinus superiorly (Figure 1.2). In postmortem examined hearts, the cavotricuspid isthmus has a mean length of 30 mm (range 10 to 40 mm). It has a lateral entry, mostly composed of muscular ramifications of the crista terminalis and a septal exit. This terminology, however, is suitable when describing the reentry circuit of counterclockwise atrial flutter. The eustachian valve/ridge is a triangular flap of fibrous or fibromuscular tissue that guards the entrance of the inferior vena cava into the right atrium [11]. The proportion of muscular component is variable and, in general, it has muscular extensions from the crista terminalis [11]. The free border of the eustachian ridge continues as a tendon in the musculature of the sinus septum

(described as the tendon of Todaro). Cabrera et al. have described three morphological sectors arranged from the posterior to anterior aspect of the isthmus. The first part is in close vicinity to the eustachian ridge and usually it is membranous in nature without muscular components. The middle part usually contains muscular trabeculations of various thickness (from 0.2 to 6 mm thick) separated by thinner areas of myocardium or membranous parts. Muscular defects between trabeculae have also been described by other authors [70]. From the geometric point of view, the posterior and middle parts of the cavotricuspid isthmus form a pouch-like inferior recess [11]. This anatomic feature of the isthmus, together with the variable degree of muscular trabeculations and thickness has implications for the ablation of atrial flutter. The most anterior part of the isthmus is the vestibular part of right atrium which represents a homogenous mass of smooth muscle in close continuity with the tricuspid annulus. Its thickness varies from 0.5 to 5 mm [11].

The cavotricuspid is a mandatory part of the reentry circuit in counterclockwise and clockwise atrial flutter and the standard target of ablative therapy of this arrhythmia. Other aspects like the relationship between isthmus size and propensity to develop atrial flutter or whether the isthmus region provides the slow conduction zone that favors the occurrence of reentry are still disputable.

▌ Triangle of Koch and atrioventricular node

Triangle of Koch is a triangular area demarcated by the tendon of Todaro, the septal leaflet of the tricuspid valve and the orifice of the coronary sinus (Figure 1.3). This area has major electrophysiological significance because it contains the atrioventricular node. The atrioventricular node is located in the anterosuperior aspect or in the apical portion of the triangle (close to the central fibrous body). The compact node is located subendocardially. The mean length, width and thickness are the following: 5.1 mm (range 3.2–6.2 mm), 5.2 mm (range 3.1–7.2 mm) and 0.8 mm (range 0.3–1.2 mm), respectively [59]. There is some variation in the location of the node in the triangle of Koch. In the study by Sanchez-Quintana et al., the compact node was located medially at the mid-level of the triangle of Koch in 82% of specimens; in the remaining 18% the node was located closer to the

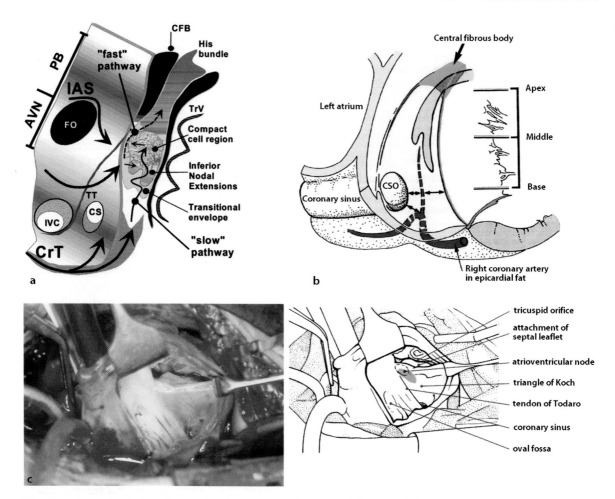

Fig. 1.3. a Schematic drawing of the region of the triangle of Koch with localization of the "fast" and "slow" pathway. *AVN* atrio-ventricular node, *CFB* central fibrous body, *CRT* crista terminalis, *CS* coronary sinus, *FO* fossa ovalis, *IVC* inferior vena cava, *PB* penetrating bundle, *TT* tendon of Todaro. Modified from Mazgalev et al. [49] with permission. **b** Schematic drawing illustrating the course of the artery to the AV node through the inferior pyramidal space and toward the central fibrous body (dark blue). The AV node and the His bundle is colored in yellow. *CSO* coronary sinus os. Modified from Sanchez-Quintana et al. [59] with permission. **c** A surgeon's view shows the landmarks of the triangle of Koch. The triangle is clearly visible, limited by the septal tricuspid leaflet and the tendon of Todaro (reproduced with permission from Hurst et al. [33])

hinge of the tricuspid valve. In 12% of specimens, the inferior parts of the node extended up to the mouth of the coronary sinus [59]. Inferiorly, the node bifurcates into rightward and leftward extensions in the majority of specimens. The atrioventricular node artery originates from the right coronary artery in 83% of specimens and from the circumflex artery in 17% of specimens. Its length from origin to the triangle of Koch is 14 to 28 mm (mean 20.5 mm). The artery ascends subendocardially from the inferior-posterior septum to the central fibrous body being closer to the coronary sinus ostium than the tricuspid valve (Figure 1.3 B) [59]. The so-called open node (or AN part; A stands for atrium and N for node) consists of transitional cells intermingled with working myocardial cells. Transitional cells extend from the compact node towards the eustachian ridge, the anterior superior rim of the fossa ovalis and the left atrial aspect of the septum. It is believed that these transitional cells, due to differences in the conduction velocity and refractory periods, constitute the electrophysiological basis for discontinuous atrioventricular conduction (fast and slow pathways) in patients with atrioventricular nodal reentrant tachycardia. However, despite electrophysiological evidence for the existence of fast and slow pathways, histological markers have never been reported. The compact node continues with the penetrating bundle of His which is located at the apical part of the triangle of Koch.

The triangle of Koch is a frequent target for ablation mostly for the treatment of atrioventricular nodal reentrant tachycardia and atrioventricular conduction modification in patients with atrial fibrillation. The putative location of fast and slow pathways is shown in Figure 1.3a. Slow pathway ablation is mostly used in the treatment of atrioventricular nodal reentrant tachycardia. In the EP laboratory, the site of recording the His bundle activity (apical region) and the os of the coronary sinus are anatomic markers for location of the triangle of Koch and for guiding the delivery of ablative energy.

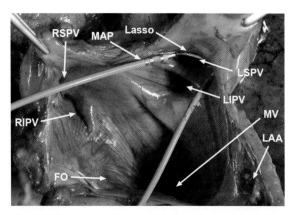

Fig. 1.4. Positioning of a lasso catheter in the left superior pulmonary vein (LSPV). The ablation catheter (MAP) approaches the ring of the lasso catheter. *FO* Fossa ovalis, *LAA* left atrial appendage, *LIPV* left inferior pulmonary vein, *RIPV* right inferior pulmonary vein, *RSPV* right superior pulmonary vein

▮ Muscle extensions into the superior and inferior vena cava

Histological studies have demonstrated the extension of right atrial muscle into the superior and inferior vena cava in both animal and human studies [34, 63, 74]. Spach et al. have reported that the excitation during sinus rhythm extends 2 to 5 cm into the superior vena cava [63]. Superior vena cava muscle and right atrial muscle have similar electrophysiological characteristics [74]. Furthermore, in rabbit preparations action potentials obtained from the muscle located at the superior vena cava show diastolic slow depolarization which may implicate the muscle in the arrhythmogenesis [34]. Human studies also have demonstrated the extension of right atrial muscle into the superior and inferior vena cava and that the length of the myocardial extension into the inferior vena cava is much shorter and has less longitudinal orientation than the muscle extension in the superior vena cava [27]. Arrhythmogenic foci initiating atrial tachycardia and atrial fibrillation have been reported in the superior [19, 69] and inferior vena cava muscle extensions [47, 60].

1.1.3 Anatomy of the left atrium

The electrophysiological importance of the left atrium increased considerably after the discovery of the dominant role of the pulmonary veins in the genesis of atrial fibrillation. The left atrium has four components: appendage, vestibule, venous component and septum. With the exception of the appendage, the inner surface of the left atrium is smooth and contains no trabeculations. The vestibular component represents the circumferential area that surrounds the orifice of the mitral valve. The posterior part of the vestibular component is thin and directly apposes the coronary sinus. The left atrial appendage is a tubular, finger-like structure that is directed superiorly relative to the left pulmonary veins and opens in the venous component through a relatively narrow mouth. The inner surface of the appendage is trabeculated. In fact, the appendage component contains nearly all pectinate muscles of the left atrium. There is only a narrow rim of muscle between the mouth of the left atrial appendage (see Figure 10.20) and the ostium of the left superior pulmonary vein (Figure 1.4). This has implications for isolation of the pulmonary veins and special stimulation protocols are used to distinguish the left superior pulmonary vein potentials from those produced by the appendage (see Chapter 10). The venous component of the left atrium is considerably larger than the venous component of the right atrium. It receives the pulmonary veins. Traditionally, the walls of the left atrium are described as superior (roof), posterior, lateral, septal and anterior. The thickness of the left atrium muscle is relatively uniform. The thickest part of the left atrial wall is found in the anterior and posterior walls (4–5 mm), while the thinnest part is found in the posterior and anterior aspects of the vestibule [31].

During the last decade, the posterior wall of the left atrium and the pulmonary veins have drawn considerable attention because of their involvement in the genesis and ablation of atrial fibrillation. In general, there are four pulmonary veins: two left-sided (superior and inferior) and two right-sided (superior and inferior) veins. However, variations in the number, diameter and the morphology of the ostial regions have been reported in postmortem examinations and EP studies. The distance between pulmonary vein orifices is reported to be 3 to 11 mm (mean 6.5 mm) for the right pulmonary veins and 3 to 16 mm (mean 8.4 mm) for the left pulmonary veins [31]. The orifice of the left superior pulmonary vein is located superior to the opening of the left atrial appendage. The orifices of the right pulmonary veins are located in close proximity to the left side of the interatrial septum. The right pulmonary veins run immediately behind the superior vena cava [31]. The close relationship between the right pulmonary veins and the interatrial septum has implications regarding the differentiation of rhythms originating in the right pulmonary veins from those originating in the posteroseptal region of the right atrium and for interpretation of the local pulmonary vein electrogram.

The most important histological characteristic of the pulmonary veins relevant to EP studies is the presence of muscle sleeves surrounding the veins [50]. Histological studies have shown that myocardial sleeves are longer in the superior pulmonary veins than in the inferior pulmonary veins. The left inferior pulmonary vein has a longer surrounding myocardial sleeve than the right inferior pulmonary vein [29, 56]. The myocardial sleeves are always separated from the medial smooth muscle cells of the pulmonary veins by fibrofatty tissue [56]. Longitudinal, circular and oblique orientations of the fibers surrounding the pulmonary veins have been described [29]. The arrangement of fibers at the ostial regions is not entirely understood. Electrophysiological studies support the concept of discrete connections between the myocardial sleeves surrounding the pulmonary veins and the muscle in the posterior wall of the left atrium giving rise to hypothesis of the existence of discrete muscle extensions spiraling around the pulmonary vein perimeter at least in some cases. Direct electrical connections by muscular

extension between the left superior and left inferior pulmonary veins have been described [68]. Furthermore, myocardial cells at the periphery of sleeves show signs of degeneration [56] which may increase their potential for abnormal impulse generation. The evidence for the existence of cells with pacemaker activity in the muscle surrounding the pulmonary veins is still incomplete.

The posterior wall of the left atrium has a complex architecture of intertwining myocardial fibers of various directions [29]. Due to this complex structure, the current opinion is that the posterior wall serves as an important arrhythmogenic substrate for maintenance of atrial fibrillation. Rotors of fibrillatory activity involving parts of the posterior wall or circular muscle at the pulmonary vein ostia have been hypothesized [36].

▌ Left atrial isthmus

The left atrial isthmus encompasses the distance from the ostium of the left inferior pulmonary vein to the mitral annulus. The distance between the ostium of the left inferior pulmonary vein and mitral annulus was reported to be 34.6 mm (range 17–51 mm). The thickness was 3 mm (range 1.4–7.7 mm) at the level of the ostium and progressively decreased to 1.2 mm (range 0–3.2 mm) at the level of the mitral annulus [6]. The current opinion is that the left atrial isthmus due to its strategic location and morphology may predispose for macroreentrant left atrial tachycardia if left intact during antiarrhythmic surgery or catheter ablation in the left atrium for the treatment of atrial fibrillation. With this understanding, linear lesions extending from the left inferior to the mitral annulus are part of current catheter ablation schemes in patients with atrial fibrillation.

1.1.4 Interatrial septum and interatrial connections

The anatomic structure of the interatrial septum is still a controversial issue among anatomists. In earlier studies, the interatrial septum viewed from the right side is described as being an extensive blade-shaped structure with three margins (posterior, anterior and inferior) and a surface area of 890 mm^2 (range 450–1542 mm^2) in adult hearts [67]. Anderson et al. describe the "septal area" as a relatively round-shaped structure extending from the orifice of the inferior vena cava to the right atrial appendage and from the mouth of the superior vena cava to the hinge of the septal leaflet of the tricuspid valve [5]. The fossa ovalis, the coronary sinus os, a part of the eustachian and the ligament of Todaro are found in this area. On the left side, the interatrial septum is a relatively featureless structure. In fact the real structure dividing the atria or the true interatrial septum is only a small portion of this area that includes the fossa ovalis and its infero-anterior rim. The round or oval-shaped fossa ovalis is located slightly posterior to the central position of the septal area. It has a surface area of 240 mm^2 (range 97–490 mm^2) in adults with no septal muscle posterior to the fossa and 146 mm^2 (range 29–452 mm^2) in adults with the septal muscle (also called the posterior isthmus) present posterior to the fossa ovalis [67]. The flap valve of the fossa ovalis is usually fibrous and contains few muscular cells. In about one-fourth of the population there is evidence for the patency of the fossa even though the valve tissue is large enough to cover the rim [28]. This happens due to incomplete adhesion of the valve to the rim. The fossa ovalis is the region in which transseptal puncture (Figure 10.5) to obtain access to the left atrium should be made because it is easy to puncture and bears low or no risk of cardiac external perforation.

The most extensive part of the "septal area" is muscular and surrounds the fossa region in all directions. The anteromedial portion in reality represents the part of the right atrium musculature that is located immediately behind the aorta. This knowledge is of crucial importance for electrophysiologists performing transseptal puncture. Puncture in this region should be avoided to prevent aortic puncture which may have grave consequences. The superior and the posterior margins are indeed infoldings of the right atrial and left atrial muscle that produce well-developed muscular rims surrounding the fossa in these directions [5]. The superior rim (or limbus) is so prominent that it can be located by catheter manipulation aimed to locate the fossa region during catheter-based transseptal puncture approaches. The inferior rim is also muscular and lies on the top of the central fibrous body and continues in the backward direction with the sinus septum which encompasses the area between the coronary sinus and the inferior vena cava. [5]

∎ **Interatrial connections**

Although anatomic and electrophysiological studies are not entirely concordant, a widely accepted idea among electrophysiologists is that three interatrial connections are particularly important for electrical connection between the atria. These connections are Bachmann's bundle, the rim of the fossa ovalis and the muscle of the coronary sinus [52]. The largest and the most important interatrial connection route is Bachmann's bundle which represents a broad, flat muscular bundle that originates rightward to the junction of the right atrium with the superior vena cava and transverses the anterior septal raphe to reach the left atrial wall [31]. It varies from a unique bundle of parallel-arranged muscular fibers to several, closely spaced bundles but has no cable-like features. Electroanatomical studies have recently revealed that the rim of the fossa ovalis represents another important electrical connection between the atria at least during left atrial pacing [52]. It has recently been reported that the coronary sinus has its own muscle and it represents the third most important interatrial connection [12, 52]. Finally, small tongues of muscles crossing the interatrial raphe on the both sides of the Bachmann's bundle as well as in multiple positions in the posterior wall of the atria have been reported [50]. However, their importance in the physiological interatrial impulse propagation or in the genesis of atrial arrhythmias remains obscure.

1.1.5 Putative consequence of anatomic differences between the atria

Although the right and the left atrium have multiple distinctive anatomic characteristics with potential electrophysiological and practical implications, one characteristic, i.e., the degree of "natural segmentation" deserves special attention. The right atrium contains several structures, anatomic (orifices of the inferior and superior vena cava, tricuspid annulus, the coronary sinus os and the fossa ovalis) and functional (the crista terminalis and potentially another zone of block at the posteromedial or sinus venosa region of the right atrium [22]) which provide barriers to impulse propagation. The presence of these structures may be supportive to macroreentrant regular rhythms in the right atrium. On the other hand, the left atrium has fewer anatomical barriers to the impulse propagation, i.e., less "natural segmentation" than the right atrium so this structure may be more suitable to maintain multiple wavelet reentry. Thus, it is not a surprise that common type atrial flutter is a "right atrial disease" and that the left atrium plays a central role in the genesis (it has the pulmonary veins) and maintenance of atrial fibrillation (more space for multiple wavelets).

1.1.6 The coronary sinus system

Apart from drainage of the cardiac blood, the coronary sinus has a central position in EP studies. The recording of a coronary sinus electrogram provides indispensable information for the diagnosis of supraventricular and ventricular tachycardias. The coronary sinus system provides a route for insertion of electrodes used for resynchronization therapy, for performing epicardial left ventricular mapping and ablation, for ablation of accessory pathways and for ablation of slow pathways extending leftwards in patients with atrioventricular nodal reentrant tachycardia. The coronary sinus provides an intraatrial connection route, and its muscle has been involved in the genesis of supraventricular tachycardia and atrial fibrillation.

The coronary sinus system consists of the coronary sinus and its ventricular tributaries, mainly the great cardiac vein, the left obtuse marginal vein and the right coronary vein. Atrial tributaries are atrial veins and the vein of Marshall which represents a small oblique vein located between the left pulmonary vein and the left atrial appendage [30]. The vein of Marshall is often a ligamentous structure (ligament of Marshall) which is rich in adrenergic endings and their firings are implicated in the genesis of atrial fibrillation [20]. The ostium of the coronary sinus is situated posteriorly at the base of the triangle of Koch and is guarded by the Thebesian valve in a way that the ostium needs to be accessed from the anterior-superior direction. The valve is highly variable in shape and often interferes with the placement of electrode catheters into the coronary sinus. In about 25% of heart specimens, fibrous bands or a filigree network of fibers (Chiari network, Figure 1.5) covers the coronary sinus entrance [30]. In rare cases, the coronary sinus may be atretic.

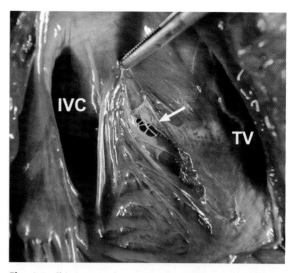

Fig. 1.5. Chiari network covering the orifice of the coronary sinus (arrow). *IVC* inferior vena cava, *TV* tricuspid valve

The recognition of this anomaly is of importance during electrophysiological studies and lead placement during implantation of resynchronization therapy devices. It prevents vigorous efforts to access the coronary sinus conventionally which may lead to prolonged X-ray exposure and cardiac perforation. In this situation access of the coronary sinus via the persistent left superior vena cava is feasible [46]. The shape of the coronary sinus is tubular with a gradual widening toward the ostium. The coronary sinus at the level of the ligament of Marshall or the valve of Vieussens continues as the great cardiac vein. Although the valve of Vieussens is a tiny structure, it may offer resistance to the catheter. Beyond the valve of Vieussens another factor leading to resistance during catheter pushing may be related to an acute band in the great cardiac vein that is reported in 46% of heart specimens [13]. Moreover, it has to be kept in mind that the course of the great cardiac vein leaves the course of the atrioventricular groove and runs along the inferior left atrial wall up to more than 15 mm above the mitral annulus [6]. Thus, a recording from the great cardiac vein does not represent the electrical activity at the level of the mitral annulus; instead it represents the activity of the posteroinferior left atrial wall. The middle cardiac vein takes its origin close to the coronary sinus ostium and runs in the groove between the right and the left ventricle on the diaphragmatic surface of the heart. The middle cardiac vein can be adjacent to the right coronary artery. It has sufficient size to insert a pacing lead in it. Other smaller venous components of the coronary system have less electrophysiological importance and are not further discussed.

One important feature of the coronary sinus is that it has its own muscle and provides and electrical connection between the right and the left atrium. The coronary sinus muscle is in continuity with right atrial muscle at the level of the coronary sinus os and continues for 25 to 51 mm along the coronary sinus wall. The muscular cuff makes contact with the left atrial muscle, at various distances from the ostial region through muscular fibers varying from a few discrete fibers to a broad interconnecting plexus [12]. Due to the anatomic structure of the interatrial septum at the level of the coronary sinus ostium, where right and left atrial muscles are divided by a small fibrofatty tissue, the activation front through the coronary sinus can not directly enter the inferoposterior left atrium, but it has to travel along the coronary sinus until there is a direct connection between the coronary sinus and the posterior left atrium. The coronary sinus muscle is implicated in the genesis of atypical left ventricular flutter, preexcitation syndromes and atrial fibrillation.

Usually the tributaries of the coronary sinus contain no muscle sleeves; however in a small percentage of the heart (2–3%) muscular fibers extend over the initial portions of the daughter veins [45]. These muscular extensions over the ventricular tributaries of the coronary sinus may enable ventricular preexcitation.

1.1.7 Anatomic differences between the left and the right atrioventricular junctions

The knowledge of the anatomic differences between the right and the left atrioventricular annuli has implications for the ablative therapy of the accessory atrioventricular pathways. The ablation of right-sided accessory pathways continues to be challenging and is associated with prolonged procedure and fluoroscopic times, lower success rates and higher rates of recurrences [42]. The worse results in the ablation of the right-sided accessory pathway compared with the results in the ablation of the left-sided accessory pathways are explained, at least in part, by differences in the anatomy of right and left atrioventricular junctions. Among these differences are:

▮ The right atrioventricular annulus is larger than the left atrioventricular annulus averaging 11 cm and 8 cm, respectively [17]. The left-sided annulus is usually thicker, well-formed and almost always complete. On the other hand, the right-sided annulus is thinner, poorly formed and is deficient (has gaps) at many sites [7]. Although these differences appear to favor the occurrence of right-sided accessory pathways, it remains puzzling why left-sided accessory pathways are encountered more often in clinical practice. However, these annular discontinuities may favor the existence of broader or multiple accessory pathways on the right side compared with thin or solitary strands on the left side.

▮ On the right side, the atrioventricular groove is much deeper than the left atrioventricular groove. In other words, the atrial musculature approaches the ventricular musculature in a narrower angle (seen from outside the heart). Therefore, accessory pathways that cross the groove on the right side are located more remote from the endocardial surface, or their insertions to the ventricular muscle are located further away from the tricuspid annulus. Occasionally, the atrial muscle hangs over the atrioventricular groove. In this situation steering the mapping/ablation catheter toward the ventricle, in reality, may move it away from the tricuspid annulus. Accessory pathways on the left side are in close proximity to the hingepoint of the mitral leaflet and, thus, they are easier mapped and ablated from the left ventricle, left atrium or coronary sinus [3]. This anatomic feature may add some technical difficulties in the catheter stabilization on the right side compared with the left side. These difficulties are additional to the difficulties in catheter positioning and stabilization during ablation on the right side.

▮ For a major portion of its circumference, the left-sided atrioventricular annulus is associated by the coronary sinus system which provides an anatomic and electrophysiological guide for mapping and an additional route for ablation of accessory pathways. The right-sided atrioventricular junction lacks such a supportive structure. Some mapping information, however, can be provided by mapping in the right coronary artery.

1.1.8 Coronary arteries

The epicardial topography of coronary arteries is close to some standard ablation sites like the slow pathway in atrioventricular nodal reentrant tachycardia (AV node artery), cavotricuspid isthmus (right coronary artery) or left atrial isthmus (circumflex artery). However, the complications related to the damage of coronary vessels are rare potentially due to the protective role of coronary blood flow (see Chapter 2).

1.1.9 The right and the left ventricle

Although ventricular arrhythmias are amenable to ablative therapy, unfortunately, anatomical markers to guide ablation comparable to those described in the atria are almost completely missing. The ventricles contain the intraventricular conduction system which is important for coordinated impulse propagation and genesis of arrhythmias. Each of the ventricles can be divided into three anatomically distinct components: the inlet, apical trabecular, and outlet portions. The ventricular muscle is thick, so in general the risk of perforation during catheter manipulation or ablation is very small. The apical trabecular portion of the both ventricles is thin so it can be vulnerable to perforation by electrode catheters and pacemaker leads. The trabeculations of the left ventricle are finer than those of the right ventricle, a fact that may have some implications for catheter manipulations or pacemaker lead placement.

As stated above, ventricles contain few anatomical landmarks to guide the ablation of ventricular arrhythmias. However, few exceptions exist. In case of channels bordered by scar tissue and the mitral or tricuspid annuli (ventricular tachycardia after myocardial infarction), the annular structures may be used to guide ablation aiming to cut the culprit isthmus. The ablation of right ventricular outflow tract tachycardias may be facilitated by anatomic landmarks; a great deal of mapping is however needed. To some extent, anatomical markers may help in ablation of fascicular tachycardias, tachycardias related to Mahaim fibers or those originating in the aortic sinus cusp.

1.2 Basic concepts for electrophysiological studies

1.2.1 Before the EP study: clinical diagnosis of arrhythmias

An ECG documentation of the patient's arrhythmia before an intracardiac EP study is very helpful as vascular access and number/types of catheters are chosen depending on the suspected diagnosis. In most chapters of this book, surface ECG criteria for diagnosis of specific arrhythmias are mentioned as a prerequisite for further invasive diagnosis. In this overview, the most important ECG features for the differential diagnosis of tachycardias are shown. The figures are adapted from the ACC/AHA/ESC guidelines [9] dealing with differential diagnostic criteria for narrow and wide QRS complex tachycardias.

▮ Differential diagnosis of narrow QRS tachycardia

Narrow QRS tachycardia (see Figure 1.6) is of supraventricular origin, but some exceptions have to be kept in mind. A ventricular tachycardia with an exit near the His bundle or with a high septal origin may present with a narrow QRS complex (about 1% of ventricular tachycardias).

The following ECG examples show two of the most common tachycardia types with a narrow QRS complex: AV nodal reentrant tachycardia (AVNRT) and atrioventricular reciprocating tachycardia (AVRT) (Figure 1.7 and 1.8).

▮ Adenosine for the differential diagnosis of tachycardia

Intravenous application of adenosine is of differential diagnostic help in *regular narrow QRS complex tachycardia* (Figure 1.9). An unchanged ongoing focal atrial tachycardia or atrial flutter can be unmasked by an intermittent AV block after adenosine application (see Figure 5.16).

▮ Differential diagnosis of wide QRS complex tachycardia

Differential diagnosis of tachycardias with a wide QRS complex is shown in Figure 1.10 and some examples of wide-complex tachycardias as are shown in Figures 1.11–1.13.

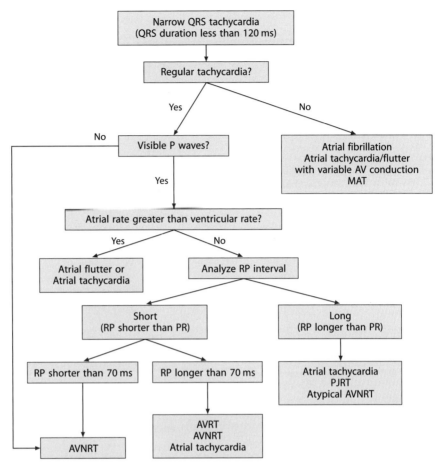

Fig. 1.6. Differential diagnosis of narrow QRS tachycardia. Focal junctional tachycardia may mimic the pattern of slow–fast AVNRT and may show AV dissociation and/or marked irregularity in the junctional rate. *AV* atrioventricular, *AVNRT* atrioventricular nodal reentrant tachycardia, *AVRT* atrioventricular reciprocating tachycardia, *MAT* multifocal atrial tachycardia, *PJRT* permanent form of junctional reciprocating tachycardia, *ms* milliseconds, *QRS* ventricular activation on ECG (legend and schema from Blomström-Lundqvist C et al. [9])

▮ Differential diagnosis of long RP tachycardia

Long RP tachycardia with a negative P wave in leads II, III and aVF often presents a challenge to the clinician. Differential diagnosis includes three types of tachycardia:

1) Atypical (fast-slow) AV nodal reentrant tachycardia,
2) focal atrial tachycardia (often inferior septal region) and
3) an atrioventricular reciprocating tachycardia using an accessory pathway with slow, decremental conduction properties.

Table 1.1 shows differential diagnostic criteria including invasive EP parameters that will be discussed in detail below.

1.2.2 Intracardiac EP studies

Intracardiac EP studies offer the unique possibility of recording the endocardial activity of the heart including 1) registration of the His bundle activity, 2) the ability to perform atrial and ventricular stimulation (for induction of supraventricular or ventricular tachycardia and for evaluation of antegrade and retrograde conduction) and 3) the mapping of endocardial activation patterns. Some basic features approaching an EP procedure will be shown in more detail in this chapter. Precise mapping and ablation techniques are discussed in the corresponding chapters of this book.

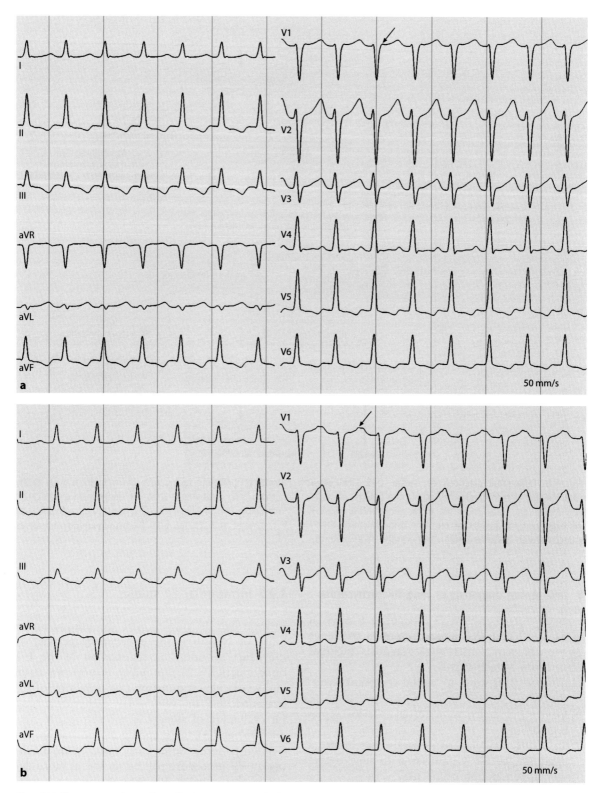

Fig. 1.7. Narrow complex tachycardia in a patient with (**a**) AV nodal reentrant tachycardia (AVNRT) and (**b**) atrioventricular reciprocating tachycardia (AVRT) due to a concealed by-pass tract. Please note r′ in V1 in AVNRT (arrow) and the long VA interval in AVRT (arrow marks the retrograde P wave)

x

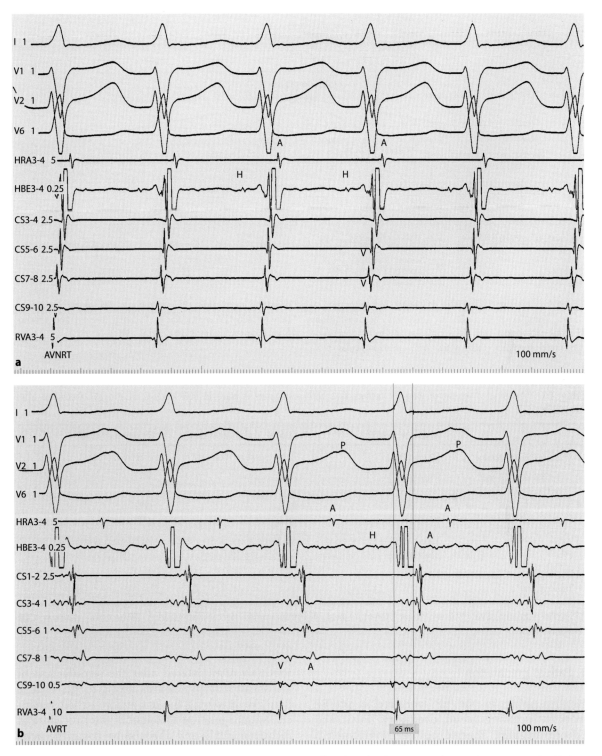

Fig. 1.8. Intracardiac recordings in a patient with (**a**) AVNRT and (**b**) AVRT (same patient as in Figure 1.7). Please note the short VA interval during AVNRT and the longer VA interval with a distal to proximal activation sequence in CS during AVRT (left-sided accessory pathway). *CS* coronary sinus, *RVA3-4* right ventricular apex

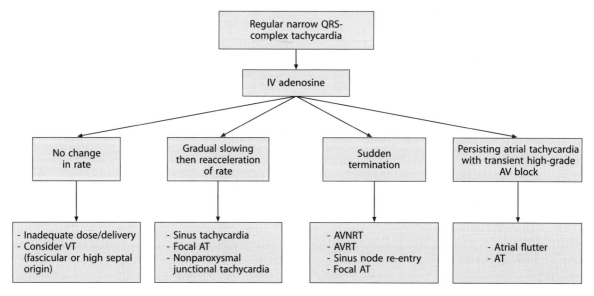

Fig. 1.9. Differential diagnosis following the response of narrow complex tachycardia to adenosine administration. *AT* atrial tachycardia, *AV* atrioventricular, *AVNRT* atrioventricular nodal reentrant tachycardia, *AVRT* atrioventricular reciprocating tachycardia, *IV* intravenous, *QRS* ventricular activation on ECG, *VT* ventricular tachycardia (legend and schema from Blomström-Lundqvist C et al. [9])

Table 1.1. Differential diagnosis of long RP tachycardias with a negative P wave in ECG leads II, III and aVF (modified after HJJ Wellens [72])

	Atypical AVNRT	Septal atrial tachycardia	Decremental AP
▌ Tachycardia occurrence	Paroxysmal	Paroxysmal or incessant	Usually incessant
▌ Tachycardia initiation	Usually VPB	APB	Sinus rate acceleration, APB, VPB
▌ Termination (PES)	APB, VPB (rare) Atrial or ventricular pacing	APB Atrial overdrive pacing	APB VPB when His is refractory
▌ Vagal maneuver	Tachycardia termination by block in the slow pathway	AV block: more P than QRS; occasionally termination	Tachycardia termination by block of AP or AV node
▌ Development of tachycardia induced CMP	No	Only if incessant	Yes

APB atrial premature beat, *VPB* ventricular premature beat, *PES* programmed electrical stimulation, *AP* accessory pathway; *CMP* cardiomyopathy

▌ Patient preparation

Patients going to the EP lab need a pre-EP workup including blood chemistry, ECG, and echocardiogram. To rule out atrial thrombi, a transesophageal echocardiogram is mandatory in patients with atrial flutter or fibrillation. Anticoagulation prior to the procedure must be considered in patients undergoing left-sided procedures (ablation of atrial fibrillation) or patients with low output hemodynamics. During the procedure, heparin 5000 IU intravenously is routinely administered after the introduction of the sheaths. In procedures taking longer than 2 hours or involving the left atrium or left ventricle, anticoagulation throughout the procedure is recommendable and checked by using the activated clotting time (ACT).

Antiarrhythmic medication is usually discontinued for five half-lives of the drug prior to the EP study. ECG recordings of the patient's arrhythmia should be available to compare the clinical with the induced arrhythmia. The diagnostic part of the EP study is usually performed

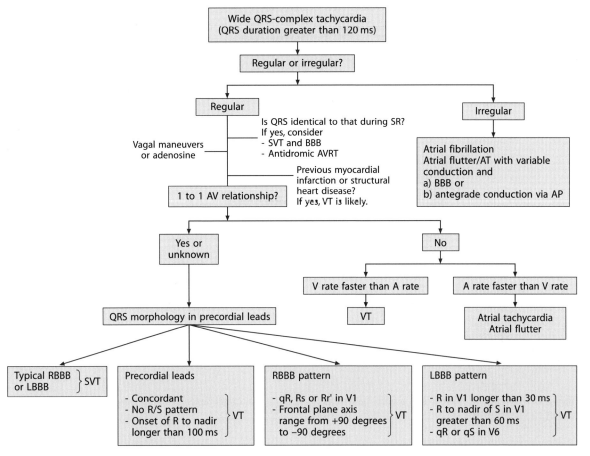

Fig. 1.10. Differential diagnosis of wide QRS-complex tachycardia (more than 120 ms). A QRS conduction delay during sinus rhythm (if available for comparison) reduces the value of QRS morphology analysis. Adenosine should be used with caution if diagnosis is unclear because it may produce VF in patients with coronary artery disease and AF with a rapid ventricular rate in preexcited tachycardias. Concordant means that all precordial leads show either positive or negative deflections. Fusion complexes are diagnostic of VT. In preexcited tachycardias, the QRS is generally wider (i.e., more preexcited) compared with sinus rhythm. *A* atrial, *AP* accessory pathway, *AT* atrial tachycardia, *AV* atrioventricular, *AVRT* atrioventricular reciprocating tachycardia, *BBB* bundle branch block, *LBBB* left bundle branch block, *ms* milliseconds, *QRS* ventricular activation on ECG, *RBBB* right bundle branch block, *SR* sinus rhythm, *SVT* supraventricular tachycardias, *V* ventricular, *VF* ventricular fibrillation, *VT* ventricular tachycardia (legend and scheme from Blomström-Lundqvist C et al. [9])

without sedation as the measurements of EP parameters and the inducibility of arrhythmias might be altered. If necessary, titrated analgosedation is used. For the therapeutic part of the EP procedure (especially during long procedures), more aggressive sedation should be administered to minimize patient discomfort. For local anesthesia at vascular entry sites, lidocaine 1% is used. The atmosphere in the EP lab should be calm and relaxed (to have music available often helps) and the patient should feel as comfortable as possible on the fluoroscopy table. Continuous monitoring of cardiac rhythm, oxygen saturation and arterial blood pressure (either by arm cuff or over a small arterial sheath) must be maintained throughout the procedure.

■ **EP laboratory personnel**

International regulations and guidelines dealing with the optimal personnel structure for an EP study differ substantially. The presence of an anesthesiologist for any kind of analgosedation in adult patients is obligatory in France and Italy but not in Germany. German guidelines recommend an anesthesiologist only for EP studies in children. The goal of optimal patient care led to

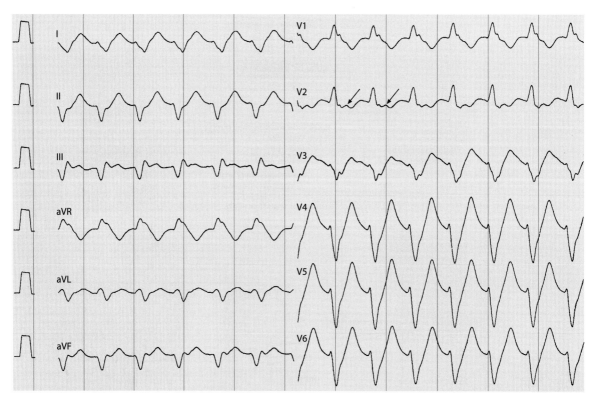

Fig. 1.11. Ventricular tachycardia with a RBBB pattern, Rr' in lead V1 and a right superior frontal plane axis. There is a 1:1 VA conduction (arrows in V2)

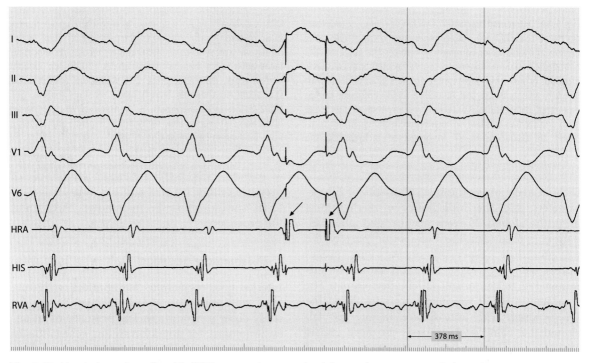

Fig. 1.12. Ventricular tachycardia with RBBB pattern (same patient as in Figure 1.11) with 1:1 VA conduction. The atrial activation can be dissociated from the ventricular activation by delivery of two extrastimuli from the HRA (arrows). This suggests a ventricular origin of the tachycardia

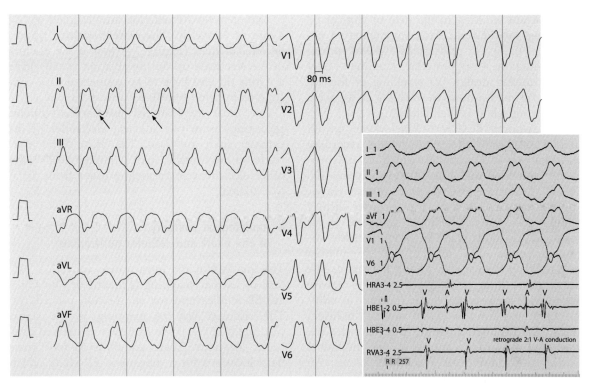

Fig. 1.13. Ventricular tachycardia with LBBB pattern. Please note R to nadir of S in V1 is greater than 60 ms. There is a 2:1 VA conduction (arrows); the V rate is faster than the A rate confirming the diagnosis of VT. The inset shows intracardiac recordings with 2:1 retrograde VA conduction

the recommendation that two physicians and one nurse (or one technician and one nurse) should be present if an EP study including ablation is intended. The "ACC/AHA Clinical Competence Statement" [65] states that a minimum of one year of specialized EP training is necessary to acquire the cognitive and technical skills required to become an EP expert. For ablation therapy an additional expertise has to be gained over a period of 1–2 years. EP training should cover the whole spectrum of ventricular and supraventricular arrhythmias on a day-to-day basis under the guidance of a senior expert in EP.

▮ Equipment

For performing diagnostic EP procedures, the following prerequisites must be available: 1) monoplane (for complex procedures better biplane) fluoroscopy, 2) a multichannel electrogram recorder, 3) a programmable stimulator and 4) an external defibrillator. For the ablation procedure, a RF or cryo-energy generator is added (see Chapter 2). More advanced non-fluoroscopic or electroanatomical mapping systems are of substantial help in complex ablation procedures (see Chapter 3).

The use of fluoroscopy in EP procedures demands special consideration. Introduction and guidance of catheters is currently performed with the use of fluoroscopy. It is a requirement of the Ionizing Radiation (Medical Exposure) Regulations 2000 [1] that doses to patients undergoing radiological procedures "are kept as low as reasonably practicable consistent with the intended purpose". It should be remembered that the risk of a new fatal malignancy of a patient ranges between 0.0002% and 0.03% per 60 minutes of fluoroscopy depending on the exposed organ [41]. Especially therapeutic procedures including ablation may be associated with higher doses and prolonged fluoroscopy times. A successful outcome of an EP procedure is feasible with low patient and investigator dosages. Low dose rate pulsed fluoroscopy should be a feature offered in every EP lab, reducing the dose-area product in comparison to continuous fluoroscopy to about 50% [40]. The use of moving grids should be made whenever possible to reduce the exposed area.

Physicians working in the field of clinical EP including ablation and device implantation are on top of the list of professions exposed to ionizing radiation. X-ray protective clothing of adequate size and design (as shielding of the left upper arm) and protective shielding at the table (fixed or movable) is mandatory.

The required ECG recording system for EP studies involves digital multichannel recording of usually up to 32 channels which are independently amplified and filtered (typically 0.5–100 Hz for the surface ECG channels, 30–500 Hz for the intracardiac signals). The recorder display should allow an oscilloscopic sweep or paper speed of 25–400 mm/s. The programmable stimulator must offer programmed stimulation and back-up bradycardia pacing if needed. The stimulator output is delivered as brief square waves with variable amplitude (current in milliamperes) and duration (pulse width in milliseconds). Usually the amplitude is set at twice the threshold value for capture at the individual pacing site and the pulse width is 2.0 ms. An external DC defibrillator is always connected to the patient over adhesive defibrillator pads attached to the anterior chest and back of the patient. This enables the prompt termination of unstable tachycardias without compromising the sterile catheter field. The commercially available RF energy generators allow controlled heating of the ablation catheter tip during power application (see Chapter 2).

∎ Vascular access and EP catheters

The availability of catheters and sheaths should be routinely checked before starting the procedure. Venous access is achieved preferentially by puncture and introduction of a guidewire (modified Seldinger technique) of the femoral vein on one or both sides. A single femoral vein can usually accommodate up to three standard (6 F) catheters. The jugular or subclavian vein are alternative routes for specific indications and accompanied by specific risks. For some procedures, placing an arterial line or catheter after puncture of the femoral artery is necessary.

A variety of different EP catheters for diagnostic and therapeutic use are commercially available. Diagnostic catheters are usually non-lumen catheters with a size of 2–8 French. They are made of woven Dacron or polyurethane and have a variable number of platinum-coated electrodes (1–2 mm) at the top.

Catheters for RF ablation are designed with a 4 mm or 8 mm tip. The newer irrigated tip ablation catheters (Figure 2.5) that allow cooling of the electrode tip during ablation usually have a 4 mm tip and have to be connected to a continuous infusion of saline.

For most applications, intracardiac bipolar recordings from two adjacent electrodes of the catheter shaft are used. The most distal electrode on the catheter shaft is numbered "1", the other electrodes in ascending order from distal to proximal.

∎ Radiological anatomy of the heart and catheter positioning

The analysis of the intracardiac activation pattern by cardiac mapping is mandatory for clinical EP studies and for all ablation procedures. The simplest way of mapping is the stable placement of electrode catheters at defined anatomic locations. There are three to four standard locations for a diagnostic EP study which

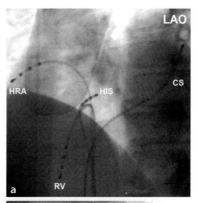

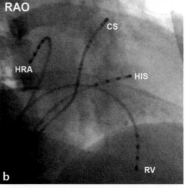

Fig. 1.14. Fluoroscopic image (**a** LAO 45° and **b** RAO 30° projection) of catheter positions during a standard EP study. The four catheter locations are high right atrium (HRA), His bundle region (HIS), coronary sinus (CS) and right ventricular apex (RV)

Table 1.2. Differential topographic use of different fluoroscopic projections

Catheter target location	First choice	Second choice	Differentiation
▌His bundle	PA	(LAO 45°)	Septal from supero-anterior in LAO
▌HRA	PA		Septal from lateral in LAO
▌RVA	PA	RAO 30°	AV-ring in RAO
▌RVOT	PA	(RAO 30°)	Septal from lateral in LAO
▌CS	LAO 45°	(PA)	Septal ostial area and ventricular side branches of vena cordis magna
▌Right free wall (Halo catheter)	PA	LAO 45°	Anterior/posterior of crista terminalis in LAO
▌TV-IVC-Isthmus (Ablation)	LAO 45°	PA	Septal, midisthmus and lateral TV-IVC-isthmus in LAO
▌Left-sided AP	LAO 45°	RAO 30°	Inferior-anterior and inferior-superior in LAO, differing distance to MV RAO
▌Septal AP	LAO 45°	RAO 30°	Anteroseptal, midseptal, inferoseptal in LAO
▌Right-sided AP	LAO 45°	PA	Superior, inferior, lateral in LAO; differing distance to TV in RAO
▌Slow pathway (ANVRT)	LAO 45°	PA/RAO 30°	Anteroseptal, midseptal, inferoseptal and CS-os in LAO
▌Left-sided PV	LAO 45°	(PA)	Distance of PV-ostium to left atrial contour in LAO
▌Right-sided PV	RAO 20°	(PA)	Distance of PV-ostium to right/left atrial contour in RAO
▌RVOT-VT	PA	LAO 45° / RAO 30°	Septal from lateral outflow tract / Anterior from posterior outflow tract
▌LV-VT	PA	LAO 45° / RAO 30°	Septal, apical and lateral LV / Anterolateral, apical, inferior and MV-ring

include the "high" right atrium (HRA), His bundle region (HIS), coronary sinus (CS) and right ventricular apex (RVA). In our lab, we routinely use three diagnostic EP catheters: an octapolar steerable catheter placed in the CS for the recording of atrial activity and for atrial pacing (usually over electrodes 7/8), a His bundle catheter and a catheter in the right ventricular apex.

A three or four catheter EP study including CS recording will reveal an abnormal retrograde atrial activation sequence during ventricular pacing as with the presence of a left-sided accessory pathway (Figure 1.8). The timing of recorded signals from a moving mapping/ablation catheter has to be integrated in the activation pattern and individual anatomy of a patient. This method of "conventional" mapping is used in most ablation procedures for supraventricular tachycardias.

Usually EP procedures are performed without the application of contrast media. Guiding and positioning of the EP catheters is done with the help of fluoroscopic landmarks. Standard projections are posterior-anterior (PA), right anterior oblique (RAO 30°) and left-anterior oblique (LAO 45°). Depending on the target location,

the optimal catheter position can be performed using specific projections. Some examples are listed in Table 1.2. In should be kept in mind that a PA projection offers the lowest radiation exposure [44, 54].

▌ Basic EP measurements and maneuvers

Prior to any pacing maneuvers, intracardiac activation sequences and baseline intervals are evaluated and measured during normal sinus rhythm. Figure 1.15 shows and explains these measurements.

The atrial activation sequence is derived from the surface P wave in conjunction with atrial electrograms from RA, His and CS (left atrial activation) catheter. As mentioned above, we do not routinely use a HRA catheter anymore. The initial deflection of the P wave on the surface ECG is followed by the atrial signal of the His recording (24–50 ms after P wave onset). Left atrial activation (recorded on the CS catheter) begins thereafter and spreads from proximal to distal along the CS catheter. Details of the AV conduction are analyzed from the His recording. The AH interval (normal range 50–120 ms) reflects conduction time within the AV node

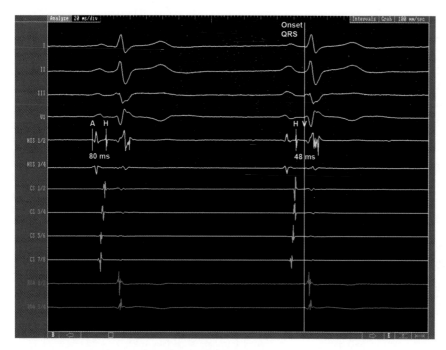

Fig. 1.15. Baseline intervals and intracardiac activation sequence during sinus rhythm (standard 3 catheter EP study). Shown are surface leads I,II, III and V1 and bipolar intracardiac recordings from a His catheter (yellow), coronary sinus (CS) catheter (green) and right ventricular apex (RVA) catheter (pink). Atrial activation (A) on the His catheter occurs slightly after P wave onset and spreads proximal (7/8) to distal (1/2) on the length of the CS catheter. *Ventricular activation* times are measured against a line which marks the earliest ventricular activation on any ECG (onset QRS complex). The RVA activates quickly after onset of QRS with subsequent activation along the right ventricular septum (seen on the His catheter) and latest ventricular activation at the left ventricular base (seen on the CS catheter). The *AH interval* (80 ms) is measured from the onset of local activation on the His catheter to the onset of rapid His deflection. The *HV interval* (48 ms) is measured from the onset of the rapid His deflection to the earliest ventricular activity on the ECG

and might be prolonged in AV nodal disease or with antiarrhythmic drugs. It usually shortens with the administration of catecholamines. The HV interval (normal range 30–55 ms) reflects the conduction time from the proximal His bundle over the bundle branches/Purkinje system to the ventricular myocardium. It is prolonged with intrinsic His-Purkinje disease or with specific antiarrhythmic medication. A short HV interval will be observed in patients with antegrade conduction over an accessory pathway as in WPW syndrome or with Mahaim fibers (see Chapter 4). If the His catheter is advanced into the right ventricle, a sharp signal from the right bundle rather than from the His bundle will be recorded, leading to an artificially short HV time (Figure 1.16)

The ventricular activation sequence is analyzed by examining the surface QRS complex in conjunction with local activation times at the RVA, His (right side of upper ventricular septum) and CS (left ventricular base) catheters.

The normal ventricular sequence of RVA-HIS-CS might also be lost in patients with preexcitation. With a left-sided pathway, the ventricular signal on the CS catheter (representing left atrial and ventricular activity) will precede the ventricular signals on the other catheters. In patients with right (RBBB) – or left (LBBB) bundle branch block, ventricular activation is distorted by conduction delay within the His-Purkinje system. In RBBB (due to interruption of conduction within the main right bundle), RVA activation time in relation to the surface QRS complex is prolonged by 50 ms or more. In LBBB, ventricular activation times are usually normal at the RVA and HBE locations, but very delayed at the CS catheter. Table 1.3 shows the normal conduction times for atrial activation times (PA), conduction within the AV node (AH) and conduction time from the proximal His bundle over the bundle branches/Purkinje system to the ventricular myocardium (HV).

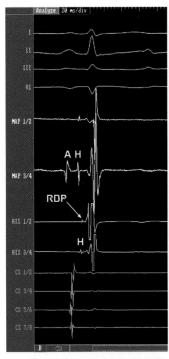

Fig. 1.16. EP study with the mapping catheter (MAP) placed in the His position. A sharp His deflection (H) is seen on the MAP catheter. The His catheter (HIS) is advanced into the right ventricle, showing a sharp right bundle potential (RBP) on electrode pair His 1/2 and a His potential on electrode pair His 3/4

Table 1.3. Normal conduction intervals in adults [8, 15, 16, 38, 53, 62]

Author	PA (ms)	AH (ms)	HV (ms)
Damato	24–45	50–120	35–45
Schuilenburg		85–150	30–55
Bekheit	10–50	50–125	35–45
Rosen	9–45	54–130	31–55
Josephson		60–125	35–55

See text for explanation of abbreviations

■ Evaluation of sinus node function

As the evaluation of sinus node function is only relevant for the decision about pacemaker implantation, it will not be discussed in further detail. In short, a relatively simple technique called sinus node recovery time can be applied to patients with selected indications. With this technique, the atrium is paced with a constant cycle length of the intrinsic rhythm (e.g., 700 ms) for one minute, followed by a 1-minute pacing pause and then pacing is started again

with a shorter cycle length. The decremental step size is 50 ms between the bursts and the shortest pacing interval is usually 400 ms.

By definition, the uncorrected sinus nodal recovery time is the longest first postpacing interval until the sinus node starts driving the rhythm again. The upper value for a normal sinus nodal recovery time (SNRT = interval between last pacing spike and begin of the first sinus rhythm P wave) is 1400 ms. To standardize the data, the corrected sinus nodal recovery time (CSNRT) was introduced. It is calculated as follows: CSNRT – SNRT – intrinsic interval during sinus rhythm. The upper limit of the CSNRT is 450 ms.

■ Evaluation of atrial, AV nodal and His-Purkinje conduction by pacing maneuvers

The most important pacing maneuver evaluating atrial, AV nodal or His-Purkinje conduction is the determination of refractory periods. The "effective" refractory period (ERP) used in clinical electrophysiology is the longest coupling interval that fails to propagate through a given tissue at a stimulation amplitude of twice the diastolic threshold. This ERP is determined using an eight-beat-basic train of a standard cycle length called "S1" (usually 600, 500 or 400 ms) followed by premature extrastimuli (attributed "S2") to a particular site (Figure 1.17).

S2 is progressively shortened (in 10 ms intervals) until it fails to excite or conduct through tissue (corresponding to the ERP of this site). The example of AV nodal and atrial ERP is shown in Figure 1.18, while the normal ranges in the adult population are shown in Table 1.4.

When performing this maneuver with atrial stimulation (in our case performed over the proximal electrodes of the CS catheter), the typical response to extrastimuli introduced at 500(S1)/490(S2) ms is capture of atrium, AV node and His-Purkinje system. With progres-

Table 1.4. Normal refractory periods in adults [2, 18, 38, 62]

Author	ERP atrium (ms)	ERP AV node (ms)	ERP ventricle (ms)
Denes	150–360	250–365	
Akhtar	230–330	280–430	190–290
Schuilenburg		230–390	
Josephson	170–300	230–425	170–290

ERP effective refractory period

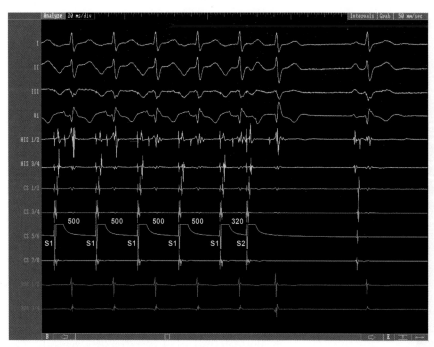

Fig. 1.17. A standard pacing protocol during an EP study (see text) includes programmed atrial pacing; here performed over the CS catheter (green). A basic train of a standard cycle length (S1; 500 ms) is followed by a premature extra- stimulus (S2) with a cycle length of 320 ms. Besides the CS catheter, a His (HIS) catheter and a catheter at the right ventricular apex (RVA) had been introduced

sively premature S2, conduction delay within the AV node is noticed and the AH interval lengthens. This lengthening is usually gradual and progressive. In patients with "dual AV nodal physiology" (see Chapter 5), a sudden "jump" of the AH interval of at least 50 ms is observed in response to a 10 ms decrease in S2 timing (Figures 1.19 and 1.20).

The HV interval usually remains constant during the process of AH prolongation. With further premature S2, there is a point at which block occurs within the AV node (AVNERP; normal range 230–430 ms), which corresponds to a paced atrial signal without subsequent His or ventricular deflection. In very rare cases (mostly with infranodal conduction pathology), the first signs of AV block occur below the His bundle, reflected by an atrial signal followed by a His signal without ventricular deflection (indicating His bundle ERP).

With progressive shortening of the premature interval, a point is reached where atrial muscle will not be captured by the impulse anymore defining atrial ERP (normal range 150–360 ms).

Another pacing technique to evaluate AV conduction is to pace the atrium at progressively shorter basic lengths and to monitor the pacing cycle length at which AV block (usually second degree AV block Wenckebach type) occurs (Figure 1.21). The Wenckebach interval is defined as the longest cycle length that does not result in a 1:1 conduction during constant pacing. This maneuver evaluates the functional capacity of the AV node and can be used for comparison before/after an ablation (see also Chapter 5).

▮ Measurements during ventricular stimulation

During a routine EP study, measurement of the ventricular ERP is performed similarly to the determination of atrial ERP. Pacing over the RVA catheter is performed with an eight-beat train of S1 (600, 500 or 400 ms) and decremental steps of 10 ms of S2 are delivered until failure of ventricular capture (ventricular ERP). During the ERP determination, the presence or absence of ventriculoatrial (VA) conduction is assessed. Interestingly, retrograde conduction via the His bundle and the AV node is observed in about 50% of patients. If VA conduction over the AV node is present during extrastimulus testing, this conduction follows a decremental pattern and the earliest atrial activation occurs at the His location (Figure 1.22).

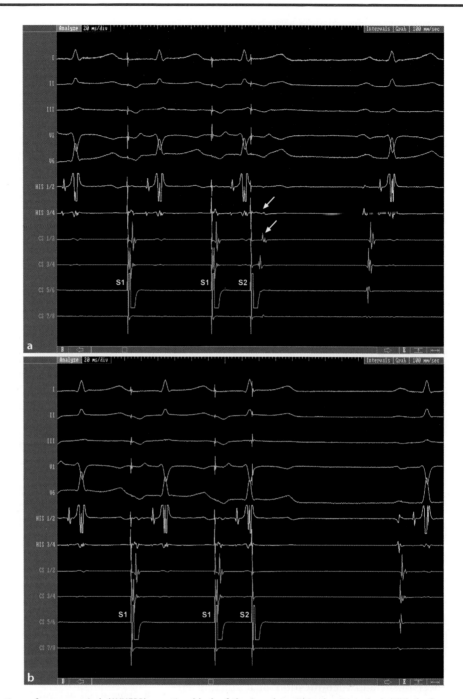

Fig. 1.18. a AV nodal effective refractory period (AVNERP): With programmed atrial pacing (over the CS catheter) and progressively premature atrial extrastimuli (S2), the impulse is captured by the atrium, but no further His signal is observed on the His catheter (yellow) corresponding to conduction block of the impulse within the AV node. **b** With further shortening of the premature impulse, the atrium is not captured (no atrial signal following the pacing spike on the CS catheter) corresponding to the atrial effective refractory period (AERP)

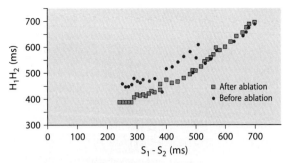

Fig. 1.19. AV nodal conduction curve with programmed atrial stimulation before and after ablation of the slow pathway in a patient with AVNRT. The red dots depict a continuous shortening of the H1H2 interval with decremental atrial extrastimulation before ablation, until at S1S2 = 520 ms a sudden prolongation of H1H2 interval is found indicating dual nodal conduction properties of the AV node. The red squares (after ablation) demonstrate a steady shortening of the H1H2 interval, until the AV node is refractory, demonstrating the existence of a single functional AV nodal pathway

These features help to distinguish an accessory pathway as the reason for retrograde conduction, which will show an "eccentric" activation sequence (see Chapter 4). Dual AV nodal physiology as described above with a sudden jump in the VA conduction time can also be observed in the retrograde direction, then mostly associated with the atypical (fast-slow) form of AVNRT (see Chapter 5). If retrograde VA conduction is present, the retrograde Wenckebach sequence is also assessed with ventricular pacing at progressively faster pacing cycle lengths.

▪ Evaluation of supraventricular tachycardia

The primary goal of an SVT study is to record multiple intracardiac signals during baseline and/or during an episode of tachycardia, which will allow definition of the precise tachycardia mechanism and identification of a suitable target for ablation. Each EP lab should have a standardized protocol for SVT studies providing the following information:

- Measurement of the PR, QRS, QT, CL, AH and HV intervals during spontaneous rhythm
- *Retrograde conduction properties*: To start with pacing on the ventricular level makes the induction of atrial fibrillation less likely, and even if this happens later during atrial pacing, retrograde conduction properties have already been assessed

- Programmed stimulation in the RV with two different basic cycle lengths (for example, 600 ms and 400 ms) and one extrastimulus. The basic cycle length should be shorter than the intrinsic cycle length. The finding of a retrograde dual AV nodal pathway physiology, atypical retrograde activation of the atria (accessory pathway) and the induction of tachycardia might result
- Fixed stimulation with a continuous decrease of the pacing cycle length by 10 ms until the retrograde conduction meets the retrograde Wenckebach interval.
- *Antegrade conduction properties:*
- Programmed atrial stimulation with two different basic cycle lengths (for example, 600 ms and 400 ms) and one extrastimulus. The finding of a dual nodal pathway, an antegrade conducting accessory pathway causing ventricular preexcitation, the potential site of AV block and the induction of tachycardia might result from this maneuver
- Fixed stimulation with continuous decrease of the pacing cycle length by 10 ms until the antegrade Wenckebach interval is reached

If these standard pacing maneuvers fail to induce a clinically documented SVT, atrial burst pacing or programmed stimulation with up to four extrastimuli is introduced. A pharmacological intervention with orciprenaline (or atropine) is often useful for tachycardia induction but also increases the risk of inducing atrial fibrillation.

Once sustained SVT has been induced, specific tachycardia behavior and electrocardiograms should be analyzed including the most critical points:
- Mode of tachycardia initiation and termination
- The relationship of atrial and ventricular activity during SVT
- The atrial activation sequence during SVT
- The response of tachycardia to ventricular premature stimuli/entrainment maneuvers
- The response of tachycardia to adenosine
- Evaluation of the P wave morphology

The specific pacing maneuvers to assess tachycardia mechanisms are discussed in the corresponding chapters of this book, especially in Chapter 5. A repeated EP study after an ablation should use the same stimulation protocol as un-

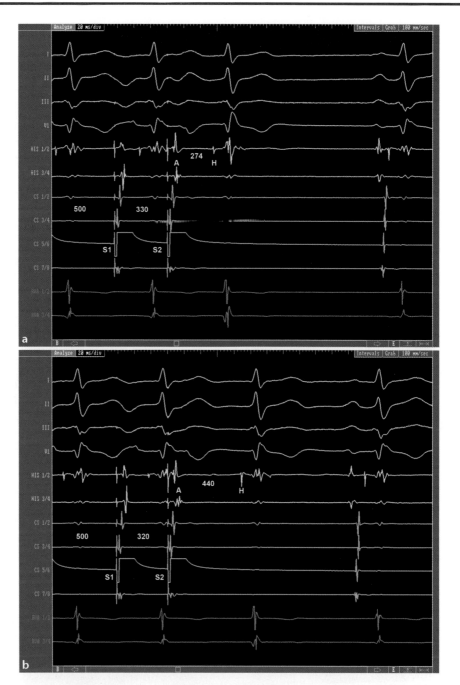

Fig. 1.20. Dual AV nodal physiology. **a**: Programmed atrial pacing (S1= 500 ms) with one extrastimulus (S2) of 330 ms is leading to an A2H2 interval of 274 ms. **b** with a 10 ms decrement in the coupling interval of S2 (320 ms), a sudden "jump" of the A2H2 interval to 440 ms is observed corresponding to a change of conduction from the "fast" to the "slow" AV nodal pathway

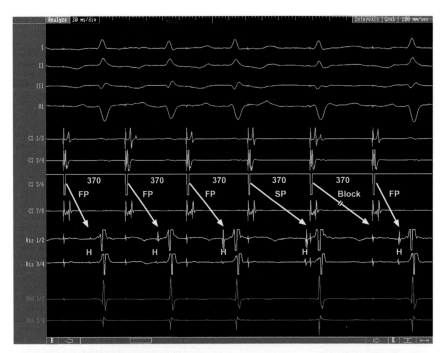

Fig. 1.21. Evaluation of AV conduction by pacing the atrium (over the CS catheter). The pacing cycle length is 370 msec. AV conduction steadily prolongs and switches from the fast pathway (FP) to the slow pathway (SP) after the fourth paced beat. The fifth paced beat is blocked in the AV node (above the His bundle). Conduction over the fast pathway is started again with the next paced beat

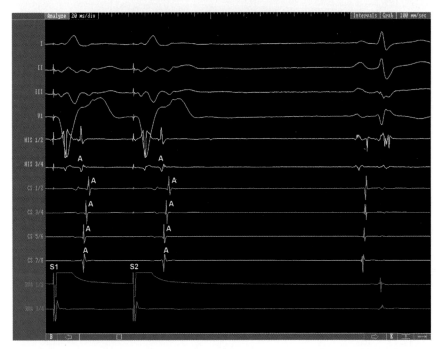

Fig. 1.22. Programmed ventricular stimulation with one extrastimulus (S2) over the right ventricular (RVA) catheter. Following S2, the earliest atrial activity (A) is recorded on the His catheter, followed by a proximal to distal atrial activation sequence on the CS catheter. This corresponds to retrograde conduction over the AV node

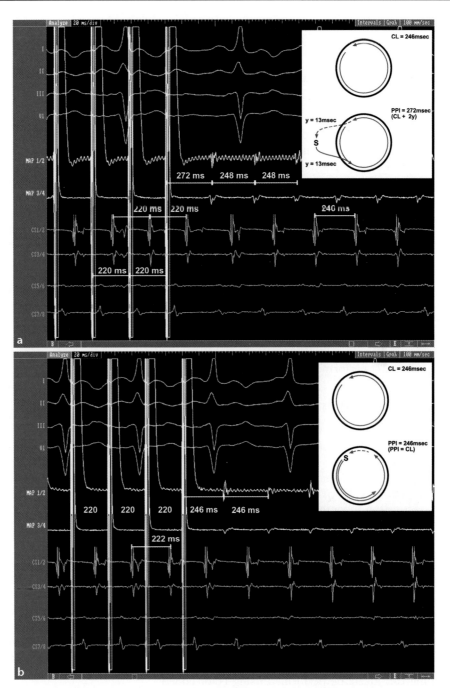

Fig. 1.23. Entrainment maneuver during intraatrial reentrant tachycardia (IART) in a patient after Fontan operation. **a** the postpacing interval (PPI) on the distal Map catheter (272 ms) is 24 ms longer than IART cycle length (CL) of 248 ms con- sistent with negative entrainment (Map catheter placed out- side the reentrant circuit). **b** the PPI is similar (246 ms) to the IART-CL (246 ms) consistent with positive entrainment (MAP catheter placed in or close to the reentrant circuit)

der baseline conditions to allow comparison of the parameters.

■ Evaluation of ventricular tachycardia

The precise evaluation of VT by various techniques is discussed in Chapter 9 of this book. In general, for EP studies the following ventricular pacing protocol is recommended:

■ Ventricular pacing with at least two basic cycle lengths (for example, 600 ms and 400 ms) in RVA (right ventricular apex) and RVOT (right ventricular outflow tract) with up to three extrastimuli until the effective ventricular refractory period is met or the extrastimulus interval reaches 180 ms
■ In a small subset of patients ventricular side branches of the coronary sinus or the left ventricle can be chosen as an additional pacing site
■ For completion of the study, assessment of atrial conduction properties, as discussed above, is performed

■ General principles of cardiac mapping

Different mapping techniques are essential for successful catheter ablation of atrial and ventricular arrhythmias.

The following mapping modes have been developed:
■ activation mapping
■ pace mapping
■ entrainment mapping
■ voltage mapping

The technique of *activation mapping* is based on the localization of the earliest electrical activation of an arrhythmia. This is of greatest importance for ablation of focal arrhythmias such as focal atrial tachycardia and will be discussed in greater detail in Chapter 8. Activation mapping can nicely be performed using color coded maps such as in electroanatomical mapping systems (Chapter 3).

The technique of *pace mapping* is rather simple: If (in sinus rhythm) the paced P wave or paced QRS complex morphology exactly matches all leads in the surface ECG (see Figure 9.6) during tachycardia, it can be presumed that pacing is performed from the site of origin of an arrhythmia. Pace mapping has certain limitations which will be further discussed in Chapter 9.

■ **Entrainment mapping** is the most important technique to characterize a reentrant circuit. In case of a macroreentrant tachycardia the determination of "earliest" activity is variable. This group of arrhythmias includes scar-related arrhythmias such as monomorphic ventricular tachycardia (after myocardial infarction) but also subgroups of atrial macroreentrant tachycardias such as typical and atypical flutter or atrial tachycardia occurring after repair of congenital heart disease. In order to abolish the reentry, it is important to identify the reentrant circuit, to delineate the zone of slow conduction and preferentially to delineate a narrow isthmus which is amenable to catheter ablation. Entrainment mapping is used most often to characterize the reentry circuit. Various examples are given in the chapters dealing with ablation of typical and atypical atrial flutter (Chapters 6 and 7) as well as in the ablation of ventricular tachycardia (Chapter 9). Briefly, the technique proves if a given stimulus or train of extrastimuli are in or outside the reentrant circuit. Entrainment mapping requires an excitable gap in a presumed reentrant circuit. Resetting the tachycardia (acceleration of the tachycardia to a paced cycle length slightly shorter than the tachycardia cycle length) without any alteration of the P wave or the QRS complex is evidence for (concealed) entrainment. In addition, it is required that after cessation of pacing the return cycle length should equal the tachycardia cycle length within limits of 20–30 ms (see Figures 1.23 and 9.18).

■ **Voltage mapping** allows the determination of local electrogram amplitudes in the atrium or ventricle. This is done with the help of 3D mapping systems and helps to identify viable and scar regions in a presumed reentry circuit and is gaining increasing importance in modern ablation concepts (see Chapters 7 and 9).

■ References

1. Department of Health (2000) The Ionizing Radiation (Medical Exposure) Regulations 2000, with supplementary guidance on good practice (http://www.doh.gov.uk/irmer.htm)
2. Akhtar M, Damato AN, Batsford WP, Ruskin JN, Ogunkelu JB (1975) A comparative analysis of antegrade and retrograde conduction patterns in man. Circulation 52:766–778
3. Anderson RH, Ho SY (1997) Anatomy of the atrioventricular junctions with regard to ventri-

cular preexcitation. Pacing Clin Electrophysiol 20:2072–2076

4. Anderson RH, Razavi R, Taylor AM (2004) Cardiac anatomy revisited. J Anat 205:159–177
5. Anderson RH, Webb S, Brown NA (1999) Clinical anatomy of the atrial septum with reference to its developmental components. Clin Anat 12:362–374
6. Becker AE (2004) Left atrial isthmus: anatomic aspects relevant for linear catheter ablation procedures in humans. J Cardiovasc Electrophysiol 15:809–812
7. Becker AE, Anderson RH, Durrer D, Wellens HJ (1978) The anatomical substrates of wolff-parkinson-white syndrome. A clinicopathologic correlation in seven patients. Circulation 57:870–879
8. Bekheit S, Murtagh JG, Morton P, Fletcher E (1971) Measurements of sinus impulse conduction from electrogram of bundle of His. Br Heart J 33:719–724
9. Blomstrom-Lundqvist C, Scheinman MM, Aliot EM, Alpert JS, Calkins H, Camm AJ, Campbell WB, Haines DE, Kuck KH, Lerman BB, Miller DD, Shaeffer CW, Stevenson WG, Tomaselli GF, Antman EM, Smith SC, Jr, Alpert JS, Faxon DP, Fuster V, Gibbons RJ, Gregoratos G, Hiratzka LF, Hunt SA, Jacobs AK, Russell RO, Jr, Priori SG, Blanc JJ, Budaj A, Burgos EF, Cowie M, Deckers JW, Garcia MA, Klein WW, Lekakis J, Lindahl B, Mazzotta G, Morais JC, Oto A, Smiseth O, Trappe HJ (2003) ACC/AHA/ESC guidelines for the management of patients with supraventricular arrhythmias – executive summary. A report of the American college of cardiology/American heart association task force on practice guidelines and the European society of cardiology committee for practice guidelines (writing committee to develop guidelines for the management of patients with supraventricular arrhythmias) developed in collaboration with NASPE-Heart Rhythm Society. J Am Coll Cardiol 42:1493–1531
10. Borggrefe M, Budde T, Podczeck A, Breithardt G (1987) High frequency alternating current ablation of an accessory pathway in humans. J Am Coll Cardiol 10:576–582
11. Cabrera JA, Sanchez-Quintana D, Ho SY, Medina A, Wanguemert F, Gross E, Grillo J, Hernandez E, Anderson RH (1999) Angiographic anatomy of the inferior right atrial isthmus in patients with and without history of common atrial flutter. Circulation 99:3017–3023
12. Chauvin M, Shah DC, Haissaguerre M, Marcellin L, Brechenmacher C (2000) The anatomic basis of connections between the coronary sinus musculature and the left atrium in humans. Circulation 101:647–652
13. Corcoran SJ, Lawrence C, McGuire MA (1999) The valve of Vieussens: an important cause of difficulty in advancing catheters into the cardiac veins. J Cardiovasc Electrophysiol 10:804–808
14. Cosio FG, Anderson RH, Kuck KH, Becker A, Borggrefe M, Campbell RW, Gaita F, Guiraudon GM, Haissaguerre M, Rufilanchas JJ, Thiene G, Wellens HJ, Langberg J, Benditt DG, Bharati S, Klein G, Marchlinski F, Saksena S (1999) Living anatomy of the atrioventricular junctions. A guide to electrophysiologic mapping. A Consensus Statement from the Cardiac Nomenclature Study Group, Working Group of Arrhythmias, European Society of Cardiology, and the Task Force on Cardiac Nomenclature from NASPE. Circulation 100:e31–37
15. Damato AN, Lau SH, Helfant R, Stein E, Patton RD, Scherlag BJ, Berkowitz WD (1969) A study of heart block in man using His bundle recordings. Circulation 39:297–305
16. Damato AN, Lau SH, Patton RD, Steiner C, Berkowitz WD (1969) A study of atrioventricular conduction in man using premature atrial stimulation and His bundle recordings. Circulation 40:61–69
17. Davies MJ (1980) Pathology of cardiac valves. Butterworthes, London
18. Denes P, Wu D, Dhingra R, Pietras RJ, Rosen KM (1974) The effects of cycle length on cardiac refractory periods in man. Circulation 49:32–41
19. Dong J, Schreieck J, Ndrepepa G, Schmitt C (2002) Ectopic tachycardia originating from the superior vena cava. J Cardiovasc Electrophysiol 13:620–624
20. Doshi RN, Wu TJ, Yashima M, Kim YH, Ong JJ, Cao JM, Hwang C, Yashar P, Fishbein MC, Karagueuzian HS, Chen PS (1999) Relation between ligament of Marshall and adrenergic atrial tachyarrhythmia. Circulation 100:876–883
21. Ernst S, Ouyang F, Linder C, Hertting K, Stahl F, Chun J, Hachiya H, Bansch D, Antz M, Kuck KH (2004) Initial experience with remote catheter ablation using a novel magnetic navigation system: magnetic remote catheter ablation. Circulation 109:1472–1475
22. Friedman PA, Luria D, Fenton AM, Munger TM, Jahangir A, Shen WK, Rea RF, Stanton MS, Hammill SC, Packer DL (2000) Global right atrial mapping of human atrial flutter: the presence of posteromedial (sinus venosa region) functional block and double potentials: a study in biplane fluoroscopy and intracardiac echocardiography. Circulation 101:1568–1577
23. Gallagher JJ, Svenson RH, Kasell JH, German LD, Bardy GH, Broughton A, Critelli G (1982) Catheter technique for closed-chest ablation of the atrioventricular conduction system. N Engl J Med 306:194–200

24. Haissaguerre M, Jais P, Shah DC, Gencel L, Pradeau V, Garrigues S, Chouairi S, Hocini M, Le Metayer P, Roudaut R, Clementy J (1996) Right and left atrial radiofrequency catheter therapy of paroxysmal atrial fibrillation. J Cardiovasc Electrophysiol 7:1132–1144

25. Haissaguerre M, Jais P, Shah DC, Takahashi A, Hocini M, Quiniou G, Garrigue S, Le Mouroux A, Le Metayer P, Clementy J (1998) Spontaneous initiation of atrial fibrillation by ectopic beats originating in the pulmonary veins. N Engl J Med 339:659–666

26. Haissaguerre M, Shah DC, Jais P, Hocini M, Yamane T, Deisenhofer I, Chauvin M, Garrigue S, Clementy J (2000) Electrophysiological breakthroughs from the left atrium to the pulmonary veins. Circulation 102:2463–2465

27. Hashizume H, Ushiki T, Abe K (1995) A histological study of the cardiac muscle of the human superior and inferior venae cavae. Arch Histol Cytol 58:457–464

28. Ho SY, Anderson RH, Sanchez-Quintana D (2002) Atrial structure and fibres: morphologic bases of atrial conduction. Cardiovasc Res 54: 325–336

29. Ho SY, Cabrera JA, Tran VH, Farre J, Anderson RH, Sanchez-Quintana D (2001) Architecture of the pulmonary veins: relevance to radiofrequency ablation. Heart 86:265–270

30. Ho SY, Sanchez-Quintana D, Becker AE (2004) A review of the coronary venous system: a road less travelled. Heart Rhythm 1:107–112

31. Ho SY, Sanchez-Quintana D, Cabrera JA, Anderson RH (1999) Anatomy of the left atrium: implications for radiofrequency ablation of atrial fibrillation. J Cardiovasc Electrophysiol 10 :1525–1533

32. Huang SK, Bharati S, Graham AR, Lev M, Marcus FI, Odell RC (1987) Closed chest catheter desiccation of the atrioventricular junction using radiofrequency energy – a new method of catheter ablation. J Am Coll Cardiol 9:349–358

33. Hurst JW, Anderson RH, Wilcox BR (1988) Atlas of the heart. McGraw-Hill Book Company, London

34. Ito M, Arita M, Saeki K, Tanoue M, Fukushima I (1967) Functional properties of sinocaval conduction. Jpn J Physiol 17:174–189

35. Jackman WM, Wang XZ, Friday KJ, Roman CA, Moulton KP, Beckman KJ, McClelland JH, Twidale N, Hazlitt HA, Prior MI et al (1991) Catheter ablation of accessory atrioventricular pathways (Wolff-Parkinson-White syndrome) by radiofrequency current. N Engl J Med 324: 1605–1611

36. Jalife J, Berenfeld O, Mansour M (2002) Mother rotors and fibrillatory conduction: a mechanism of atrial fibrillation. Cardiovasc Res 54:204–216

37. Janse MJ, Anderson RH (1974) Specialized internodal atrial pathways – fact or fiction? Eur J Cardiol 2:117–136

38. Josephson ME (1993) Electrophysiologic investigation: general concepts. In: Josephson ME (ed) Clinical Cardiac Electrophysiology. Lea & Febiger, Philadelphia/London, pp 23–70

39. Kalman JM, Olgin JE, Karch MR, Hamdan M, Lee RJ, Lesh MD (1998) "Cristal tachycardias": origin of right atrial tachycardias from the crista terminalis identified by intracardiac echocardiography. J Am Coll Cardiol 31:451–459

40. Kotre CJ, Charlton S, Robson KJ, Birch IP, Willis SP, Thornley M (2004) Application of low dose rate pulsed fluoroscopy in cardiac pacing and electrophysiology: patient dose and image quality implications. Br J Radiol 77:597–599

41. Kovoor P, Ricciardello M, Collins L, Uther JB, Ross DL (1998) Risk to patients from radiation associated with radiofrequency ablation for supraventricular tachycardia. Circulation 98:1534–1540

42. Kugler JD, Danford DA, Houston KA, Felix G (2002) Pediatric radiofrequency catheter ablation registry success, fluoroscopy time, and complication rate for supraventricular tachycardia: comparison of early and recent eras. J Cardiovasc Electrophysiol 13:336–341

43. Lewis T, J. M, PD W (1914) The excitatory process in the Dog's heart. Part I – The auricles. Philos Trans R Soc Lond 205B:375–420

44. Lindsay BD, Eichling JO, Ambos HD, Cain ME (1992) Radiation exposure to patients and medical personnel during radiofrequency catheter ablation for supraventricular tachycardia. Am J Cardiol 70:218–223

45. Ludinghausen M, Ohmachi N, Boot C (1992) Myocardial coverage of the coronary sinus and related veins. Clin Anat 5:1–15

46. Luik A, Deisenhofer I, Estner H, Ndrepepa G, Pflaumer A, Zrenner B, Schmitt C (2006) Atresia of the coronary sinus in patients with supraventricular tachycardia. PACE 29:171–174

47. Mansour M, Ruskin J, Keane D (2002) Initiation of atrial fibrillation by ectopic beats originating from the ostium of the inferior vena cava. J Cardiovasc Electrophysiol 13:1292–1295

48. Mayer AG (1906) Rhymical pulsation in scyphomedusae. Publication 47 of the Carnegie Institution, Washington, pp 1–62

49. Mazgalev TN, Ho SY, Anderson RH (2001) Anatomic-electrophysiological correlations concerning the pathways for atrioventricular conduction. Circulation 103:2660–2667

50. Nathan HaME (1966) The junction between the left atrium and the pulmonary veins. An anatomic study of human hearts. Circulation 34: 412–422

51. Pappone C, Rosanio S, Oreto G, Tocchi M, Gugliotta F, Vicedomini G, Salvati A, Dicandia C, Mazzone P, Santinelli V, Gulletta S, Chierchia S (2000) Circumferential radiofrequency ablation of pulmonary vein ostia: A new anatomic approach for curing atrial fibrillation. Circulation 102:2619–2628

52. Roithinger FX, Cheng J, SippensGroenewegen A, Lee RJ, Saxon LA, Scheinman MM, Lesh MD (1999) Use of electroanatomic mapping to delineate transseptal atrial conduction in humans. Circulation 100:1791–1797

53. Rosen KM (1972) Evaluation of cardiac conduction in the cardiac catheterization laboratory. Am J Cardiol 30:701–703

54. Rosenthal LS, Mahesh M, Beck TJ, Saul JP, Miller JM, Kay N, Klein LS, Huang S, Gillette P, Prystowsky E, Carlson M, Berger RD, Lawrence JH, Yong P, Calkins H (1998) Predictors of fluoroscopy time and estimated radiation exposure during radiofrequency catheter ablation procedures. Am J Cardiol 82:451–458

55. Saffitz JE, Kanter HL, Green KG, Tolley TK, Beyer EC (1994) Tissue-specific determinants of anisotropic conduction velocity in canine atrial and ventricular myocardium. Circ Res 74:1065–1070

56. Saito T, Waki K, Becker AE (2000) Left atrial myocardial extension onto pulmonary veins in humans: anatomic observations relevant for atrial arrhythmias. J Cardiovasc Electrophysiol 11:888–894

57. Sanchez-Quintana D, Anderson RH, Cabrera JA, Climent V, Martin R, Farre J, Ho SY (2002) The terminal crest: morphological features relevant to electrophysiology. Heart 88:406–411

58. Sanchez-Quintana D, Cabrera JA, Farre J, Climent V, Anderson RH, Ho SY (2005) Sinus node revisited in the era of electroanatomical mapping and catheter ablation. Heart 91:189–194

59. Sanchez-Quintana D, Ho SY, Cabrera JA, Farre J, Anderson RH (2001) Topographic anatomy of the inferior pyramidal space: relevance to radiofrequency catheter ablation. J Cardiovasc Electrophysiol 12:210–217

60. Scavee C, Jais P, Weerasooriya R, Haissaguerre M (2003) The inferior vena cava: an exceptional source of atrial fibrillation. J Cardiovasc Electrophysiol 14:659–662

61. Scherlag BJ, Lau SH, Helfant RH, Berkowitz WD, Stein E, Damato AN (1969) Catheter technique for recording. His bundle activity in man. Circulation 39:13–18

62. Schuilenburg RM, Durrer D (1972) Conduction disturbances located within the His bundle. Circulation 45:612–628

63. Spach MS, Barr RC, Jewett PH (1972) Spread of excitation from the atrium into thoracic veins in human beings and dogs. Am J Cardiol 30:844–854

64. Spach MS, Miller WT, 3rd, Dolber PC, Kootsey JM, Sommer JR, Mosher CE, Jr. (1982) The functional role of structural complexities in the propagation of depolarization in the atrium of the dog. Cardiac conduction disturbances due to discontinuities of effective axial resistivity. Circ Res 50:175–191

65. Statement AACC (2000) A Report of the American College of Cardiology/American Heart Association/American College of Physicans-American Society of Internal Medicine Task Force on Clinical Competence. Circulation 102:2309–2320

66. Swartz JF, Pellersells G, Silvers J, Cervantez D (1994) A catheter-based curative approach to atrial fibrillation in humans. Circulation 90(supp I): 335

67. Sweeney LJ, Rosenquist GC (1979) The normal anatomy of the atrial septum in the human heart. Am Heart J 98:194–199

68. Takahashi A, Iesaka Y, Takahashi Y, Takahashi R, Kobayashi K, Takagi K, Kuboyama O, Nishimori T, Takei H, Amemiya H, Fujiwara H, Hiraoka M (2002) Electrical connections between pulmonary veins: implication for ostial ablation of pulmonary veins in patients with paroxysmal atrial fibrillation. Circulation 105:2998–3003

69. Tsai CF, Tai CT, Hsieh MH, Lin WS, Yu WC, Ueng KC, Ding YA, Chang MS, Chen SA (2000) Initiation of atrial fibrillation by ectopic beats originating from the superior vena cava: electrophysiological characteristics and results of radiofrequency ablation. Circulation 102:67–74

70. Waki K, Saito T, Becker AE (2000) Right atrial flutter isthmus revisited: normal anatomy favors nonuniform anisotropic conduction. J Cardiovasc Electrophysiol 11:90–94

71. Wang K, Ho SY, Gibson DG, Anderson RH (1995) Architecture of atrial musculature in humans. Br Heart J 73:559–565

72. Wellens HJ (2003) Twenty-five years of insights into the mechanisms of supraventricular arrhythmias. J Cardiovasc Electrophysiol 14:1020–1025

73. Yang Y, Wahba GM, Liu T, Mangat I, Keung EC, Ursell PC, Scheinman MM (2005) Site specificity of transverse crista terminalis conduction in patients with atrial flutter. Pacing Clin Electrophysiol 28:34–43

74. Zipes DP, Knope RF (1972) Electrical properties of the thoracic veins. Am J Cardiol 29:372–376

2 Ablation of cardiac arrhythmias – energy sources and mechanisms of lesion formation

GJIN NDREPEPA, HEIDI ESTNER

Throughout the history of the use of antiarrhythmic drugs to suppress cardiac arrhythmias, the prevailing opinion has been that this therapeutic option produces less than optimal results in terms of durable arrhythmia suppression and the magnitude and the spectrum of side effects. The era of ablative therapy of cardiac arrhythmias began in 1968 when Cobb et al. reported successful surgical interruption of the Kent bundle in a patient with Wolff-Parkinson-White syndrome [9]. The profoundly invasive character of antiarrhythmic surgery involving open thoracotomy limited the widespread use of such therapy and accelerated the efforts for development of closed-chest, catheter-based ablative therapy.

In general, all ablative-type therapies for cardiac arrhythmias consist of the delivery of some source of energy within the heart at such a magnitude that it causes local myocardial destruction of anatomic regions critical for abnormal impulse generation and/or propagation. The ultimate aim of these destructive lesions is either silencing the foci responsible for abnormal automaticity or interruption of the reentry circuits responsible for arrhythmia genesis or continuation. The first energy form used for ablation was high voltage, direct current catheter ablation [74]. With this technique, internal shocks were applied to specific regions in the heart which led to local destruction through a combination of electrical, thermal and mechanical (barotrauma) factors. Catheter-based direct current ablation had a limited use due to its uncontrolled character, reported serious side effects and the fear of using it on thin-walled atrial or coronary sinus structures for ablation of supraventricular tachycardias. Soon after the introduction of the direct current ablation technique, several other sources of ablative energy such as radiofrequency [3, 31], cryothermal [22], microwave [87], laser [49] and intracoronary alcohol infusion [6] were used for ablation

of cardiac arrhythmias. However, only catheter-based radiofrequency (RF) ablation and to some extent cryothermal ablation found the widest clinical applications, and they are currently the most commonly used and the most standardized catheter-based ablation techniques for ablation of cardiac arrhythmias. In this Chapter, only catheter-based ablation procedures will be described.

2.1 Radiofrequency ablation

2.1.1 Physical aspects

Radiofrequency ablation (RF) is the most widely accepted catheter-based treatment for supraventricular and ventricular arrhythmias and is the energy source most familiar to cardiologists. The frequency of the RF current, mostly used in ablation of cardiac arrhythmias is 300 to 1000 kHz. Lower frequency alternating currents (<100 kHz) usually stimulate excitable cells and produce pain and muscle contractions or ventricular fibrillation when applied to myocardium. RF current is delivered to specific regions within the heart through transvenous electrode catheters with a catheter tip between 4 and 10 mm (Figure 2.1). As the high-frequency current passes through the living tissues, electrically charged carriers (ions) tend to follow the changes in the direction of the alternating current. This leads to conversion of the electromagnetic energy into the mechanical energy of ions and heat production. This type of current-mediated heat production is called Ohmic or resistive heating. Resistive heating is the primary mechanism by which cardiac lesions are produced. The RF energy is emitted from the catheter tip over a very small area and, thus, has high current density. This high-density cur-

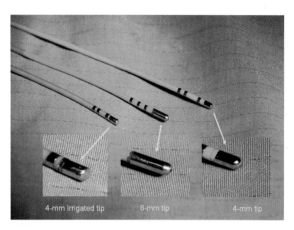

Fig. 2.1. Catheters mostly used for RF ablation

rent encounters the tissue, which acts as a resistor leading to heat generation. RF current may be delivered in the unipolar or bipolar mode. In the unipolar mode which is most commonly used, the RF is concentrated at the ablation surface (catheter tip-tissue contact), disperses throughout the body and exits to a large surface electrode (indifferent, groundpad or dispersive electrode) positioned distally on the body surface. The surface area of the groundpad electrode should be 100 to 250 cm^2. The electrode geometry and size as well as the close skin contact helped by applying electrocardiographic gels produce a very low density current avoiding any substantial local heating and potential skin burning. The groundpad electrode may be placed in any convenient place on the patient's skin; however, the placement on the posterior aspect of the chest is preferred. Since the RF current is alternating, the selection of polarity of the connections with the generator source has no importance.

2.1.2 Factors that influence lesion formation

The effects the RF energy on myocardial tissue depend on multiple factors such as the current density, the surface area of the active electrode, the quality of electrode-tissue contact, the duration of current application, histological characteristics of the tissue including blood supply and proximity to major blood vessels, the degree of tissue heating and the degree of heat dissipation (proximity to intramyocardial major blood vessels or ablating in cardiac regions with rapid blood flow).

As stated above the main mechanism of lesion formation with RF current ablation is by resistive heating. However, the resistive heating is effective only for distances less than 2 mm from the RF current source (electrode tip). This is due to the fact that current density, the main driving force of resistive heating, is diminished markedly with the increase in the distance from RF current source. Deeper penetration of heat within the myocardium is enabled by thermal conduction or heat transfer from the zone with higher temperature to zones with lower temperatures. While resistive heating in myocardial regions close to the RF current source is rapid, passive heat transfer to deeper layers is a slow process. An experimental study by Wittkampf et al. showed that the intramyocardial temperature at a distance 3 mm from the catheter tip increases progressively with the increase in the time during which RF current is applied from 10 to 60 seconds [91]. This study showed that in order to produce an effective RF ablation lesion the current should be applied for at least 60 seconds because a steady state is not achieved until 40–50 seconds of RF energy application. Another factor that conditions the amount of heat transferred to deeper layers is the temperature at the zone of resistive heating. The greater the temperature in the resistive heating zone the greater is the amount of heat transfer to deeper myocardial layers. The heat transfer continues even after discontinuation of RF current delivery. This may result in lesion volume expansion after RF current cessation which may have clinical consequences (i.e., arrhythmia termination or side effects seconds after current delivery interruption) [90]. The optimal temperature for human RF ablation is not entirely clear. In general catheter-based endocardial ablation is performed for 60 seconds at a target temperature of 50 to 70 °C (Table 2.1). However, there is great variability in the tissue characteristics according to the nature of structural heart disease. As a general rule, however, temperatures greater than 95 °C should be avoided due to risk of tissue disruption.

The dimensions and the volume of the ablated tissue are proportional to the delivered power [89]. The increase of power invigorates the heat production and results in deeper penetration of heat with destructive capability. Energy delivery is regulated by temperature control that is based on fixing a target temperature and adjusting the RF energy to maintain the

Table 2.1. Catheter use and ablation settings (as used at the Deutsches Herzzentrum München)

	Type of RF catheter			Ablation parameter settings		
	4 mm	8 mm	4 mm irrigated tip	Maximal temperature	Maximal power	Remarks
∎ Supraventricular tachycardias						
∎ Focal atrial tachycardia	×		(×)	60 °C	30 W	Irrigation recommended in LA
∎ WPW	×		(×)	60 °C	30 W	Irrigation recommended in epicardial AP
∎ AVNRT	×			60 °C	30 W	Cryo energy might be used
∎ Common type atrial flutter		×	×	55 °C/48 °C	55 W/45 W	Both catheters with similar results
∎ Non isthmus-dependent atrial flutter		×	×	55 °C/48 °C	55 W/45 W	Irrigation recommended in LA
∎ Atrial fibrillation			×	48 °C	30 W (35 W)	
∎ Ablation in pediatric patients	×		(×)	60 °C	30 W	Cryo energy might be used
∎ Ablation in congenital heart disease		(×)	×	48 °C	Up to 40 W	
∎ Ventricular tachycardias						
∎ Idiopathic VT (e.g., RVOT)	×		(×)	60 °C	30 W	
∎ Ischemic VT		(×)	×		Up to 40 W	

AP accessory pathway; *AVNRT* atrioventricular nodal reentrant tachycardia; *LA* left atrium; *RF* radiofrequency current; *RVOT* Right ventricular outflow tract tachycardia; *VT* ventricular tachycardia; *WPW* Wolff-Parkinson-White syndromes. × indicates recommended catheter; (×) indicates the second choice

target temperature. However, power delivery has limits. A temperature increase at the electrode-tissue surface close to or in excess of 100 °C may result in denaturation of plasma proteins and blood coagulation factors may stick to the electrode tip together with blood cells leading to charring or coagulum formation (Figure 2.2). Accumulation of the char or coagulative material on the ablating surface of the catheter tip serves as an insulator and prevents optimal lesions from being created. Charring or coagulum formation is associated with sudden increase in the impedance instead of gradual impedance decrease that accompanies successful RF energy delivery resulting in lesion formation. The coagulum formation increases the risk of thromboembolism.

Electrode size is another factor that influences the dimensions and volume of the ablation lesion as well as the clinical efficacy of RF ablation. Initially, electrode catheters with a 2 mm tip were used. However, Jackman et al.

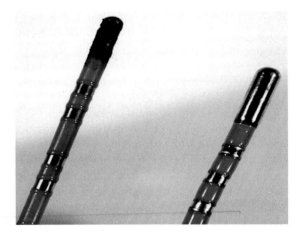

Fig. 2.2 Charring with 8 mm tip electrode catheters

demonstrated that larger electrodes (4 mm versus 1.25 mm) allowed a 3-fold increase in delivered power and markedly decreased the number of current applications required to produce atrioventricular block [36]. It was subsequently recognized that larger electrodes produce larger ablation lesions and yield better clinical results. Larger electrodes produce larger lesions for at least two reasons: first, for a given electrode-tissue interface temperature, the size of the lesion is proportional to the size of RF current source (electrode tip) [25]; and second, larger electrodes have more extensive contact with circulating blood which leads to a greater passive convective cooling and an augmentation of the amount of energy that is injected into the myocardial tissue [28]. Presently, electrode catheters with 4 mm, 8 mm and 10 mm are used in ablation studies in the adult population. Although larger electrodes produce larger ablative lesions, they bear the risk of nonuniformity of heating and spots of high temperature along the electrode tip (the so-called edge effect) [54]. It has been shown that in larger electrodes the regions of greatest heating are located at the electrode-insular boundary [54]. A temperature rise up to 100 °C may occur due to the edge effect and hot spots located remote from the detection thermocouple may go undetected. Furthermore, in contrast to smaller electrodes in which such an increase in the temperature results in a sudden increase in the electrical impedance, the increase in impedance with larger electrodes is small (at least initially). Nonuniformity in temperature rise with larger electrodes is dangerous because higher temperatures along the electrode tip may result in charring or coagulum formation (see below). In principle, the use of electrode catheters with high thermal conductivity, the use of perfused electrodes or multisite temperature monitoring may help in preventing edge effect heating and related complications [24].

Heat dissipation is another factor that may influence optimal lesion formation. Convective heat dissipation from circulating blood flow acts both at the level of the tissue and at the electrode tip. At the tissue level, convective heat dissipation due to circulating blood flow removes heat from the tissue reducing its temperature and thus opposing the thermal action of RF current. Heat dissipation from the circulating blood is more pronounced at the endocardial surface of the ablation lesion and this is the reason why ablative lesions have a smaller perimeter at the endocardial surface than on intramyocardial sections. In the case of optimal electrode-tissue contact, convective cooling may positively affect lesion formation by optimizing

energy delivery to the tissue (see irrigated tip catheters below). Particularly convective cooling from epicardial coronary arteries located adjacent to lesion sites is worth mentioning. Intramyocardial arteries with rapid blood flow enable heat dissipation by serving as heat sinks. A recent study in rabbit right ventricular preparations demonstrated that blood flow even through small intramyocardial vessels may prevent transmural lesion formation, thus, preserving conduction across RF lesions [17]. By opposing temperature rise adjacent to coronary arteries, apart from a negative impact on lesion formation, this mechanism may protect coronary arteries from excessive heat.

The efficacy of RF current ablation on scarred tissue as compared with normal myocardium is still a matter of debate. It has been previously postulated that scarred tissue may interfere with lesion formation by RF current and may lead to decreased efficacy of RF current ablation [1]. Other studies [46] including a recent one [47] have concluded that scar does not affect the lesion size or intramyocardial temperature profile during RF current ablation given that the electrode size, tissue contact and the catheter tip temperature are optimal and controlled.

Optimization of lesion formation by irrigated tip catheters is discussed later in this Chapter.

2.1.3 Mechanism of lesion formation by RF current

The effect of RF current on myocardial tissue is mediated by two factors: current itself and the thermal effect. The effects of current on myocardial tissue are largely unknown. Experimental studies in chick atrial myocytes have demonstrated that direct current shocks cause cellular depolarization and loss of automaticity [38]. A graded response, in a sense that higher energy shocks cause more pronounced and more prolonged electrophysiological changes, has been observed. When shocks with a 200 V/cm field were applied, micropores in the sarcolemmal membrane potentially reflecting dielectric breakdown were observed with electron microscopy [39]. Micropores are transient and are closed by self-reparatory properties of the plasma membrane so that viability is restored. It is not known, however, whether nonspecific pore formation in the sarcolemmal membrane takes place or to what extent it participates in lesion formation during RF ablation.

Hyperthermia, as a result of the thermal effect of RF current application, has a multitude of metabolic, electrophysiological and structural effects on cells. Metabolic effects of hyperthermia are mediated primarily by sensitivity of various enzymes to temperature. It is well known that the activity of most enzymes shows a bell-shaped curve depending on milieu temperature, which means that initial increases of temperature increase enzyme activity, whereas with a further increase of temperature enzymatic activity is diminished up to complete inactivation. Because profound metabolic effects are not observed up to temperatures at which cell death occurs, it is believed that metabolic changes are not the main mechanism for cell death and lesion formation. Electrophysiological effects surrounding RF ablative lesions have also been described [20]. Microelectrode studies in epicardial left ventricular cells have shown that action potential duration, maximal action potential amplitude and conduction time were reduced in the tissue surrounding the RF-created lesions [20, 92]. These electrophysiological changes resolved within 22 ± 13 days following lesion formation [92].

The recognition of the impact of hyperthermia on cellular calcium metabolism is important because it may be directly involved in cell death. Studies in perfused guinea pig papillary muscles exposed to rapid temperature change from $38\,°C$ to $56\,°C$ for 60 seconds with returning to $37\,°C$ showed that the increase in the fibers' resting tension was reversible up to $50\,°C$ and became irreversible at temperatures greater than $50\,°C$ [14]. The heat-induced increase in the resting tension was associated with an increase in the intracellular calcium content. An early increase in the intracellular calcium content caused by modest increases in temperature may be buffered by the sarcoplasmic reticulum. However, at higher temperatures, calcium retention by the sarcoplasmic reticulum is inhibited which results in cytoplasmic calcium overload, irreversible contracture and cell death [24].

Hyperthermia has profound electrophysiological effects on excitable cells. Perfused canine epicardial myocardial strips were used to study the effect of RF current ablation [20]. The tissue that underwent RF ablation showed reduced negativity of resting membrane potential and action potentials of shorter duration and with decreased dV/dt. The observed changes were more severe in layers close to the RF current source (within 2 mm from the electrode tip) than in deeper layers [20]. Nath et al. studied the effects of hyperthermia on isolated guinea pig papillary muscle [63]. This study has shown that

■ hyperthermia produces a progressive depolarization of the resting membrane potential at temperatures greater than $40\,°C$ which becomes more prominent for temperatures greater than $45\,°C$;

■ hyperthermia decreases the amplitude of action potential and shortens the action potential duration in a temperature-dependent manner;

■ hyperthermia causes a reversible loss of excitability in the temperature range 42.7 to $51.8\,°C$ and a irreversible loss of excitability for temperatures greater that $50\,°C$;

■ hyperthermia induces abnormal automaticity for temperatures greater than $45\,°C$ [63].

Ultrastructural changes at the cellular level are important associates of thermal injury. Hyperthermia increases the membrane fluidity [13] and cause a host of temperature-dependent electrophysiological phenomena (see above). Hyperthermia-induced changes in ionic transport and in the ionic content of the cells have also been reported [93]. The architecture and spatial relationship of various fibrilar components that compose cellular cytoskeleton are sensitive to hyperthermia. Although studies with cardiac myocytes are lacking, experiments with red cells have shown that spectrin, the major component of the cytoskeleton of erythrocytes denatures at $50\,°C$. Immediately after hyperthermic exposure, exposed erythrocytes change their shape from a biconcave disk to a spherical shape and cellular fragmentation is observed [8]. Apart from denaturation, hyperthermia-induced calcium overload may contribute to cytoskeleton changes. Increased calcium concentration induces coalescence of microfilaments into cytoplasmic bundles. One consequence of intracytoplasmic calcium overload may be its interaction with intracytoplasmic microfilaments that form cytoskeleton and provide mechanical support for the sarcolemmal membrane. Once the microfilaments contract, mechanical support for the membrane is lost. Membrane segments that have lost microfilament mechanical support become vulnerable to disruption which, if large enough, may result in immediate cell death. This may be an important mechanism through which cells are killed by the thermal effect. Although in noncardiac cells, hyperthermia has effects on DNA content and replication and in the increased protein content in the nucleus, comparative studies in cardiac myocytes have not been performed, so their relevance to RF ablation in cardiac tissue is unknown [24].

Finally, with regard to pathophysiological mechanisms that produce the ablative lesions by RF current, two conclusions may be drawn: first, in order to produce irreversible cellular changes/death, the tissue must be heated up to at least 50 °C and second, sarcolemmal disruption seems to be a major mechanism through which cell death occurs and lesion formation takes place during RF ablation.

2.1.4 Histological characteristics of the RF ablative lesions

Macroscopically RF ablative myocardial lesions appear pale and may be covered by a thin layer of fibrin adherent to the endocardial surface (Figure 2.3). Occasionally, lacerations of the endocardial surface, adherent coagulative or charring material may be observed. These phenomena are observed more often when an increase in impedance occurred during the RF ablation procedure [25]. An example of impedance rise and charring is shown in Figure 2.4. The loss of color may result from denaturation of myoglobin which is the red pigment of muscle.

The endocardial surface covering the RF ablation lesions is slightly under the level of surrounding endocardial surface reflecting the volume loss of the ablated tissue due to heat-induced desiccation. However, since myoglobin denaturation occurs at temperatures in excess of 60 °C, dead cells are found outside pale spots since cell death occurs in temperatures less than 60 °C. In histological sections, RF ablative have two distinct morphological features: a central zone of coagulation necrosis (central pale re-

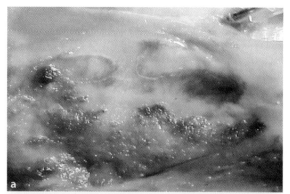
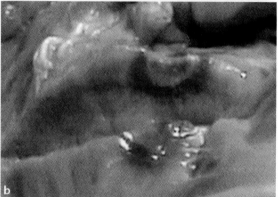
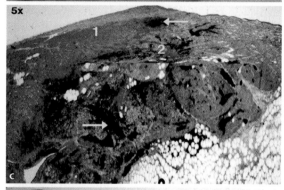
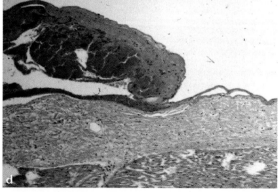

Fig. 2.3. Morphologic and histological characteristics of RF ablation lesions. **a** Endocardial surface view showing pale spots. **b** Section of the ablation lesion showing central coagulum necrosis surrounded by a hemorrhagic zone. **c** Histological view of a transmural lesion extending from the endocardium to fat issue (white matter) in sheep right atrium 1 week after ablation. Hematoxylin-eosin stain; magnification X5. Shown are: (1) granulation tissue, (2) necrosis, and hemorrhagic spots (yellow arrows). **d** Microscopic endocardial adhesion of thrombotic material by RF application. Hematoxylin-eosin stain; magnification X20

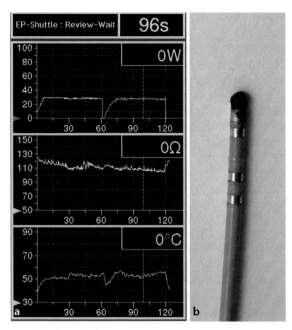

Fig. 2.4. An example of impedance rise (**a**) associated with catheter charring (**b**)

gion) and a surrounding zone of hemorrhagic tissue [27, 65]. Hemorrhagic spots may also be observed within the area of necrosis [75]. Myocardial tissue under the effect of RF current loses its typical fiber orientation and shows evidence of disrupted cellular architecture [69, 73]. Cells within the central region show nuclear pyknosis, basophylic stippling and prominent contraction band necrosis due to calcium overload [24, 73]. Hemorrhage occurs due to disruption of endothelial cells and erythrocyte passage [62, 64]. Mononuclear cells are observed in the transition hemorrhagic zone and represent an early inflammatory response. Studies in mongrel dogs have shown that RF ablation results in marked reduction in the blood flow within the acute lesion as well as beyond the borders of the lesion due to microvascular injury [64]. Among microscopic findings underlying microvascular injury were loss of basement membrane, disruption of plasma and nuclear membranes and extravasation of erythrocytes [64]. Studies using electron microscopy have identified a series of ultrastructural abnormalities involving the plasma membrane, mitochondria, sarcomeres, sarcoplastic reticulum and gap junctions as well as microvasculature extending up to 6 mm outside the lesion edge [64]. These findings may explain electrophysiological alterations that are observed beyond the lesion bor-

der. Although the definitive evidence describing the evolution of transitional hemorrhagic zone is missing, due to profound cellular alterations observed in this zone it is believed that most of it ends in necrosis within a few days after RF ablation. Specimens obtained several days after the ablation procedure show the presence of coagulation necrosis in the center of the lesion, a nearly complete disappearance of the hemorrhagic transitional zone and the surrounding granulation tissue [89]. Chronic evolution of the RF ablation lesion goes through stages of inflammation, fatty infiltration and fibrosis and is believed to be completed within 8 weeks [32, 73]. Chronic appearance of RF ablation lesions is that of patchy fibrosis. However, recently, a mixture of fibrosis, osseous and bone marrow metaplasia has been described in RF ablation lesions 1 year after the ablation procedure, potentially related to recruiting circulating stem cells by the ablation lesions [52].

2.1.5 Electrode size and design

In recent years, various electrode designs have been tested in experimental and clinical settings such as longer tip, balloon, coil and perfused or irrigated tip electrodes. The increase in the electrode tip size as a means to increase the efficacy of RF current ablation has been mentioned earlier in this Chapter (see: *Factors That Influence Lesion Formation*). In the clinical setting, electrode catheters with 4 and 8 mm tips are mostly used. Although it has been proven that the use of large tip electrodes definitively increases the lesion size and results in better clinical results [36], large electrodes have several disadvantages such as reduction in the electrogram resolution which reduces the quality of mapping and identification of ablation targets, greater variability in the electrode-tissue coupling depending on catheter tip orientation relative to the endocardium and reduced flexibility and mobility of the catheter. The use of large tip electrodes carries the risk of nonuniform heating (edge effect) which potentially may result in charring or coagulum formation, increasing the risk of thromboembolism which causes serious concern when ablating in the left heart chambers. Since the lesions created by large tip electrodes are more extensive than lesions created with smaller tip electrodes, a close temperature and power control should be pursued. Long coil electrodes have been used to create long linear lesions in experimental and clinical setting such as intraoperative ablation of atrial fibrillation [55, 57, 75]. Creation of long linear lesions is possible with these electrodes; however, poor electrode tissue contact and the frequent observation of discontinuities allowing conduction across the lesions cause serious concerns [57, 75]. Electrodes with other designs have limited clinical use and are not discussed further.

2.1.6 Cooled and perfused-tip RF ablation

Initial experience with the use of 2 mm tip electrodes for RF ablations showed limited efficacy of these electrodes [3, 35] due to coagulum formation and impedance rise at a relatively low power level, which was explained, at least, in part, by limited convective cooling by circulating blood. Although, improved convective cooling with 8 mm tip electrodes contributes to creation of more extensive ablation lesions and better clinical outcomes, these electrodes have also inherent limitations related primarily to their large size. Another way to increase power delivery to myocardial tissue is by active cooling via within catheter circulating cooled saline. Experimental studies have shown that active cooling allows transmission of a greater fraction of RF power to the tissue via smaller electrodes that results in higher tissue temperature, larger lesions and less dependency of lesion size on the electrode orientation or extrinsic cooling [59]. Technically, active cooling is accomplished by two systems. One system uses the electrode tip perfusion in which cooled saline circulates inside the catheter including the tip through closed channels (closed loop cooling). The second system infuses cooled saline which exits the catheter through small perfusion holes located in the catheter tip (open irrigated cooling;

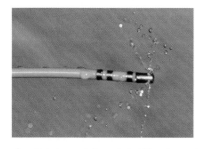

Fig. 2.5. 4-mm irrigated tip RF catheter (open system)

Figure 2.5). The rate of saline infusion is controllable. Both systems result in effective cooling and several studies have demonstrated that cooled tip ablation produces larger ablation lesions compared with conventional RF ablation [11, 23, 60]. Cooled tip ablation (closed system) has been used in patients with ventricular tachycardia and eliminated all mappable tachycardias in 106 of 146 patients (75%) with an incidence of major complications of 8% and 2.7% mortality [7]. Other studies have shown that cooled tip and larger tip ablation have similar efficacy in ablation of common type atrial flutter [10, 76]. A recent study has reported that cooled ablation may offer particular benefit in ablating areas with overlying epicardial fat [11].

Guidance of energy delivery with cooled tip ablation (both closed and open systems) is difficult because catheter tip temperatures are reduced by the continuously circulating saline. Thus, with cooled tip ablation, tissue temperatures are higher than the catheter tip temperature and are not accurately represented or extrapolated by monitoring temperature at the electrode-tissue interface. As a result higher tissue temperatures, and sudden boiling with steam production, can occur and may be audible (steam pops). In most cases steam pops are released in the endocardial space. However, when RF ablation is performed in thin-walled structures, such as atria or the coronary sinus, perforation may occur. A recent experimental study in dogs showed that catheter tip and tissue temperatures are markedly discrepant during cooled tip ablation [5]. Thus, for a power delivery of 5 W, tissue temperature was 14 °C (46 °C versus 32 °C, on a mean basis) greater than the electrode tip temperature. The difference in temperature increased to 38 °C (75 °C versus 37 °C on a mean basis) for a power delivery of 45 W [5]. In 19 of 72 energy titrations, bubble formation did not occur despite reaching tissue temperatures from 49 °C to 104 °C and a power delivery range of 15 to 45 W making the authors conclude that bubble formation can not be seen as a straightforward surrogate for tissue heating [5]. Another aspect of cooled tip ablation that may predispose for complications pertains to the deeper than expected heat penetration which may damage intramyocardial structures such as coronary arteries. Although coronary arteries are protected by coronary blood flow [17, 81], this mechanism may not be effective for high temperatures and coronary injury may ensue. Finally, prolonged procedures with the irrigated tip catheter may result in volume overload which may be problematic to patients with reduced left ventricular systolic function.

2.2 Cryothermal catheter ablation

Cryoablation has a long history of use in the treatment of cardiac arrhythmias, particularly in the setting of open surgery procedures. In the late 1990s, technological advances enabled catheter-based cryothermal ablation. Currently, cryothermal ablation is used for the treatment of a wide spectrum of cardiac arrhythmias and is second only to RF current ablation as a percutaneous transcatheter ablation approach for ablation of cardiac arrhythmias. With the recent advances in the percutaneous cryocatheters, cryoablation has become a viable alternative option to RF current ablation.

2.2.1 Mechanism of tissue injury by cryoablation

The application of a cryoprobe to tissue results in the formation of a hemispherical block of frozen tissue or iceball (Figure 2.6). Cells within the iceball are irreversibly damaged and are replaced by fibrous tissue within a few weeks after the cryoablation procedure. With the use of cryoablation catheters, tissue cooling is achieved by delivery of a refrigerant through an infusion channel to an evaporation chamber in the thermally conductive catheter tip (Joule-Thompson expansion of gas through a capillary

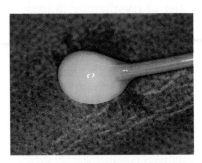

Fig. 2.6. Iceball surrounding the cryocatheter tip produced outside the myocardial tissue by applying cryoenergy with the catheter tip submerged in saline

tube) which results in heat removal from the catheter tip and surrounding tissue. Catheter tip temperature and system pressure are measured throughout the energy delivery to ensure consistent catheter tip performance. Traditional cryoablation systems use liquid nitrogen (or N_2O) as a refrigerant. However, argon-based and helium-based systems have been developed.

Mechanisms by which cryothermal ablation result in tissue injury and cell death have been studied particularly in the setting of cryosurgery [2, 18]. Cryothermal ablation induced lesion can be categorized into the following phases: freeze/thaw phase, hemorrhagic and inflammatory phase and fibrosis replacement phase [50].

■ **Freeze/thaw cycle.** Depending on the temperature achieved and the rate of cooling, extracellular or intracytoplasmic ice formation occurs [2, 18]. At temperatures up to $-20\,°C$ extracellular ice formation occurs which produces a hyperosmotic extracellular environment and cell-shrinkage due to water movement from the intracellular to extracellular space. This may cause damage to the plasma membrane and other cellular constituents. Upon rewarming, the reversal of these phenomena results in cell swelling which may disrupt plasma membranes. If tissue cooling reaches the temperature $-40\,°C$ or beyond, intracytoplasmic ice formation occurs which is lethal to the cells. Intracytoplasmic ice formation disrupts cellular membranes and intracytoplasmic organelles and is the major mechanism of cell death by cryoablation. Early in the rewarming phase, small ice crystals coalesce into larger ones deepening the tissue destruction by causing further damage to cellular membranes and organelles [2, 18]. In the perfused muscle, intracytoplasmic ice crystals are found in the tissue close to the cryoprobe, whereas crystals at the periphery of the iceball tend to be more often extracellular [50, 88]. This is consistent with the intralesion temperature gradient and has implications regarding the reversibility of tissue damage depending on the distance from the cryothermal source. Immediately after thawing, skeletal muscle cells (frozen for 1 minute to $-70\,°C$) show a variety of structural abnormalities [88]. The Z and I lines lose linearity and may even disappear. Mitochondria and microfilaments seem to be particularly sensitive to cryothermal injury. In the postthawing phase mitochondria are enlarged, have decreased matrix density and show cristae disruption. Within one hour of thawing, glycogen stores are depleted. By 2 hours, myofibril structure is almost entirely absent. Experimental studies have shown that a freeze/thawing cycle results in the loss of mitochondrial membrane integrity and increased permeability. Furthermore, due to membrane damage and other alterations oxidative function of the mitochondria is drastically reduced [66]. Myocardial reaction to cryothermal ablations seems to be similar to that of skeletal muscle. After 30 minutes of thawing, mitochondria in the iceball appear swollen and their matrix seems inhomogeneous. By this time myofilaments appear to be extremely stretched [34]. Following thawing, alterations in the structure of mitochondria and microfilaments progress to further damage in the hours to come.

▮ **Hemorrhagic and inflammatory phase.** Cryothermal ablation is known to have a profound effect on the microvasculature of frozen tissue. During the cooling phase, vasoconstriction occurs, and upon freezing circulation is interrupted. Upon re-warming, a hyperemic vasodilatation with increased vascular permeability resulting in tissue hemorrhage, local stasis and edema is observed. Damage to endothelium results in microthrombi formation and microcirculation compromise demonstrable 30 to 45 minutes after thawing. By 4 hours, small vessels within the lesion are occluded and the loss of blood supply results in ischemic necrosis which completes the lesion creation. Although the relative importance of ischemic necrosis as compared with other mechanisms of tissue damage by cryoablation is unknown, ischemic necrosis due to vascular injury is accepted as a major mechanism of lesion formation by cryothermy [79].

Histologically, the cryothermal lesion is characterized by a central uniform coagulation necrosis surrounded by a peripheral zone in which only partial cell death has occurred. The extent of necrosis becomes evident about 2 days after thawing. Near the cryoprobe (cryocatheter tip) cell death is uniform, whereas the peripheral zone represents a mixture of dead and damaged but still viable cells. This reflects the intralesion gradient of temperature which results in less cooling and less tissue destruction at the periphery of lesions. Apoptotic cells are seen in the peripheral zone. It has recently been recognized that apoptosis plays an important role in cell death after cryothermy [2]. Importantly, due to less destruction, the periphery of lesions may recover function which may have clinical implications. At 1 week after thawing, the periphery of lesions is surrounded by an inflammatory infiltrate containing macrophages, lymphocytes and fibroblasts as well as fibrin, collagen stranding and new capillary formation [56]. Hemorrhagic spots may still be observable and foci of dystrophic calcification are occasionally seen.

▮ **Fibrosis replacement phase.** The process of lesion repair begins in the peripheral zone and progresses slowly in the weeks after cryoablation procedure. Inflammatory cells, new blood vessels, dense collagen and fat infiltration are seen within the cryothermal lesion. At 1 months the lesion is marked by dense fibrosis [4]. By 3 months, cryothermal lesions undergo further maturation, ending in small patchy fibrosis with normal distribution of the blood vessels and considerable tensile strength [50].

The size of cryothermal lesions depends on several factors such as, achieved temperature, size of the cryothermal probe, duration of application of cryothermal energy and number of freeze/thaw cycles. For any given duration of cryothermal exposure, lower temperatures generate larger lesions. On the other hand, at a given temperature lesion size reaches a plateau after 5 minutes [21, 53]. Furthermore, repetitive freeze/thaw cycles increase the thermal conductivity of the tissue and may explain progressive damage with the increase in the freeze/thaw cycles [21]. As with RF current ablation, larger cryoprobes produce more extensive cryothermal lesions.

2.2.2 Characteristics of cryothermal lesions

Cryothermal lesions have several characteristics with important clinical implications. The degree of endothelial disruption with cryothermy is known to be less than with RF current lesions. Khairy et al. have compared temperature-controlled RF lesions with catheter-based cryothermal lesions and found that cryothermal lesions had substantially less endothelial disruption and overlying thrombotic material than RF current lesions [42]. This characteristic has important clinical implications for at least three reasons: first, limited endothelial disruption implies that cryothermal lesions are less thrombogenic; second it is likely that cryoablation may be safer than RF current ablation for ablation close to the coronary arteries [78], and third, less endothelial disruption may result in less reaction which may lead to a lesser propensity to develop pulmonary vein stenosis following cryoablation of pulmonary vein tissue than RF current ablation. Likewise, cryothermal ablation may be safer than RF ablation for creation of linear lesions in the left atrium.

Another characteristic of cryothermal lesions pertains to the maintenance of the extracellular collagen matrix without collagen denaturation and collagen contracture which is observed with RF current ablation. Consequently, even acute cryothermal lesions still possess considerable tensile strength which may reduce the chances of tissue rupture particularly when ablating in the atria. Furthermore, necrosis by cryothermal injury is of shorter duration (evolves faster) than necrosis following coronary occlusion [37].

The cryothermal lesions have a sharp and well-demarcated border with preserved blood flow [30]. Due to these characteristics, cryothermal lesions appear to have low arrhythmogenic potential [29, 33, 44]. Experimental studies have demonstrated that creation of cryothermal lesions is associated with a reduction in the amplitude of electrical signals, probably reflecting ice insulation or inhibition of myocardial electrical potential. A greater than 70% absolute reduction of the amplitude relative to control pre-ablation values is predictive of cell death in histological analyses performed 2 days to 2 weeks after the procedure [29]. Klein et al. have reported that epicardial electrograms recorded above cryothermal lesions showed amplitude loss; however, electrograms recorded in close vicinity to the lesions were unaffected. This observation was evident 4 weeks after the cryothermal lesion formation. Recordings with the use of plunge electrodes demonstrated the same fact, i.e., preserved normal electrical activity in close vicinity to the cryothermal lesions. Furthermore, programmed electrical stimulation with up to three ventricular extrastimuli performed immediately after, and 2, 7, 14, and 28 days after cryothermal procedure did not induce any sustained ventricular tachycardia [44]. All these facts lend credit to the possibility that cryothermal lesions have a low arrhythmogenic potential.

Finally, the ability of cryothermal energy to reversibly block electrical conduction at less severe temperatures not causing irreversible tissue damage has enabled performance of cryo-mapping (or icemapping) [19]. Experimental studies have demonstrated that cooling prolongs the refractory period causing conduction delay and transient conduction block [84]. These phenomena are short-lived and reversible. Cryomapping has clinical implications for at least three reasons: first, cryomapping allows focal tachycardia or reentrant circuit mapping by reversibly interrupting them; second cryomapping avoids inadvertent targeting of structures that may be close to ablation targets, i.e., atrioventricular node-His bundle axis in patients with paraseptal location of accessory pathways; and third, by allowing selective cryothermal energy delivery to appropriate targets only, cryomapping may allow less extensive tissue damage and economization of cryothermal energy with destructive power to the myocardium. Upon freezing, the catheter tip becomes adherent to the endocardium securing a very stable catheter positioning, which is helpful for accurate mapping and energy delivery. Cryothermal lesions are painless so may be more tolerable to the patients.

2.2.3 Clinical applications of cryoablation

The ability of cryothermal energy to create, circumvented, well-demarcated structurally homogeneous lesions with low arrhythmogenicity, the optimal safety margin of its use in the clinical setting and the option of cryomapping have made cryoablation a useful therapeutic modality in the percutaneous transcatheter ablation of a wide spectrum of cardiac arrhythmias. Extensive experience exists in the cryothermal ablation of supraventricular and ventricular tachycardias. A general feeling is that whenever ablation is required in close proximity to the atrioventricular node or within venous structures like the pulmonary veins, or distal coronary sinus, cryoablation offers advantages. Unique features of cryoablation make it an approach of choice for targeting arrhythmogenic substrates in close vicinity to the atrioventricular node-His bundle axis including slow pathway ablation in patients with atrioventricular nodal reentrant tachycardia [16, 77] and septal accessory pathways particularly those of parahisian location

[16]. In a recent study, Friedman et al. used cryoablation in 154 patients with AVNRT and accessory pathways [16]. Acute success was achieved in 91% of the patients. At 6 months 94% of the patients were without tachycardias. Importantly transient atrioventricular block was observed in 11 patients and all of them recovered within 6 minutes of the postablation period (most of them within the first 10 seconds after cryoablation energy interruption). This trial showed also that cryoablation interrupted successfully only 69% of accessory pathways. Very recently Zrenner et al. performed a randomized study comparing RF with cryoablation in patients with atrioventricular nodal reentrant tachycardia [94]. The study showed that transvenous cryoablation using a 4 mm tip cryocatheter produces comparable acute results but a higher recurrence rate as compared with RF ablation in patients with atrioventricular nodal reentrant tachycardia [94]. Several recent studies have attempted pulmonary vein isolation by cryothermal ablation [70, 82]. Because, cryothermal ablation is associated with less lesion shrinkage and consequently has a lower potential to produce pulmonary vein stenosis than RF ablation, this ablation modality seems to be promising for pulmonary vein isolation in patients with atrial fibrillation. In a series of 52 patients with paroxysmal or persistent atrial fibrillation undergoing pulmonary vein isolation, with cryoablation, both acute (97%) and long-term (56%) success rates were comparable to those of RF ablation [82]. This study, however, reported long procedure duration (mean 7.5 hours) and prolonged fluoroscopy time (mean 114 minutes). Thus, although the procedures have been reported to be safe in terms of complications, modest success rates and long procedure durations cause concerns. The latter is related to the fact that each cryothermal energy application has to last for 4 minutes. Several electrode types such as circular ablation electrodes allowing circular energy delivery and balloon cryothermal balloons have been designed to optimize cryothermal energy aiming at pulmonary vein isolation; experience with these newly designed balloons is lacking. Cryoablation has also been successfully used to ablate common type atrial flutter [51]. Although experience is limited, the use of cryoablation to treat arrhythmias in pediatric patients seems promising due to potential advantages in small hearts related to size constraints [12, 43, 58].

2.3 Ultrasound ablation

Ultrasound ablation uses ultrasound energy to achieve tissue heating and lesion formation. The mechanism of ultrasound ablation is mechanical hyperthermia. Ultrasound is produced when a transducer with a piezoelectric crystal vibrates at a fixed frequency when alternating electrical energy is applied to the crystal. In analogy with sound, ultrasound (frequency >20 000 Hz) propagates as a cyclical displacement of atoms/molecules around their average position (compression and decompression of the medium) in the direction of propagation. In a similar manner, when propagating through the tissue, ultrasound transmits to the tissue kinetic energy which results in increased particle movement and heat production. The degree of heat production depends on the ultrasound frequency and the characteristics of the transmitting medium. One favorable feature of an ultrasound beam is that it travels through blood (with minimal energy loss) or through saline with almost no energy loss. Furthermore, optical geometric manipulation allowing ultrasound focusing (ultrasonic lenses) and collimation (minimization of beam convergence and divergence) enable direction of an ultrasound beam toward confined distant tissue volume. These features are crucial for the use of ultrasound energy for ablative purposes.

In an experimental in vitro and in vivo study, He et al. applied ultrasound (10 MHz transducer) to create ablative lesions in canine hearts [26]. The lesion depth increased progressively up to 90 seconds of energy delivery, whereas a linear time of energy delivery/lesion depth relationship was observed for the first 50 seconds. Lesion depth also had a linear relationship to acoustic power with applications of 1.1 Watts producing lesions of 11 mm depth. Epicardial or endocardial applications produced equivalent results [26].

The ability of ultrasound to remain collimated as it passes through saline fluids enabled the development of transvenous through-the-balloon ablation systems. The balloon delivery system (equipped with an 8 MHz transducer mounted in a saline filled balloon) has been used to isolate pulmonary veins in two small series of patients with atrial fibrillation [61, 72]. This device was designed to heat the pulmonary vein wall in a circular fashion in order to achieve complete isolation of the pulmonary vein from the left atrium. In one of these studies, a median of four applications per vein was required. The chronic cure rate was about 30%. The variability in pulmonary vein anatomy was accused as a major factor for the modest results. Two major complications were also reported: one periprocedural stroke and one phrenic nerve pulsy [61]. Pulmonary vein stenosis was not observed on the 3-month CT scans [61].

Currently there is an increased interest in epicardial ablation. However, the existence of epicardial fat is considered to be an obstacle for RF ablation as well as minimally invasive surgical procedures. Because ultrasound can be focused at specific depths as well as it has the feature of remaining collimated over distance and is contact independent, ultrasound ablation shows promise as an alternative to standard RF current ablation for epicardial ablation [80]. Clinical experience is, however, lacking.

2.4 Laser ablation

Laser (light amplification by stimulated emission of radiation) has a powerful potential to destroy tissues by a photothermal mechanism (optical heating). A laser is a monochromatic, phase-coherent beam of specific wavelength that can be delivered for a specific duration and intensity. The wavelengths of commonly used lasers are shown in Table 2.2 [40].

As a laser beam penetrates the tissue, it is absorbed and scattered. The absorption of photon energy excites chromophore molecules resulting in vibrations and heat production. Power amplitude and light frequency are determinants of the depth of volume heating. In earlier studies, high-energy lasers were used which

Table 2.2. Wavelengths of commonly used lasers

Laser	Medium	Wavelength	Band
▌ Excimer	Gas	308 nm	Ultra violet
▌ Argon	Gas	630 nm	Visible light
▌ Diode	Semi-conductor	700–1500 nm	Near infrared
▌ Nd-YAG	Solid state	1064 nm	Infrared
▌ Holmium	Solid state	2000 nm	Infrared

carried the risk of crater formation and extensive endothelial damages. Lee et al. used neodymium-yttrium-aluminum-garnet (Nd-YAG) lasers to produce ablative lesions in canine hearts. The study showed that ablative lesions were composed of a central crater of vaporized tissue surrounded by a rim of necrotic tissue [48]. Clinical use of laser ablation is limited. Saksena et al. used an argon laser (a water-cooled argon gas laser with a power setting of 15 Watts) to ablate ventricular tachycardia in patients with ischemic heart disease undergoing coronary artery bypass graft surgery [71]. Tachycardia had a septal location in 90% of patients. With endocardial laser application 82% of 38 tachycardias (20 patients) were treated, whereas the remaining 18% required surgical resection. Only one patient had postoperative ventricular tachycardia, while in 19 patients tachycardia remained noninducible at postoperative testing. No sudden cardiac death occurred during one year of follow-up [71]. In another study by Pfeiffer et al., a Nd-YAG laser was used to ablate epicardial free wall ventricular tachycardia. Laser energy was applied epicardially at sites corresponding to mid or late diastolic potentials during ongoing ventricular tachycardia. The authors were able to terminate tachycardia in 6 of 7 patients; 6 patients remained arrhythmia-free during a 14-month follow-up [67]. The results of both studies were encouraging regarding the use of laser technology to treat ventricular tachycardias in the setting of surgery.

The use of lasers with transcatheter approaches has been hindered by the dispersion of light by red blood cells and by difficulties in achieving adequate breadth of tissue heating. Weber et al. used a special catheter system (strut structure to hold the fiberoptic source off the endocardial surface) to perform laser coagulation of myocardium in dogs [86]. The development of a continuous lower energy diode laser enabled the creation of controlled and precisely located lesions. Ware et al. advanced a sharp tipped linear optical fiber diffuser into the mid myocardium from the tip of an endocardial catheter [85]. Laser energy was delivered by a diode source. The authors were able to produce lesions with well-defined edges without endocardial damage. The disadvantage of the system was that the fiberoptic device had to be advanced intramurally through the endocardial puncture. With the development of linear diffuser, laser energy may be delivered through the entire active element. This is achieved by the inclusion of titanium particles along the active element. Titanium particles scatter laser light allowing uniform linear laser ablation. With the use of linear diffusers (equipped with diodes serving as the laser source) applied endocardially, Keane and Ruskin were able to produce continuous transmural conduction block in the trabeculated right atrial anterior wall in a goat model [41]. Transmural linear lesions have also been demonstrated in the canine right ventricle using a 50 Watt Nd-YAG laser 81064 nm) without charring or endocardial disruption [15]. The use of a beam splitter has enabled development of laser balloons for the purpose of pulmonary vein isolation. The technology creates a ring of laser energy at the pulmonary vein ostium aiming at circumferential linear lesion creation. Good contact with the pulmonary vein ostium throughout the balloon circumference is a prerequisite for optimal results in pulmonary vein isolation [68]. Laser balloons have entered clinical trial phases in Europe and the United States. Currently, however, the clinical use of laser energy is rather limited.

2.5 Microwave ablation

Microwave ablation uses microwave energy to produce tissue heating and lesion formation. Microwave ablation can be performed at either 915 MHz or 2450 MHz which are frequencies allowed for medical use. Over recent years, microwave ablation has been extensively used for ablation of cardiac arrhythmias during surgical procedures. Although the ultimate means of tissue destruction by microwave is thermal, the mechanism of heat production is different from RF ablation. Microwave creates a field that stimulates oscillation of dipoles (mostly water molecules) producing kinetic energy and heat. Microwave delivery catheter systems have antennae mounted in their tips. Although, the microwave energy is transmitted by radiation and not by conduction, power transmission to tissues is optimal when microwave antennae are parallel to the endocardium (or epicardium). Antennae of several designs have been developed to optimize microwave energy delivery to tissues. Although theoretically microwave ablation may have advantages over RF current ablation for producing

larger lesions, there are several setbacks that may limit its use. One problem is that current flow from the probe is omnidirectional, so that all present microwave antennae are side-firing antennae. To overcome this limitation end-firing antennae or antennae favoring forward radiation have been designed. Whayne et al. using an end-firing monopole antenna produced lesions of 1 cm depth without endocardial disruption in porcine ventricles [87]. The authors also demonstrated that the depth of the lesion increased exponentially with the increase in time of microwave application. Penetration of microwaves into the tissue declines exponentially with the increase of the distance from the probe. Thus, although direct contact is not needed, distance is still an important consideration. The length and the impedance of transmission should be carefully matched with the microwave generator since impedance mismatch and power reflection may occur. In order to optimize lesion size and avoid side effects, temperature feedback power control has been used with helical antennae [83].

The main current application of microwave ablation is intraoperative use during surgical Maze procedures to treat chronic atrial fibrillation [45]. In one series of 90 patients with chronic atrial fibrillation, Knaut et al. performed a microwave Maze procedure during open heart surgery. Microwave ablation time lasted 13 minutes. At one year follow-up, 67% of patients remained in sinus rhythm. Currently microwave ablation is being evaluated as an ablation tool in epicardial ablation in the context of minimally invasive surgery.

2.6 Short summary

As a result of technological progress in the last two decades, several energy sources have become available to clinical electrophysiologists for transcatheter ablation of cardiac arrhythmias. Considerable progress has also been made in the delivery systems of such energy sources to myocardium. The currently used ablation systems differ with respect to clinical experience and safety aspects (Table 2.3).

These technological advancements as well as major progress that have been made in cardiac mapping, particularly with the development of

Table 2.3. Energy sources and their characteristics. Modified from Keane [40]

Energy source	Clinical experience	Endocardial thrombogenicity	Mapping option	Transmural efficacy/ contact independence
▮ Radiofrequency	++++	++	+	-
▮ Cooled ablation	+++	+	+	-
▮ Cryoablation	++	+	++	-
▮ Ultrasound	+	++	-	++++
▮ Laser	+	++	-	+
▮ Microwave	+	++	-	+++

several computer-based 3D mapping systems have transformed ablation therapy from experimental to the therapy of choice in almost all sustainable cardiac arrhythmias.

▮ References

1. An HL, Saksena S, Janssen M, Osypka P (1989) Radiofrequency ablation of ventricular myocardium using active fixation and passive contact catheter delivery systems. Am Heart J 118:69–77
2. Baust JG, Gage AA (2005) The molecular basis of cryosurgery. BJU Int 95:1187–1191
3. Borggrefe M, Budde T, Podczeck A, Breithardt G (1987) High frequency alternating current ablation of an accessory pathway in humans. J Am Coll Cardiol 10:576–582
4. Brown NJ, Pollock KJ, Bayjoo P, Reed MW (1994) The effect of cryotherapy on the cremaster muscle microcirculation in vivo. Br J Cancer 69:706–710
5. Bruce GK, Bunch TJ, Milton MA, Sarabanda A, Johnson SB, Packer DL (2005) Discrepancies between catheter tip and tissue temperature in cooled tip ablation: relevance to guiding left atrial ablation. Circulation 112:954–960
6. Brugada P, de Swart H, Smeets JL, Wellens HJ (1989) Transcoronary chemical ablation of ventricular tachycardia. Circulation 79:475–482
7. Calkins H, Epstein A, Packer D, Arria AM, Hummel J, Gilligan DM, Trusso J, Carlson M, Luceri R, Kopelman H, Wilber D, Wharton JM, Stevenson W (2000) Catheter ablation of ventricular tachycardia in patients with structural heart disease using cooled radiofrequency energy: results of a prospective multicenter study. Cooled RF Multi Center Investigators Group. J Am Coll Cardiol 35:1905–1914
8. Coakley WT, Deeley JO (1980) Effects of ionic strength, serum protein and surface charge of membrane movements and vesicle production in heated erythrocytes. Biochim Biophys Acta 602:355–375
9. Cobb FR, Blumenschein SD, Sealy WC, Boineau JP, Wagner GS, Wallace AG (1968) Successful surgical interruption of the bundle of Kent in a patient with Wolff-Parkinson-White syndrome. Circulation 38:1018–1029
10. Da Costa A, Cucherat M, Pichon N, Messier M, Laporte S, Romeyer-Bouchard C, Mismetti P, Lopez M, Isaaz K (2005) Comparison of the efficacy of cooled tip and 8 mm-tip catheters for radiofrequency catheter ablation of the cavotricuspid isthmus: a meta-analysis. Pacing Clin Electrophysiol 28:1081–1087
11. d'Avila A, Houghtaling C, Gutierrez P, Vragovic O, Ruskin JN, Josephson ME, Reddy VY (2004) Catheter ablation of ventricular epicardial tissue: a comparison of standard and cooled tip radiofrequency energy. Circulation 109:2363–2369
12. Drago F, De Santis A, Grutter G, Silvetti MS (2005) Transvenous cryothermal catheter ablation of reentry circuit located near the atrioventricular junction in pediatric patients: efficacy, safety, and midterm follow-up. J Am Coll Cardiol 45:1096–1103
13. Dynlacht JR, Fox MH (1992) The effect of 45 degrees C hyperthermia on the membrane fluidity of cells of several lines. Radiat Res 130:55–60
14. Everett THt, Nath S, Lynch C, 3rd, Beach JM, Whayne JG, Haines DE (2001) Role of calcium in acute hyperthermic myocardial injury. J Cardiovasc Electrophysiol 12:563–569
15. Fried NM, Lardo AC, Berger RD, Calkins H, Halperin HR (2000) Linear lesions in myocardium created by Nd:YAG laser using diffusing optical fibers: in vitro and in vivo results. Lasers Surg Med 27:295–304
16. Friedman PL, Dubuc M, Green MS, Jackman WM, Keane DT, Marinchak RA, Nazari J, Packer DL, Skanes A, Steinberg JS, Stevenson WG, Tchou PJ, Wilber DJ, Worley SJ (2004) Catheter cryoablation of supraventricular tachycardia: results of the multicenter prospective "frosty" trial. Heart Rhythm 1:129–138
17. Fuller IA, Wood MA (2003) Intramural coronary vasculature prevents transmural radiofrequency

lesion formation: implications for linear ablation. Circulation 107:1797–1803

18. Gage AA, Baust J (1998) Mechanisms of tissue
injury in cryosurgery. Cryobiology 37:171–186

19. Gallagher JD, Del Rossi AJ, Fernandez J, Maran-
hao V, Strong MD, White M, Gessman LJ (1985)
Cryothermal mapping of recurrent ventricular
tachycardia in man. Circulation 71:732–739

20. Ge YZ, Shao PZ, Goldberger J, Kadish A (1995)
Cellular electrophysiological changes induced in
vitro by radiofrequency current: comparison
with electrical ablation. Pacing Clin Electrophysiol 18:323–333

21. Gill W, Fraser J, Carter DC (1968) Repeated
freeze-thaw cycles in cryosurgery. Nature 219:
410–413

22. Gillette PC, Swindle MM, Thompson RP, Case
CL (1991) Transvenous cryoablation of the bundle of His. Pacing Clin Electrophysiol 14:504–
510

23. Haines D (2004) Biophysics of ablation: application to technology. J Cardiovasc Electrophysiol
15:S2–S11

24. Haines DE (2002) Pathophysiology of radiofrequency lesion formation and the role of new
energy modalities. In: Zipes DP, Haissaguerre
M (Eds) Catheter Ablation of Arrhythmias, 2nd
Edition, Futura Publishing, Inc, Armonk, NY,
pp 67–88

25. Haines DE, Watson DD, Verow AF (1990) Electrode radius predicts lesion radius during radiofrequency energy heating. Validation of a proposed thermodynamic model. Circ Res 67:124–
129

26. He DS, Zimmer JE, Hynynen K, Marcus FI, Car-
uso AC, Lampe LF, Aguirre ML (1995) Application of ultrasound energy for intracardiac ablation of arrhythmias. Eur Heart J 16:961–966

27. Hindricks G, Haverkamp W, Gulker H, Rissel U,
Budde T, Richter KD, Borggrefe M, Breithardt G
(1989) Radiofrequency coagulation of ventricular myocardium: improved prediction of lesion
size by monitoring catheter tip temperature.
Eur Heart J 10:972–984

28. Hogh Petersen H, Chen X, Pietersen A, Svendsen
JH, Haunso S (1999) Lesion dimensions during
temperature-controlled radiofrequency catheter
ablation of left ventricular porcine myocardium:
impact of ablation site, electrode size, and convective cooling. Circulation 99:319–325

29. Holman WL, Ikeshita M, Douglas JM, Jr., Smith
PK, Lofland GK, Cox JL (1983) Ventricular
cryosurgery: short-term effects on intramural
electrophysiology. Ann Thorac Surg 35:386–393

30. Holman WL, Ikeshita M, Lease JG, Smith PK,
Ungerleider RM, Cox JL (1986) Cardiac cryosurgery: regional myocardial blood flow of ventricular cryolesions. J Surg Res 41:524–528

31. Huang SK, Bharati S, Graham AR, Lev M, Marcus FI, Odell RC (1987) Closed chest catheter
desiccation of the atrioventricular junction
using radiofrequency energy–a new method of
catheter ablation. J Am Coll Cardiol 9:349–358

32. Huang SK, Bharati S, Lev M, Marcus FI (1987)
Electrophysiologic and histologic observations
of chronic atrioventricular block induced by
closed-chest catheter desiccation with radiofrequency energy. Pacing Clin Electrophysiol 10:
805–816

33. Hunt GB, Chard RB, Johnson DC, Ross DL
(1989) Comparison of early and late dimensions
and arrhythmogenicity of cryolesions in the
normothermic canine heart. J Thorac Cardiovasc Surg 97:313–318

34. Iida S, Misaki T, Iwa T (1989) The histological
effects of cryocoagulation on the myocardium
and coronary arteries. Jpn J Surg 19:319–325

35. Jackman WM, Kuck KH, Naccarelli GV, Carmen
L, Pitha J (1988) Radiofrequency current directed across the mitral anulus with a bipolar epi-
cardial-endocardial catheter electrode configuration in dogs. Circulation 78:1288–1298

36. Jackman WM, Wang XZ, Friday KJ, Fitzgerald
DM, Roman C, Moulton K, Margolis PD, Bow-
man AJ, Kuck KH, Naccarelli GV, et al (1991)
Catheter ablation of atrioventricular junction
using radiofrequency current in 17 patients.
Comparison of standard and large-tip catheter
electrodes. Circulation 83:1562–1576

37. Jensen JA, Kosek JC, Hunt TK, Goodson WH,
3rd, Miller DC (1987) Cardiac cryolesions as an
experimental model of myocardial wound heal-
ing. Ann Surg 206:798–803

38. Jones JL, Lepeschkin E, Jones RE, Rush S (1978)
Response of cultured myocardial cells to counter-
shock-type electric field stimulation. Am J Physiol 235:H214–222

39. Jones JL, Proskauer CC, Paull WK, Lepeschkin
E, Jones RE (1980) Ultrastructural injury to
chick myocardial cells in vitro following "electric countershock". Circ Res 46:387–394

40. Keane D (2002) New catheter ablation techniques for the treatment of cardiac arrhythmias.
Card Electrophysiol Rev 6:341–348

41. Keane D, Ruskin JN (1999) Linear atrial ablation with a diode laser and fiberoptic catheter.
Circulation 100:e59–e60

42. Khairy P, Chauvet P, Lehmann J, Lambert J, Macle L, Tanguay JF, Sirois MG, Santoianni D, Dubuc M (2003) Lower incidence of thrombus formation with cryoenergy versus radiofrequency
catheter ablation. Circulation 107:2045–2050

43. Kirsh JA, Gross GJ, O'Connor S, Hamilton RM
(2005) Transcatheter cryoablation of tachyarrhythmias in children: initial experience from
an international registry. J Am Coll Cardiol
45:133–136

44. Klein GJ, Harrison L, Ideker RF, Smith WM, Kasell J, Wallace AG, Gallagher JJ (1979) Reaction of the myocardium to cryosurgery: electrophysiology and arrhythmogenic potential. Circulation 59:364–372

45. Knaut M, Tugtekin SM, Spitzer S, Gulielmos V (2002) Combined atrial fibrillation and mitral valve surgery using microwave technology. Semin Thorac Cardiovasc Surg 14:226–231

46. Kottkamp H, Hindricks G, Horst E, Baal T, Fechtrup C, Breithardt G, Borggrefe M (1997) Subendocardial and intramural temperature response during radiofrequency catheter ablation in chronic myocardial infarction and normal myocardium. Circulation 95:2155–2161

47. Kovoor P, Daly MPJ, Pouliopoulos J, Byth K, Dewsnap BI, Eipper VE, Yung T, Uther JFB, Ross DL (2006 (In Press)) Comparison of radiofrequency ablation in normal versus scarred myocardium. J Cardiovasc Electrophysiol 17:80–86

48. Lee BI, Gottdiener JS, Fletcher RD, Rodriguez ER, Ferrans VJ (1985) Transcatheter ablation: comparison between laser photoablation and electrode shock ablation in the dog. Circulation 71:579–586

49. Littmann L, Svenson RH, Tomcsanyi I, Hehrlein C, Gallagher JJ, Bharati S, Lev M, Splinter R, Tatsis GP, Tuntelder JR (1991) Modification of atrioventricular node transmission properties by intraoperative neodymium-YAG laser photocoagulation in dogs. J Am Coll Cardiol 17:797–804

50. Lustgarten DL, Keane D, Ruskin J (1999) Cryothermal ablation: mechanism of tissue injury and current experience in the treatment of tachyarrhythmias. Prog Cardiovasc Dis 41:481–498

51. Manusama R, Timmermans C, Limon F, Philippens S, Crijns HJ, Rodriguez LM (2004) Catheter-based cryoablation permanently cures patients with common atrial flutter. Circulation 109:1636–1639

52. Matsuyama TA, Inoue S, Kobayashi Y, Sakai T, Saito T, Miyoshi F, Tanno K, Katagiri T, Ota H (2005) Bone marrow observed in radiofrequency ablation scar tissue. J Cardiovasc Electrophysiol 16:354–355

53. Mazur P (1970) Cryobiology: the freezing of biological systems. Science 168:939–949

54. McRury ID, Panescu D, Mitchell MA, Haines DE (1997) Nonuniform heating during radiofrequency catheter ablation with long electrodes: monitoring the edge effect. Circulation 96:4057–4064

55. Melo J, Adragao P, Neves J, Ferreira M, Timoteo A, Santiago T, Ribeiras R, Canada M (2000) Endocardial and epicardial radiofrequency ablation in the treatment of atrial fibrillation with a new intraoperative device. Eur J Cardiothorac Surg 18:182–186

56. Mikat EM, Hackel DB, Harrison L, Gallagher JJ, Wallace AG (1977) Reaction of the myocardium and coronary arteries to cryosurgery. Lab Invest 37:632–641

57. Mitchell MA, McRury ID, Haines DE (1998) Linear atrial ablations in a canine model of chronic atrial fibrillation: morphological and electrophysiological observations. Circulation 97:1176–1185

58. Miyazaki A, Blaufox AD, Fairbrother DL, Saul JP (2005) Cryo-ablation for septal tachycardia substrates in pediatric patients: mid-term results. J Am Coll Cardiol 45:581–588

59. Nakagawa H, Wittkampf FH, Yamanashi WS, Pitha JV, Imai S, Campbell B, Arruda M, Lazzara R, Jackman WM (1998) Inverse relationship between electrode size and lesion size during radiofrequency ablation with active electrode cooling. Circulation 98:458–465

60. Nakagawa H, Yamanashi WS, Pitha JV, Arruda M, Wang X, Ohtomo K, Beckman KJ, McClelland JH, Lazzara R, Jackman WM (1995) Comparison of in vivo tissue temperature profile and lesion geometry for radiofrequency ablation with a saline-irrigated electrode versus temperature control in a canine thigh muscle preparation. Circulation 91:2264–2273

61. Natale A, Pisano E, Shewchik J, Bash D, Fanelli R, Potenza D, Santarelli P, Schweikert R, White R, Saliba W, Kanagaratnam L, Tchou P, Lesh M (2000) First human experience with pulmonary vein isolation using a through-the-balloon circumferential ultrasound ablation system for recurrent atrial fibrillation. Circulation 102:1879–1882

62. Nath S, Haines DE (1995) Biophysics and pathology of catheter energy delivery systems. Prog Cardiovasc Dis 37:185–204

63. Nath S, Lynch C, 3rd, Whayne JG, Haines DE (1993) Cellular electrophysiological effects of hyperthermia on isolated guinea pig papillary muscle. Implications for catheter ablation. Circulation 88:1826–1831

64. Nath S, Whayne JG, Kaul S, Goodman NC, Jayaweera AR, Haines DE (1994) Effects of radiofrequency catheter ablation on regional myocardial blood flow. Possible mechanism for late electrophysiological outcome. Circulation 89:2667–2672

65. Oeff M, Langberg JJ, Franklin JO, Chin MC, Sharkey H, Finkbeiner W, Herre JM, Scheinman MM (1990) Effects of multipolar electrode radiofrequency energy delivery on ventricular endocardium. Am Heart J 119:599–607

66. Petrenko A (1992) A mechanism of latent cryoinjury and reparation of mitochondria. Cryobiology 29:144–152

67. Pfeiffer D, Moosdorf R, Svenson RH, Littmann L, Grimm W, Kirchhoff PG, Luderitz B (1996) Epicardial neodymium. YAG laser photocoagulation of ventricular tachycardia without ventriculotomy in patients after myocardial infarction. Circulation 94:3221–3225

68. Reddy VY, Houghtaling C, Fallon J, Fischer G, Farr N, Clarke J, McIntyre J, Sinofsky E, Ruskin JN, Keane D (2004) Use of a diode laser balloon ablation catheter to generate circumferential pulmonary venous lesions in an open-thoracotomy caprine model. Pacing Clin Electrophysiol 27:52–57

69. Ring ME, Huang SK, Graham AR, Gorman G, Bharati S, Lev M (1989) Catheter ablation of the ventricular septum with radiofrequency energy. Am Heart J 117:1233–1240

70. Rodriguez LM, Geller JC, Tse HF, Timmermans C, Reek S, Lee KL, Ayers GM, Lau CP, Klein HU, Crijns HJ (2002) Acute results of transvenous cryoablation of supraventricular tachycardia (atrial fibrillation, atrial flutter, Wolff-Parkinson-White syndrome, atrioventricular nodal reentry tachycardia). J Cardiovasc Electrophysiol 13:1082–1089

71. Saksena S, Gielchinsky I, Tullo NG (1989) Argon laser ablation of malignant ventricular tachycardia associated with coronary artery disease. Am J Cardiol 64:1298–1304

72. Saliba W, Wilber D, Packer D, Marrouche N, Schweikert R, Pisano E, Shewchik J, Bash D, Fanelli R, Potenza D, Santarelli P, Tchou P, Natale A (2002) Circumferential ultrasound ablation for pulmonary vein isolation: analysis of acute and chronic failures. J Cardiovasc Electrophysiol 13:957–961

73. Saul JP, Hulse JE, Papagiannis J, Van Praagh R, Walsh EP (1994) Late enlargement of radiofrequency lesions in infant lambs. Implications for ablation procedures in small children. Circulation 90:492–499

74. Scheinman MM, Morady F, Hess DS, Gonzalez R (1982) Catheter-induced ablation of the atrioventricular junction to control refractory supraventricular arrhythmias. JAMA 248:851–855

75. Schneider MA, Ndrepepa G, Vallant A, Gayk U, Richter T, Henke J, Zrenner B, Karch MR, Erhardt W, Schomig A, Schmitt C (2002) Application of right atrial contiguous linear lesions: an in vivo efficacy validation of multipolar ablation catheters in an animal model. Pacing Clin Electrophysiol 25:1459–1466

76. Schreieck J, Zrenner B, Kumpmann J, Ndrepepa G, Schneider MA, Deisenhofer I, Schmitt C (2002) Prospective randomized comparison of closed cooled tip versus 8 mm-tip catheters for radiofrequency ablation of typical atrial flutter. J Cardiovasc Electrophysiol 13:980–985

77. Skanes AC, Dubuc M, Klein GJ, Thibault B, Krahn AD, Yee R, Roy D, Guerra P, Talajic M (2000) Cryothermal ablation of the slow pathway for the elimination of atrioventricular nodal reentrant tachycardia. Circulation 102:2856–2860

78. Skanes AC, Jones DL, Teefy P, Guiraudon C, Yee R, Krahn AD, Klein GJ (2004) Safety and feasibility of cryothermal ablation within the mid- and distal coronary sinus. J Cardiovasc Electrophysiol 15:1319–1323

79. Skanes AC, Yee R, Krahn AD, Klein GJ (2002) Cryoablation of atrial arrhythmias. Card Electrophysiol Rev 6:383–388

80. Soejima K, Stevenson WG, Sapp JL, Selwyn AP, Couper G, Epstein LM (2004) Endocardial and epicardial radiofrequency ablation of ventricular tachycardia associated with dilated cardiomyopathy: the importance of low-voltage scars. J Am Coll Cardiol 43:1834–1842

81. Solomon AJ, Tracy CM, Swartz JF, Reagan KM, Karasik PE, Fletcher RD (1993) Effect on coronary artery anatomy of radiofrequency catheter ablation of atrial insertion sites of accessory pathways. J Am Coll Cardiol 21:1440–1444

82. Tse HF, Reek S, Timmermans C, Lee KL, Geller JC, Rodriguez LM, Ghaye B, Ayers GM, Crijns HJ, Klein HU, Lau CP (2003) Pulmonary vein isolation using transvenous catheter cryoablation for treatment of atrial fibrillation without risk of pulmonary vein stenosis. J Am Coll Cardiol 42:752–758

83. VanderBrink BA, Gilbride C, Aronovitz MJ, Lenihan T, Schorn G, Taylor K, Regan JF, Carr K, Schoen FJ, Link MS, Homoud MK, Estes NA, 3rd, Wang PJ (2000) Safety and efficacy of a steerable temperature monitoring microwave catheter system for ventricular myocardial ablation. J Cardiovasc Electrophysiol 11:305–310

84. Wallace AG, Mignone RJ (1966) Physiologic evidence concerning the reentry hypothesis for ectopic beats. Am Heart J 72:60–70

85. Ware DL, Boor P, Yang C, Gowda A, Grady JJ, Motamedi M (1999) Slow intramural heating with diffused laser light: A unique method for deep myocardial coagulation. Circulation 99: 1630–1636

86. Weber H, Enders S, Keiditisch E (1989) Percutaneous Nd:YAG laser coagulation of ventricular myocardium in dogs using a special electrode laser catheter. Pacing Clin Electrophysiol 12: 899–910

87. Whayne JG, Nath S, Haines DE (1994) Microwave catheter ablation of myocardium in vitro. Assessment of the characteristics of tissue heating and injury. Circulation 89:2390–2395

88. Whittaker DK (1984) Mechanisms of tissue destruction following cryosurgery. Ann R Coll Surg Engl 66:313–318

89. Wittkampf FH, Hauer RN, Robles de Medina EO (1989) Control of radiofrequency lesion size by power regulation. Circulation 80:962–968

90. Wittkampf FH, Nakagawa H, Yamanashi WS, Imai S, Jackman WM (1996) Thermal latency in radiofrequency ablation. Circulation 93:1083–1086

91. Wittkampf FH, Simmers TA, Hauer RN, Robles de Medina EO (1995) Myocardial temperature response during radiofrequency catheter ablation. Pacing Clin Electrophysiol 18:307–317

92. Wood MA, Fuller IA (2002) Acute and chronic electrophysiologic changes surrounding radio-frequency lesions. J Cardiovasc Electrophysiol 13:56–61

93. Yi PN, Chang CS, Tallen M, Bayer W, Ball S (1983) Hyperthermia-induced intracellular ionic level changes in tumor cells. Radiat Res 93:534–544

94. Zrenner B, Dong J, Schreieck J, Deisenhofer I, Estner H, Luani B, Karch M, Schmitt C (2004) Transvenous cryoablation versus radiofrequency ablation of the slow pathway for the treatment of atrioventricular nodal reentrant tachycardia: a prospective randomized pilot study. Eur Heart J 25:2226–2231

3 Three-dimensional electroanatomic mapping systems

Gjin Ndrepepa

3.1 Introduction

Radiofrequency (RF) catheter ablation has become the therapeutic option of choice for a wide spectrum of cardiac arrhythmias. Currently nearly every known cardiac arrhythmia is considered amenable to RF current ablation. The improvement in the catheter and RF current generation and delivery technology and particularly the recent advances in the three-dimensional mapping techniques have played a crucial role in expanding the spectrum of cardiac tachyarrhythmias treated by catheter ablation. Catheter ablation has achieved a high degree of success in the treatment of tachycardias related to accessory pathways (overt or concealed), atrioventricular nodal reentrant tachycardia, atrioventricular junction ablation for rate control in atrial fibrillation and common type atrial flutter. Other arrhythmias, such as atrial arrhythmias maintained by intraatrial reentry, tachyarrhythmias after surgical correction of congenital heart disease, ventricular tachycardias in the setting of ischemic heart disease and atrial fibrillation still pose a great challenge to clinical electrophysiologists. The increase in the efficacy of RF catheter ablation and the expansion of the spectrum of treatable arrhythmias have gone in parallel with the refinements in the mapping techniques with the greatest impact made by computer-based electroanatomic mapping systems.

3.2 The conventional mapping technique

The conventional mapping technique has great merits in the development of clinical electrophysiology and it has helped a great deal in the understanding of mechanisms of initiation and sustenance of clinical arrhythmias and in their RF ablation. In the hands of experienced operators, the conventional mapping technique produces excellent results particularly for arrhythmias with an identifiable anatomic substrate in which ablation is guided by anatomic markers such as tachycardias related to accessory pathways, atrioventricular nodal reentrant tachycardias, atrial flutter, segmental isolation of the pulmonary veins and to some extent ventricular tachycardias arising in the right ventricular outflow tract or those having distinct electrocardiographic features (i.e., ventricular tachycardia with left or right bundle branch block pattern on the surface electrocardiogram). Effective and accurate mapping of a cardiac arrhythmia requires a certain number of electrograms recorded simultaneously (by multiple electrodes) or sequentially (with a single electrode referenced to a stable surface electrocardiographic or intracardiac signal). The conventional mapping technique uses a combination of multipolar recording catheters with an ablation catheter which are positioned at selected regions of the endocardial surface of cardiac chambers under fluoroscopic guidance. Mapping with the conventional techniques, however, has serious limitations particularly when used to map arrhythmias with a complex arrhythmogenic substrate and arrhythmias that lack anatomic markers or typical electrogram patterns. Mapping with a limited number of intracardiac catheters has limitations that stem from poor resolution, lack of global view of chamber activation, beat-to-beat variability in the cardiac cycle, inability to mark ablation sites, lack of reproducibility of catheter positioning, lack of accessibility to a specific endocardial site and increased exposure to ionizing radiation posing risk for patients and physicians. The increase in the number of catheters marginally improves the resolution but is associated with other problems such as catheter stability, thrombosis, infection and vascular trauma due to multiple vascular insertions. Finally, transient arrhythmias or arrhythmias associated with hemodynamic instability are not mappable by the conventional mapping technique.

Many of the limitations of the conventional mapping technique have been overcome by new mapping techniques which are largely based on computer processing of multiple electrical signals recorded sequentially or simultaneously from the endocardial surface of cardiac chambers.

3.3 Multielectrode basket catheters

Multielectrode basket catheters represent basket-shaped arrays of electrodes distributed evenly on linear metallic structures called splines. Current basket catheters consist of 8 equidistant splines providing a total of 64 unipolar electrograms or 32 or 56 bipolar electrograms (depending on electrode combination scheme) simultaneously recorded. The electrodes are 1 to 2 mm long and 1 mm in diameter; interelectrode distance varies from 3 to 10 mm depending on the basket radii. Basket catheters can be inserted percutaneously with the help of long sheaths. The size of the basket is selected based on the echocardiographic dimensions of the cardiac chamber in which the basket will be deployed. Femoral or internal jugular veins may be used for vascular access. During introduction, the basket is collapsed. Once it reaches the cardiac chamber, the sheath is retracted and the basket expands resulting in contact with the endocardial surface. If uneven spline distribution occurs, the basket is retracted, rotated within the sheath and repositioned. After basket catheter deployment, other catheters are inserted and positioned where needed. Anticoagulation should be performed to keep activated clotting time close to 300 seconds. RF ablation is performed with the basket in place. At the end of the procedure, the sheath is readvanced over the basket to collapse it. The relationship between basket catheter splines and endocardial contour can be defined by various criteria:
∎ fluoroscopically identifiable markers;
∎ recording of large ventricular signal identifies splines facing tricuspid or mitral annuli;

∎ for a basket catheter deployed in the right atrium, His bundle recording is possible and can serve as an identifier for other splines [85].

The mapping system consists of an acquisition module connected to a computer, which is capable of simultaneously processing the unipolar or bipolar electrograms from the basket catheter, other intracardiac recordings (i.e., coronary sinus or ablation catheter) and surface electrocardiographic leads. Electrograms are continuously displayed on the computer monitor and stored on an optical disk for off-line analysis. Computer programs have been developed to allow three-dimensional color-coded maps of activation (Figure 3.1). Activation marks on electrograms are generated automatically using either peak or slope (dV/dt) algorithms with the option of manual correction if needed [87].

3.3.1 Clinical experience with basket catheters

In the clinical setting, multielectrode basket catheters have been used to map and guide ablation in patients with ventricular tachycardia in coronary artery disease [58], right ventricular outflow tract tachycardia [1], atrial tachycardia [62] atrial flutter [86] and supraventricular tachyarrhythmias after palliation of congenital heart disease [88]. Furthermore, basket catheters have been used to characterize conduction patterns in pulmonary veins [39], guide pulmonary vein ablation [2] in patients with atrial fibrillation or map extra pulmonary vein foci initiating atrial fibrillation [61]. All these studies have stressed the feasibility and advantages of mapping with a multielectrode basket catheter.

3.3.2 Strengths and limitations of mapping with basket catheters

The multielectrode basket catheters allow simultaneous recording of electrical impulses from multiple sites and construction of activation maps of the chamber in which the basket is deployed. Multielectrode catheters have proven effective in rapidly detecting the zones of early activity in patients with right atrial tachycardias [62] and in detecting zones of slow conduction

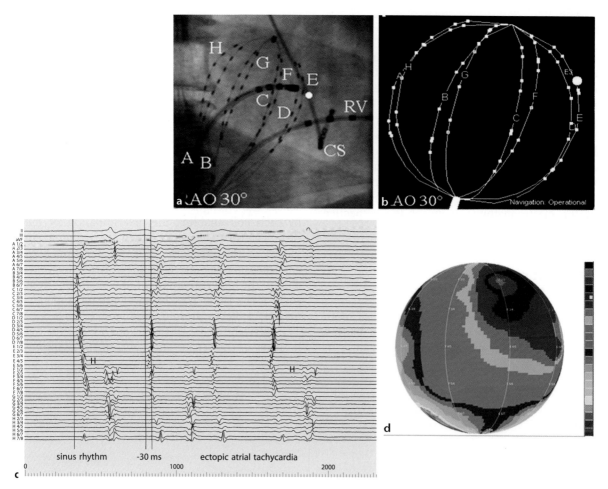

Fig. 3.1. Mapping with multielectrode basket catheters. Fluoroscopic view of multielectrode basket and other catheters in the right atrium of a patient with focal atrial tachycardia (**a** upper left panel). Visualization of the virtual orientation of the basket catheter and the roving catheter in the RAO 30° view using the navigation system (**b** upper right panel). Three surface electrocardiographic leads and intracardiac recordings from the basket catheter. Electrode pair E 2/3 shows the earliest electrical activity (**c** lower left panel). Animation view showing the earliest activity at the electrode pair 2/3. Isochrones are drawn every 10 ms (**d** lower right panel). *CS* coronary sinus, *RAO* right anterior oblique, *RV* right ventricle

that may be a suitable target for ablation in patients with ventricular tachycardia [58]. This limits the time needed to map a tachycardia compared to the conventional mapping technique and, thus, facilitates mapping of hemodynamically unstable tachycardias.

Multielectrode basket catheters have a series of limitations related to poor resolution, need for multichannel recordings systems, quality of electrode-endocardium contact, maneuverability, interpretation of activation based on multiple electrograms, and spatial relationship between basket catheter electrodes (splines) and endocardial contour [85]. To overcome these limitations, steerable sector baskets to improve resolution in patients with ventricular tachycardia, homing devices to facilitate steering of the ablation catheters to electrodes of interest and computer programs to enable 3D activation mapping have been developed (Figure 3.1) [58, 85]. However, the clinical utility of basket catheters has remained rather limited and the place of basket catheters as mapping tools in clinical arrhythmias remains uncertain.

3.4 Electroanatomical mapping

Electroanatomical or CARTO mapping system is a nonfluoroscopic mapping system that uses electromagnetic principles to accurately determine the location and orientation of the mapping and ablation catheter along with simultaneous recording of local electrical signals (bipolar or unipolar local electrograms). Sequentially acquired information at multiple locations of the catheter within the heart chamber coupled with local electrograms enables reconstruction of the electroanatomic maps of the respective heart chamber [3, 23].

3.4.1 Basic principles of electroanatomic mapping

The CARTO mapping system is composed of an ultra-low magnetic field emitter (locator pad), a miniature passive magnetic field sensor em-

bedded in the mapping and ablation catheter and a data processing unit with graphical display. The magnetic field emitter placed beneath the operating table at the level of patient's chest generates an ultra-low magnetic field in the range 0.05 to 0.2 Gauss (the magnetic field generated by a magnetic resonance imaging machine is up to 250 000 Gauss). The magnetic field emitter consists of three coils generating a magnetic field that decays in strength as a function of the distance from the coil. The sensor embedded in the mapping and ablation catheter senses the strength of magnetic fields produced by each coil enabling the determination of the distance from each coil. When the catheter tip moves in the magnetic field, the location sensors measure the strength of the field, thus, enabling the determination of the distance from each of the coils. The distances are radii of theoretical spheres around each coil (Figure 3.2). The intersection of all three spheres defines the location of the sensor and, thus, of the mapping

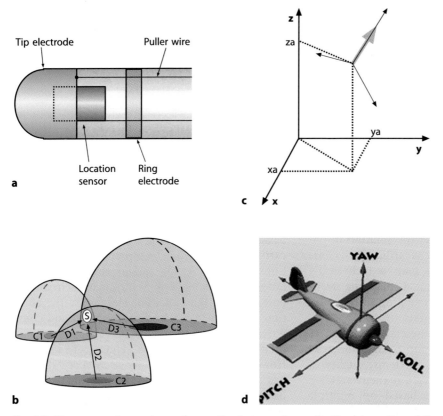

Fig. 3.2. Electroanatomic mapping. **a** Constructive features of the catheter tip used to perform mapping/ablation. **b** Location pad with three coils (C1, C2 and C3) generating magnetic fields that decay as a function of the distance from the

coils. The intersection of the three theoretical spheres' radii (D1, D2 and D3) determines the catheter tip location in space. **c** Spatial orientation in the x, y, z coordinates of the catheter tip. **d** Rotation orientation of the catheter tip

catheter tip in space. The accuracy of determination of the catheter position is highest for the locations in the center of the magnetic field implying that the locator pad should be placed under the patient's chest. The accuracy of the sensor position has been shown to be less than 1 mm in both in vitro and in vivo studies [24]. The spatial and temporal characteristics of the sensed magnetic field contain information about position (x, y, z axes) and rotation (roll, pitch and yaw) (Figure 3.2). The position and orientation of the catheter tip can be seen on the screen and monitored in real-time as it is moved in the cardiac chamber.

3.4.2 Practical aspects of electroanatomic mapping

To perform electroanatomic (CARTO, Biosense) mapping, the mapping catheter is introduced percutaneously and positioned within the cardiac chamber of interest. The catheter position is recorded relative to a reference back patch which compensates for patient movement. The CARTO mapping system continuously calculates the position of the mapping catheter relative to the anatomic reference which compensates for motion artifacts. The system enables nonfluoroscopic catheter navigation and point collection; in general, however, fluoroscopy is used to mark a certain number of known anatomic structures which will serve as references to create an anatomic model of the chamber. The mapping procedure involves dragging the catheter tip sequentially over the endocardial contour of the chamber. Once the stable positioning at a certain point is achieved, the location and electrophysiological information (unipolar or bipolar electrogram from the catheter tip) are simultaneously acquired for every point in the endocardial contour of the chamber. The system allows the operator to continuously check the quality of catheter-tissue contact as well as local activation time stability, a feature that ensures the validity and reproducibility of each measurement. The timing of each recorded unipolar or bipolar electrogram is then calculated relative to a reference electrogram which serves as a fiducial point. Any electrical signal from the surface ECG or from intracardiac recordings may serve as a reference electrogram. A coronary sinus electrogram (due to stability of the catheter placed in the coronary sinus) is preferred by

the majority of operators. In the reference electrogram itself, the fiducial point may be maximum or minimum slope. When mapping with unipolar electrograms, the fiducial point is relatively precise because it consists of the steepest part of the electrogram (the negative peak of the first temporal derivative dV/dt of the unipolar electrogram). However, quality of unipolar electrograms is reduced when mapping areas of scar tissue which may provide an unfavorable signal-to-noise ratio. In this situation, bipolar electrograms are preferred by the majority of operators even though local activation is less precisely defined. Once the criterion for local activation is selected it should not be changed throughout the mapping procedure [10, 21, 74].

Apart from selection of the reference electrogram and fiducial point in it, another prerequisite for CARTO mapping is definition of the *window of interest* which is the time interval relative to the fiducial point during which the local electrogram is required and its local activation time is determined. The length of the window of interest depends on the arrhythmia cycle length and should not exceed it. Window of interest consists of two intervals, one before the reference signal and the other after it. Usually boundaries of the window of interest are selected to cover 90% of the cycle length of the arrhythmia under consideration. Within the window of interest, the local activation time is calculated as the interval between the electrogram recorded at a given site to the fiducial point of the reference electrogram [10, 21, 74].

Electroanatomic mapping is performed by navigating the mapping catheter at multiple sites within the endocardial surface of the chamber. Once the location and electrogram are acquired by the system, the catheter is moved to another site and information is acquired without the use of fluoroscopy. Selected points are connected with each other on the principle of triangulation in which points are connected by lines to form several adjoining triangles in the global model of the chamber. The number of acquired points and, thus, the resolution of the reconstructed map depends on the operator. The regions of interest (i.e., those related to site of arrhythmia, critical parts of reentry circuits or candidate sites for ablation) may contain more closely spaced points, i.e., higher resolution. During map reconstruction, the image may be rotated at any degree including conventional views, the size of image may be increased or reduced and selected standard views may be displayed on the screen while continuing the map reconstruction. After finishing the point collection, the system allows the operator to review the accuracy of the collected points in terms of location and quality of electrogram, delete them if considered inaccurate as well as annotate every structure and tag ablation sites on the reconstructed map [10, 21, 74].

The CARTO system generates different types of maps to facilitate three-dimensional impulse propagation for precise definition of focal onsets or reentrant circuits and identification of the candidate regions for RF ablation. In the activation map, electrophysiological information derived from local activation times is superimposed on the anatomic map. In the activation map, regions are color-coded with red denoting the earliest activation; other colors such as orange, yellow, green, blue and purple are used to denote activation which occurs progressively later (in reference to the fiducial point of the reference signal). Interpolation is used to fill in the colors between the points. The extent of interpolation is programmable (the triangle-fill threshold) and can be adjusted if considered necessary. If points are too remote, no interpolation is applied. A propagation map is another option to view electrical propagation of the reconstructed geometry of the chamber. In the propagation map, the whole chamber is colored with blue and electrical activation is seen in red spreading throughout the chamber as a continuous animated loop. Apart from animated propagation activation, the propagation map assists in the validation of the procedural end point by delineation of the ablation-created lines of block or in depicting the gaps in ablation lines. In the voltage map, instead of local activation times, voltage amplitudes of the signals acquired from each of the points are superimposed on the anatomic map. The lowest voltage amplitude is marked with red, whereas orange, yellow, green, blue and purple mark progressively increasing voltage amplitudes. This option enables definition of areas of scarring and electrically diseased myocardial tissue and is crucial for so-called substrate mapping (i.e., in ventricular tachycardia). The mesh map is another option that displays the reconstruction based on the actually sampled location points during the procedure and is used to view inside the chamber or to determine the exact anatomical relationships (Figure 3.3). Finally, electroanatomic map-

ping coupled with the recording of monophasic action potentials allows reconstruction of repolarization maps which may be useful for detection of the repolarization differences in various regions of the atria or ventricles.

Each of the maps can be rotated freely to best visualize anatomy and electrophysiology. Key anatomic landmarks can be precisely defined using the system.

3.4.3 Clinical experience with electroanatomic mapping

Theoretically, electroanatomic mapping may be used to guide mapping and ablation of every known cardiac arrhythmia and, in fact, there is ample evidence on the advantages of electroanatomic mapping for mapping and ablation of various arrhythmias. The conventional mapping/ablation approach produces optimal results particularly for arrhythmias with an anatomically identifiable substrate. Thus, it might be prudent and cost-effective to use electroanatomic mapping for those arrhythmias in which results of conventional mapping are less than optimal. The main indications for the use of electroanatomic mapping are atrial tachycardias (ectopic focal or with intraatrial reentry) including atrial tachycardias after palliation of congenital heart disease, atrial fibrillation and ventricular tachycardia.

∎ **Atrial tachycardia and common type atrial flutter.** Although the conventional technique has been shown to be effective in guiding ablation of atrial tachycardias [42, 55], prolonged procedures and fluoroscopy times have been reported [42, 82]. Difficulties in localizing the regions of earliest activity due to broad areas of early activity, rapid conduction with nonuniform spread of global activation, difficulties in catheter manipulation using fluoroscopy and lack of reproducibility in catheter position particularly during repeated RF current applications are well known problems with the conventional mapping technique. Atrial tachycardias after surgical correction of congenital heart disease have proven even more challenging for the conventional technique due to the complex arrhythmogenic substrate and intricate macroreentrant circuits involving critical channels of slow conduction bordered by scattered scar tissue and/or anatomic boundaries [12, 43, 50]. Instrumental to

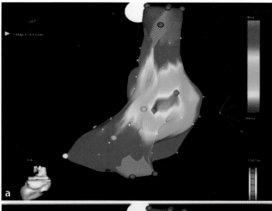

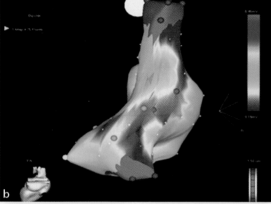

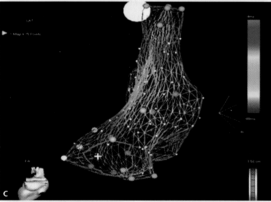

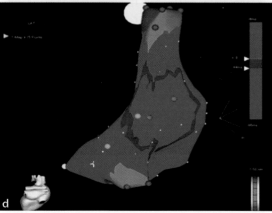

successful mapping and ablation has been identification of isolated early diastolic potentials and entrainment maneuvers. Widespread areas of slow or fractionated potentials of low amplitude, electrically silent scar zones distant from anatomic landmarks, and multiple loop reentrant circuits appear to limit long-term success independent of primary success.

Electroanatomic mapping has facilitated the mapping and ablation of atrial tachycardias. The system has been highly effective in ablating atrial tachycardia with a limited number of RF current applications and reduced fluoroscopy time [28, 37]. In the presence of structural heart disease, the system provides three-dimensional maps with useful annotations of crucial anatomic structures. The system offers detailed and high resolution mapping of the regions of interest (areas of earliest activation or zones of slow conduction critical to reentrant circuits). Furthermore, ablation sites can be tagged and if needed the mapping and ablation catheter can be renavigated to the areas already mapped or ablated. The voltage map option and the system's ability to depict scar regions allow delineation and estimation of the zones of the diseased tissue (slow conduction) and protected zones of diastolic activity. Electroanatomic mapping has demonstrated the presence of multiple isolated channels between scars usually located in the right free wall which were responsible for macroreentrant atrial tachycardias after correction of congenital heart disease [50]. Ablation within these channels resulted in a higher success in terminating tachycardias compared with the conventional technique.

Although the general feeling is that the conventional mapping/ablation technique performs well in the case of common type atrial flutter, electroanatomic mapping has been used to confirm the anatomic location of reentry circuit and to guide linear lesion creation and evaluate bidirectional isthmus block [72]. The system facilitates application of both activation and local criteria for isthmus conduction block assess-

Fig. 3.3. Map options using the electroanatomic mapping system. The electroanatomic map of the right atrium in a patient with focal atrial tachycardia in the posterior wall of the right atrium is shown. The focus was located in the mid section of the posterior wall. The postero-anterior view is shown. **a** Activation map. **b** Voltage map. **c** Mesh map. **d** Propagation map

ment, and it can identify the gaps in the linear lesion if arrhythmia relapses occur after ablation. In addition, the system offers advantages in recognizing other arrhythmias that may co-exist with atrial flutter and in guiding their ablation. In patients with atypical atrial flutters, the reentry circuit has been delineated using the electroanatomic mapping system [32].

Electroanatomic mapping has been shown to offer advantages in delineating mechanisms and in guiding ablation of tachycardias after atrial septal defect repair [71], tachycardias after Mustard or Senning operations [84] and left atrial tachycardia or flutter [29].

▊ **Atrial fibrillation.** Electroanatomic mapping can guide catheter-based creation of linear lesions mimicking surgical Maze. However, the process is time-consuming, possesses the risk of systemic embolism and cardiac perforation, and completeness of linear lesions is difficult to ascertain. Currently, two ablation approaches are most commonly used to treat atrial fibrillation by ablation techniques: 1) segmental pulmonary vein isolation by inserting discrete ablation lesions at the ostial region of the pulmonary veins aiming at their electrical isolation from the left atrium [26] and 2) circumferential pulmonary vein ablation which rather modifies the pulmonary vein-posterior left atrial wall by creation of circular lesions in the left atrium around the venous ostial regions [53]. Due to the sequential nature of electroanatomic mapping, the system is of limited value for localizing discharging foci which are transient. The technique of circumferential pulmonary vein ablation is enabled by the electroanatomic mapping system, particularly by its ability to reconstruct an anatomic map of the left atrium, to precisely mark pulmonary vein ostia and to tag ablation sites. Nonfluoroscopic navigation of the catheter close to prior ablation sites enables the creation of encircling linear lesions around the pulmonary vein ostia. Although the system offers possibilities to test completeness of ablation lines through voltage and activation criteria, the utility of such criteria remain dubious. A recent study that assessed the ability to create linear lesions to prevent atrial fibrillation concluded that creation of contiguous linear lesions in the septal and inferior pulmonary vein regions is technically difficult, leading authors to state that electroanatomically guided creation of linear lesions is feasible only in the right atrium [17].

Other authors have demonstrated that using the electroanatomically guided anatomic approach pulmonary veins were isolated in only 40% of the mapped veins; however, the approach prevented atrial fibrillation in 80% of patients, leading the authors to conclude that isolation of the pulmonary veins is not crucial for curing atrial fibrillation [75]. It is generally accepted that incomplete lesions, however, pose the risk of favoring reentrant left atrial flutters after ablation. In the latter situation, electroanatomic mapping helps in delineating the culprit reentry circuits and in closing conduction gaps through ablation lines [8].

▊ **Ventricular tachycardia.** Ventricular tachycardia, particularly in the setting of structural heart disease (most often in the setting of ischemic heart disease), is considered difficult to treat by ablation techniques, due to widespread scarring and diseased tissue that favors multiple reentrant circuits underlying multiple electrocardiographic interchanging forms, poor reproducibility of clinical forms and hemodynamic instability. In fact, RF ablation of ventricular tachycardia after myocardial infarction has had only moderate success [76].

Theoretically, electroanatomic mapping seems to be noticeably advantageous for ablation of ventricular tachycardia. However, in order to define reentry circuits and critical areas for RF current application, electroanatomic mapping should be performed during ongoing tachycardia. In order to acquire a sufficient number of points to enable reconstruction of optimal electroanatomic maps, tachycardia should be stable and tolerable by the patient for a certain amount of time. Most ventricular tachycardias particularly in the setting of structural heart disease with extensive myocardial damage and reduced left ventricular function are nonsustained or associated with multiple circuits or hemodynamic instability. Electroanatomic mapping during nonsustained or tachycardia associated with hemodynamic instability is very difficult, if possible at all. In the latter situation, the electroanatomic mapping system offers so-called "substrate mapping" which characterizes the arrhythmogenic substrate [45]. In a group of patients with drug-refractory unmappable ventricular tachycardia with frequent shock deliveries by implanted cardioverter-defibrillator, Marchlinski et al. were able to define areas of diseased endocardium by reconstructing voltage (substrate) maps in sinus rhythm [45]. Zones of "dense scars" were those that displayed local voltages < 0.5 mV. A median of four linear lesions with an average of 3.9 cm were placed from scar regions to anatomic boundaries or normal myocardium under the guidance of electroanatomic and pace mapping. The substrate mapping-guided ablation effectively controlled arrhythmia in 12 of 16 patients over a median of 8.5 months of follow-up [45]. Once the voltage mapping is completed, pace mapping may be performed by placing the catheter at the border of scar regions deemed to serve as protected isthmus or exit points for tachycardia in an at tempt to replicate clinical tachycardia. Recently, voltage mapping has been used successfully to diagnose right ventricular dysplasia by demonstrating low voltage areas associated with fibrofatty myocardial replacement [9] and to guide ablation of ventricular tachycardia in arrhythmogenic right ventricular dysplasia with good short-term success [81].

Electroanatomic mapping has been used to guide ablation in patients with focal ventricular tachycardia [49] and ventricular tachycardia that occurs after surgical correction of congenital heart disease [56].

3.4.4 Advantages and limitations of electroanatomic mapping

The greatest advantage of electroanatomic mapping relies on its ability to integrate anatomic and electrophysiological information in the form of electroanatomic maps, so that it links origin of arrhythmia to discrete anatomic structures. High resolution of anatomic and electric mapping is achievable. This has been a great help for delineation of arrhythmia mechanisms and in selecting candidate regions for RF ablation. The second advantage of electroanatomic mapping has to do with its ability to visualize the ablation catheter, tag precisely the ablation sites and renavigate the ablation catheter to the sites of prior current application or close to it. This feature enabled creation of linear ablative lesions which are a validated approach of ablation in supraventricular and ventricular tachycardias. Third, with its capability to characterize normal and diseased tissue (voltage or substrate mapping) and thus the potential arrhythmogenic substrate, electroanatomic mapping has enabled ablation of hemodynamically un-

stable arrhythmias. Due to these advantages electroanatomic mapping has improved the results of RF ablation and has expanded the spectrum of arrhythmias that can be subjected to this therapeutic modality.

Electroanatomic mapping relies on sequential mapping, so that multiple beats are required for creation of maps. Thus, stable rhythm and hemodynamic tolerance are required during the time of point collection. Short-lived arrhythmias (i.e., firing foci initiating atrial fibrillation) are not mappable with electroanatomic mapping. Beat-to-beat changes affect the quality of mapping. Rapidly changing or unstable arrhythmias can not be accurately mapped; however, in the latter situation the system offers substrate mapping option. Finally, in order to reconstruct high-resolution maps or to assess the integrity of linear lesions (i.e., those encircling the pulmonary veins in patients with atrial fibrillation) a great number of points should be acquired leading to prolongation in the procedure time (Table 3.1).

3.4.5 Recent advances in electroanatomic mapping

∎ **Magnetic electroanatomic mapping.** In an attempt to reduce the time needed for point-by-point data acquisition, the recently introduced CARTO XP (Biosense) uses a novel 26-electrode mapping catheter (Qwikstar, Biosense) to acquire multiple points simultaneously from each electrode. The electrode consists of a 4 mm tip electrode and a 2 mm ring electrode (spacing 1 mm) to acquire unipolar or bipolar electrograms. The other 24 electrodes are positioned on the catheter shaft in 6 arrays, each containing 4 electrodes (2 orthogonal pairs); arrays are separated from each other by a distance of 9 mm. Unipolar or bipolar electrograms are recorded. The software compares electrograms with each other to determine the proximity to the endocardial surface. Local activation times are automatically determined by the maximal negative slope dV/dt of bipolar electrograms filtered at 30 to 400 Hz. Anatomic data are derived from electrodes being within 8 mm from the endocardial surface. With the increase in the number of points acquired by tip and shaft electrodes, geometry and activation are continuously updated by the software. Two additional location sensors placed close to the tip and

Table 3.1. Comparison of computed-based three-dimensional mapping systems

Feature/mapping system	Electroanatomic mapping	Noncontact mapping	NavX	RPM	LocaLisa*
▐ Replicates anatomy without distortion	+++	++	++	++	–
▐ Multiple chamber/structure rendering (simultaneous)	+++	–	++	–	–
▐ Pulmonary vein, SVC/IVC display	Rendered anatomy or pulled tubes	Cut outs/juxta-posed spheres	Cut outs/ juxtaposed spheres	–	–
▐ Esophagus annotation	No	Direct localization	Direct localization	–	+
▐ Interstructure delineation without interpolation obliteration	++	Fixed points required	Fixed points required	Snap points required	No surface geometry
▐ Spatial accuracy (mm)	1	<1	<1	2	2
▐ Temporal accuracy (sampling rate)	0.1K	1.2 K	1.2 K	3 K	
▐ Simultaneous onscreen map view windows	2	2	2	2	2
▐ Virtual cardioscope views	+++	+++	+++	+	–
▐ Ease of map display user interface	+++	++	++	++	+
▐ "Transparency" view	No	Yes	Yes	Yes	–
▐ Activation time mapping	+++	++	++	+++	Annotation by hand
▐ Voltage mapping	+++	++++	+++	+	Annotation by hand
▐ High-resolution electrogram mapping	+	+++	+	+	No
▐ Nonsustained AT/VT-APC/VPC mapping	With effort	++++	With effort	With effort	–
▐ Unstable AT/VT mapping	No	+++	No	No	No
▐ Robust intervention annotation (ablation dots)	++++	+++	+++	++	++
▐ Detection of low-amplitude signals	++	++	++	+++	+
▐ Repolarization mapping	+	+++	No	+	–
▐ Mapping using alternative signal content	In development	In development	In development	In development	No
▐ Mechanical/contraction mapping	Yes NOGA	No	+No	No	No
▐ Preablation map-based intervention planning	+++	+	+	+	No
▐ Click and point electrogram recall	+++	+++	++	+++	No
▐ Catheter tip/tissue contact visualization	+++	++	+	+	++
▐ Multiple chamber mapping (synchronized)	+++	–	++	–	–
▐ Geometry "learning" during mapping and ablation	+++	+	+	–	–

Table 3.1 (continued)

Feature/mapping system	Electroanatomic mapping	Noncontact mapping	NavX	RPM	LocaLisa*
■ Ablation catheter use	Specific	Any	Any	Specific	Any
■ Navigation/electrograms during ablation	Yes	Yes	Yes	No	Yes
■ Respiratory compensation	+	+++	+++	-	No
■ Simultaneous electrode	26	Array +4	64	N/A	?

* Catheter localization system. *APC* Atrial premature contractions, *AT* Atrial tachycardia, *IVC* Inferior vena cava, *SVC* Superior vena cava, *VPC* Ventricular premature contractions, *VT* Ventricular tachycardia. From reference [52]

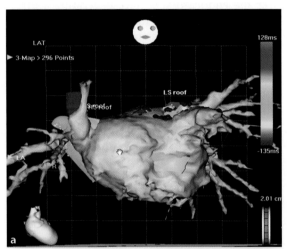

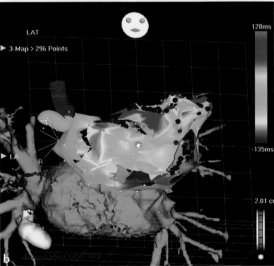

Fig. 3.4. Multislice computed tomography (CT) image of the left atrium (**a**) and merging of the CT anatomy with the electrophysiological information from electroanatomical mapping (**b**) in a patient with atrial fibrillation

proximal to the shaft electrodes allow the animated three-dimensional representation of the tip and shaft of the roving catheter. A reference signal and window of interest are selected as with the original system. Clinical experience with magnetoelectroanatomic mapping system is limited. The system has recently been used in a small group of patients with atrial and ventricular tachycardias and structural heart disease [5]. The system enables complete electroanatomic mapping with fewer point-by-point acquisitions compared with the system using the bipolar (Navistar) catheter.

Recently, the CARTOMerge™ Integration module has been introduced. The system uses anatomic images of the heart chambers reconstructed by computed tomography (CT) or magnetic resonance imaging (MRI) over which activation or voltage maps are superimposed by catheter navigation within the CT or MRI models (Figure 3.4). Apart from accuracy of information on anatomic structures, the system is supposed to offer advantages related to minimal additional point acquisition which improves the speed of the system. Clinical experience with the system is presently almost completely lacking.

3.5 The noncontact endocardial mapping system

3.5.1 Basic principles of noncontact mapping

The Noncontact mapping system (Ensite 3000™; Endocardial Solutions, Inc., St. Paul, MN, USA) consists of a catheter-mounted multielectrode array, a custom-designed amplifier system and a Silicon Graphics workstation that displays reconstructed maps. The system simultaneously reconstructs more than 3000 electrograms, and can display data as standard electro(cardio)grams, or three-dimensional graphical representation of the heart chamber in an isochronal or isopotential mode. Simultaneously up to 32 electrograms can be displayed as waveforms.

The noncontact multielectrode array consists of a 7.6-ml balloon mounted on a 9F catheter around which a braid of 64 insulated 0.003 inch diameter wires is woven. Laser technology was used to remove a single spot of insulation (0.025 inch) on each wire, producing 64 noncontact unipolar electrodes (Figure 3.5). The signals from the multielectrode array are recorded using a reference ring electrode located on the shaft of the catheter nearly 16 cm proximal to the balloon. After deployment, the balloon is inflated with a contrast-saline mixture. The system is able to locate spatially any conventional catheter with respect to the multielectrode array by applying a 5.68 kHz current (locator signal) between the catheter being located and alternately between the multielectrode array and the ring electrode. The locator signal is used in the construction of a three-dimensional model of the endocardial geometry (virtual endocardium) and for displaying and logging the position of the mapping catheter on the virtual endocardium. The three-dimensional model is acquired by moving the conventional catheter over the endocardial surface generating a three-dimensional model of the chamber. The system automatically stores only the most distant points reached by catheter and ignores those points detected when the catheter was not in close contact with the endocardium; thus, the virtual model has the end-diastolic dimensions of the chamber. A virtual model of the chamber is created at the beginning of the study independent of rhythm status (sinus rhythm or arrhythmia). In general, the virtual model of any cardiac chambers is completed in less than 5 minutes and can serve for electrogram and isopotential map display throughout the study. Relevant anatomic structures can be annotated

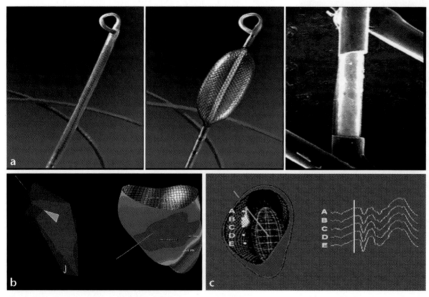

Fig. 3.5. Noncontact multielectrode array. **a** Deflated, expanded multielectrode array and one electrode produced by laser having removed a single spot of insulation. **b** Reconstruction of the virtual geometry and depolarization map. Green line shows the position of the mapping catheter. **c** Virtual unipolar electrograms obtained by dragging the mapping catheter over corresponding points on the virtual geometry map

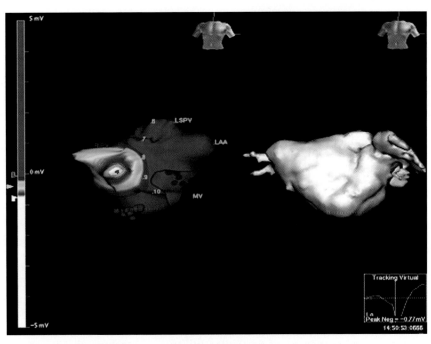

Fig. 3.6. Noncontact mapping of a focus near the right inferior pulmonary vein in a patient with atrial fibrillation (left panel). Corresponding anatomy derived from magnetic resonance imaging (right panel)

on the virtual endocardium model. Apart from geometric modeling, the locator signal serves to display and log any conventional catheter within the chamber. Importantly, the locator signal enables real-time navigation of the ablation catheter to the sites of interest on the isopotential maps and cataloging of the sites of RF deliveries on the virtual endocardium [60].

Once the virtual geometry has been reconstructed, detected signals on the surface of the multiarray electrode are used to compute endocardial electrograms. Since the cavitary potentials are lower both in amplitude and frequency than at their source on the endocardial surface, the application of inverse solution of LaPlace's equation utilizing a boundary element method improves accuracy and stability of their reconstruction [35]. The system reconstructs up to 3360 electrograms simultaneously over a computer-generated model of the entire chamber where the multielectrode array is deployed (Figure 3.5 and 3.6). The activation process is depicted by color-coded isopotential maps which graphically display regions that are depolarized and the wavefront propagation is displayed in a user-controlled way. Furthermore, unipolar or bipolar virtual electrograms can be displayed over a selected area of interest. Fidelity of vir-

tual electrograms compared with conventionally acquired contact electrograms has been validated [25].

3.5.2 Clinical experience with noncontact mapping

▮ **Atrial tachycardia and flutter.** Several studies have demonstrated that noncontact mapping facilitates mapping and ablation of atrial tachycardias and atrial flutter. Noncontact mapping provides electrophysiological images of global activation sequences over known anatomical structures obtained by virtual maps. In analogy with electroanatomic mapping, noncontact mapping enables repeated nonfluoroscopic navigation of the ablation catheter to any area of interest on the virtual geometric map of the chamber and tagging of ablation lesions. Due to simultaneous high-resolution data acquisition, the system enables mapping of transient or short-lived arrhythmias. Theoretically, single-beat analysis is feasible. The intrinsic ability of unipolar elctrograms to pinpoint the source of impulse generation (having almost entirely negative morphology at the origin of impulse), seems to be of value in localizing the origin of focal tachycardias. Noncontact mapping has been used to guide ablation in patients with ectopic atrial tachycardia [69] and atrial reentrant tachycardia after surgery for congenital heart disease [54].

In patients with tachycardias after Fontan procedure, noncontact mapping improved the identification of the anatomic and surgical substrate as well as of the exit zones and the zones of slow conduction within the reentry circuits [4]. In patients with atrial flutter, noncontact mapping has been used to confirm the anatomic location of the reentry circuit, to reduce fluoroscopy time and to evaluate isthmus conduction block [66]. Noncontact mapping facilitates identification of conduction gaps in ablation lines [63] and enables the assessment of isthmus conduction block criteria by activation mapping and local (double potentials in virtual electrograms over the isthmus region) criteria. Noncontact mapping seems to facilitate the recognition and ablation of atypical flutters [78]. Noncontact mapping may be of particular utility in patients with more than one coexisting tachycardia due to the lack of need to reperform geometric map reconstruction in case of identification of a new arrhythmia during the ongoing electrophysiological procedure [10].

∎ **Atrial fibrillation.** Ablation of initiation triggers or their isolation from the rest of the atria is considered crucial for preventing atrial fibrillation particularly its paroxysmal form. Ectopic impulses originating primarily from the pulmonary veins [26] and other atrial structures [61] have been identified as triggers for paroxysmal and persistent atrial fibrillation. Particularly the ability of the system to perform a single-beat analysis and to trace the impulse generation to its origin seem to offer real advantages in mapping the focal triggers of atrial fibrillation [27, 67]. Noncontact mapping has been used to guide linear lesion creation in the right and the left atrium in patients with chronic drug-refractory atrial fibrillation [70]. The system proved to be useful in evaluating the completeness and identifing discontinuities in the ablation lines. The right atrial approach has been reported to be safe; however, with the deployment of the multiarray electrode in the left atrium complications have been reported [70]. In spite of potential advantages, it has to be emphasized that the experience in using noncontact mapping to guide RF ablation of atrial fibrillation is still limited.

∎ **Ventricular tachycardia.** Ventricular tachycardia is difficult to ablate with conventional methods because of the hemodynamic instability that develops during tachycardia. The noncontact mapping system, due to simultaneous data acquisition and single-beat analysis, facilitates RF ablation of this arrhythmia. Furthermore, after reconstruction of the virtual geometry of the chamber, ventricular tachycardia can be induced, data acquired and terminated so that the analysis can be performed off-line with the patient in sinus rhythm. Schilling et al. were the first to demonstrate feasibility of the noncontact mapping system to map and guide ablation of human ventricular tachycardia [59]. In more than 50% of cases, the system detected at least a part of the diastolic pathway of the reentrant impulse and therefore suitable targets for ablation [59]. In other studies, isolated diastolic potentials, zones of slow conduction and exit sites have been identified in patients with ventricular tachycardia using virtual electrogram analysis and isopotential maps [77]. Noncontact mapping-guided ablation of ventricular tachycardia has had a one-year success rate of more than 75% [59]. Recently, the noncontact mapping system has successfully been used to guide mapping and ablation of right ventricular outflow tract tachycardia [22]. In case of noninducible tachycardia, extrasystolic beats with a morphology resembling that of tachycardic beats may be mapped and ablated. The system has also been used to guide ablation of extrasystolic beats inducing ventricular fibrillation [5].

3.5.3 Advantages and limitations of the noncontact mapping system

As with the electroanatomic mapping system, the noncontact mapping system offers the advantages of a global view of activation, nonfuoroscopic catheter navigation, and annotation of relevant structures on the virtual maps and tagging of ablation lesions and revisiting the points of interest by repeat catheter navigation to those areas. Noncontact mapping seems to be useful in patients with multiple or transient arrhythmias with no overt structural heart disease. The ability of the system to use the virtual geometry map for every abnormal rhythm that can be induced during the electrophysiological study seems to offer a real advantage for mapping multiple or transient arrhythmias.

Noncontact mapping system has also limitations (Table 3.1). Virtual electrograms deteriorate for distances greater than 4 cm requiring multielectrode array repositioning. Being a relatively bulky structure, the multielectrode array might be difficult to position particularly in the left atrium or in ventricles. Application of high output intracardiac stimulation may lead to virtual saturation of virtual electrograms. RF current application disturbs the emittance of the 5 kHz signal causing temporal shifts in three-dimensional localization of the roving catheter. Due to overlapping of ventricular repolarization, early diastole might be difficult to map. This is important because most triggering rhythms initiating sustained arrhythmias (i.e., atrial fibrillation) take place early in diastole. During activation mapping, it is difficult to delineate the borders of activation in zones not bordered by anatomic structures using round-shaped isopotential propagation. The effect of filter settings on noncontact mapping and ablation needs to be further studied [65]. It has recently been demonstrated that noncontact mapping does not reliably identify ventricular scaring, casting doubt on its utility in tachycardias in the setting of overt structural heart disease [79].

∎ **The EnSite NavX system** represents a recent development in the noncontact mapping system. The EnSite NavX system is a nonfluoroscopic navigation system that has the ability to generate anatomic maps and integrate in it the precise location of up to 64 electrodes (8 catheters). The system uses regular mapping and ablation catheters to sense a 5.68 kHz constant low-current locator signal generated by each of the three pairs of externally placed electrodes to

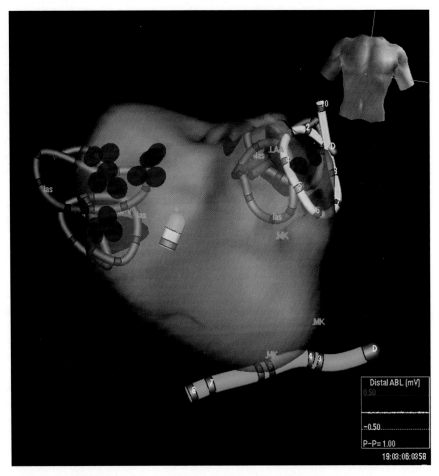

Fig. 3.7. NavX geometry of the left atrium showing the multipolar circular catheter in the left superior pulmonary vein. Shadows of the catheters at the level of the right pulmonary vein ostia as well as the mapping/ablation and the coronary sinus catheters are shown. Brown spots show ablation sites at the region of the right pulmonary vein ostia

create a transthoracic electric field. One electrode pair is placed at the back of the neck (spinous processes C3–C4) and medial upper left leg, the second pair of external electrodes is placed on the right and left lateral thoracic cage in the mid-axillary line at the level of V5–V6 and V5r–V6r precordial electrocardiographic recording places, and the third pair of electrodes is placed on the anterior and posterior of the chest at the precordial V2 lead and infrascapular paravertebral area, respectively. Thus, electrodes are organized in three orthogonal axes with the heart at their center [80]. A multiplex frequency of 93 Hz allows almost real-time navigation and visualization of catheter position. Any movement of the catheter in the heart results in a change in the measured voltage or impedance for each electrode. The accuracy of electrode location is 0.6 mm for a wide range of patient body weights. The three-dimensional geometry of the chamber is reconstructed by sweeping any conventional catheter over the endocardial surface (Figure 3.7). Relevant anatomic landmarks are annotated. A shadow can be displayed for each catheter, so that in case of displacement, the original position can be restored. The system uses the EnSite system hardware and a special catheter input module.

A recent study has demonstrated the feasibility of catheter tracking and three-dimensional cardiac chamber model reconstruction using the NavX system [38]. Another recent study demonstrated that NavX-guided ablation of common type atrial flutter and atrial fibrillation reduces total X-ray exposure compared with the fluoroscopy-guided approach [57]. Clinical experience with the system is still limited.

3.6 The LocaLisa navigation system

LocaLisa system is a real-time three-dimensional catheter localization and navigation system that uses externally applied electrical fields in three orthogonal directions to generate a transthoracic electric field [83]. In fact, the principles of the LocaLisa catheter navigation system have been integrated into the EnSite NavX system described above. The LocaLisa navigation system has been used to guide ablation of supraventricular tachycardias [36], incisional atrial tachycardias [48] junctional tachycardia

[73] and atrial flutter [64], pulmonary vein ablation [44], and ablation of atrioventricular nodal reentrant tachycardia in children [13, 34]. It is generally felt that the system reduces X-ray exposure and fluoroscopy time. Due to its simple principle and compatibility with a wide range of catheters, the system is considered attractive in terms of low costs and ease of operation. Clinical experience with the LocaLisa navigation system is limited and derived from studies with limited numbers of patients.

3.7 The real-time position management (RPM) system

The real-time position management system uses ultrasound ranging to calculate the distance between transmitting and receiving transducers mounted on intracardiac catheters. Two multitransducer catheters are positioned at the coronary sinus and the right ventricular apex in a stable position and these catheters track the location of the third catheter [11]. The system is nonfluoroscopically operated and has ability to display three-dimensional anatomy and electrical recordings on the same platform. The feasibility studies have been performed in humans and serious limitations have been identified [68]. The clinical experience of the system is limited.

Strengths and limitations of newly developed electrophysiological mapping systems have recently been reviewed (see Table 3.1) [52].

3.8 Intracardiac echocardiography

Intracardiac echocardiography is a new technology that allows high-resolution imaging of intracardiac structures and the electrode-tissue interface. Intracardiac echocardiography has been proved useful in guiding the procedures that require precise anatomical guidance such as ablation of atrial flutter [7], anatomical location of arrhythmogenic foci and ablation of atrial tachycardia [33], sinus node modification [41], ablation of atrioventricular nodal reentrant tachycardia [20], transseptal punctures [47], creation of linear lesions [14, 51], pulmonary

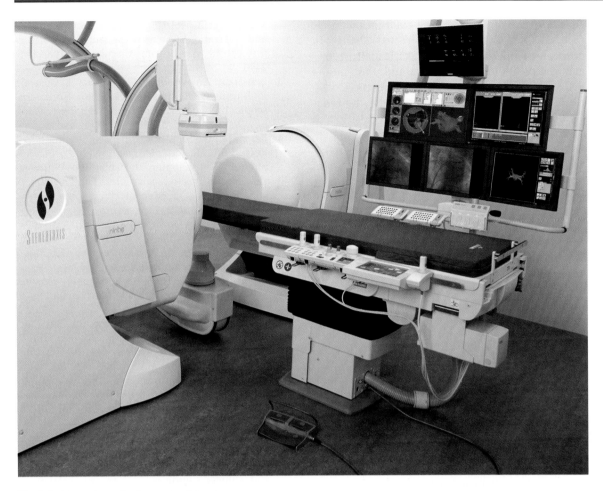

Fig. 3.8. Magnetic navigation system laboratory

vein isolation [46] and ventricular tachycardia [30, 40]. Recently the clinical implications of intracardiac echocardiography in interventional and electrophysiological procedures have been reviewed [28]. From all these studies, there is a general consensus that intracardiac echocardiography has advantages over fluoroscopy in terms of precise location of the catheter tip in relation to endocardial structures, evaluation of catheter tip-tissue contact, confirmation of lesion formation and morphological characterization, diagnosis of procedure-related complications, identification of anatomical structures that serve as foci for arrhythmogenesis and potential reduction in fluoroscopy time.

3.9 The magnetic navigation system (Stereotaxis)

Recently, a remote-controlled magnetic navigation system has been developed (Figure 3.8). The system enables navigation and positioning of soft catheters to any desired place within the heart chambers guided by magnetic fields [18]. The system currently in use (Nioobe Stereotaxis, Inc.) has two permanent magnets, placed on either side of the fluoroscopic table. The magnet positions relative to each other are computer-controlled. In the "navigate" position, the magnets generate a uniform magnetic field (0.08 Tesla) which penetrates about 15 cm inside the patient's chest. The catheter is composed of soft material and has embedded in its tip a small permanent magnet which is guided according to the external magnetic field direction. The change in the direction of the external magnetic field, enabled by computer-directed change in position of the external magnets leads to reorientation of the internal magnet and, thus, in the deflection of the catheter tip. The magnetic vectors are stored so that the catheter may be renavigated automatically to the selected position. A computer-controlled advancer system allows remote catheter navigation without manual intervention. The video workstation of the system unit allows precise orientation of the catheter with a joystick or mouse from the control room [15, 16].

Human experience with the system is still very limited. The magnetic navigation system has been used to guide ablation of the supraventricular tachycardias [19], atrioventricular nodal reentrant tachycardia and accessory pathways [15, 16].

▌3.10 Future directions

Within the last decade we have witnessed the development and clinical introduction of a number of computer-based mapping and ablation systems. Considering rapid advances in the field, the mapping and ablation system of the future is difficult to predict. However, based on the existing experience, the mapping and ablation system to be used in the near future may integrate 3 existing technologies: anatomic images reconstructed by computed tomography or magnetic resonance imaging, electroanatomic mapping which allows visualization of electrophysiological information precisely linked to discrete anatomic areas and a remote magnetic catheter navigation system. Such a system seems to be in the early stages of development (CARTO-RMT system). Presently the clinical experience with this system is lacking.

▌ References

1. Aiba T, Shimizu W, Taguchi A, Suyama K, Kurita T, Aihara N, Kamakura S (2001) Clinical usefulness of a multielectrode basket catheter for idiopathic ventricular tachycardia originating from right ventricular outflow tract. J Cardiovasc Electrophysiol 12:511–517
2. Arentz T, von Rosenthal J, Blum T, Stockinger J, Burkle G, Weber R, Jander N, Neumann FJ, Kalusche D (2003) Feasibility and safety of pulmonary vein isolation using a new mapping and navigation system in patients with refractory atrial fibrillation. Circulation 108:2484–2490
3. Ben-Haim SA, Osadchy D, Schuster I, Gepstein L, Hayam G, Josephson ME (1996) Nonfluoroscopic, in vivo navigation and mapping technology. Nat Med 2:1393–1395
4. Betts TR, Roberts PR, Allen SA, Salmon AP, Keeton BR, Haw MP, Morgan JM (2000) Electrophysiological mapping and ablation of intra-atrial reentry tachycardia after Fontan surgery with the use of a noncontact mapping system. Circulation 102:419–425
5. Betts TR, Yue A, Roberts PR, Morgan JM (2004) Radiofrequency ablation of idiopathic ventricular fibrillation guided by noncontact mapping. J Cardiovasc Electrophysiol 15:957–959
6. Chauhan VS, Nair GM, Sevaptisidis E, Downar E (2004) Magnetoelectroanatomic mapping of arrhythmias in structural heart disease using a novel multielectrode catheter. Pacing Clin Electrophysiol 27:1077–1084
7. Chu E, Kalman JM, Kwasman MA, Jue JC, Fitzgerald PJ, Epstein LM, Schiller NB, Yock PG, Lesh MD (1994) Intracardiac echocardiography during radiofrequency catheter ablation of cardiac arrhythmias in humans. J Am Coll Cardiol 24:1351–1357
8. Chugh A, Oral H, Lemola K, Hall B, Cheung P, Good E, Tamirisa K, Han J, Bogun F, Pelosi F, Jr., Morady F (2005) Prevalence, mechanisms, and clinical significance of macroreentrant atrial tachycardia during and following left atrial ablation for atrial fibrillation. Heart Rhythm 2:464–471
9. Corrado D, Basso C, Leoni L, Tokajuk B, Bauce B, Frigo G, Tarantini G, Napodano M, Turrini P, Ramondo A, Daliento L, Nava A, Buja G, Iliceto S, Thiene G (2005) Three-dimensional electroanatomic voltage mapping increases accuracy of diagnosing arrhythmogenic right ventricular cardiomyopathy/dysplasia. Circulation 111:3042–3050
10. Darbar D, Olgin JE, Miller JM, Friedman PA (2001) Localization of the origin of arrhythmias for ablation: from Electrocardiography to advanced endocardial mapping systems. J Cardiovasc Electrophysiol 12:1309–1325
11. de Groot NM, Bootsma M, van der Velde ET, Schalij MJ (2000) Three-dimensional catheter positioning during radiofrequency ablation in patients: first application of a real-time position management system. J Cardiovasc Electrophysiol 11:1183–1192
12. Delacretaz E, Ganz LI, Soejima K, Friedman PL, Walsh EP, Triedman JK, Sloss LJ, Landzberg MJ, Stevenson WG (2001) Multi atrial macro-re-entry circuits in adults with repaired congenital

heart disease: entrainment mapping combined with three-dimensional electroanatomic mapping. J Am Coll Cardiol 37:1665–1676

13. Emmel M, Sreeram N, Brockmeier K (2005) Catheter ablation of junctional ectopic tachycardia in children, with preservation of atrioventricular conduction. Z Kardiol 94:280–286

14. Epstein LM, Mitchell MA, Smith TW, Haines DE (1998) Comparative study of fluoroscopy and intracardiac echocardiographic guidance for the creation of linear atrial lesions. Circulation 98:1796–1801

15. Ernst S, Hachiya H, Chun JK, Ouyang F (2005) Remote catheter ablation of parahisian accessory pathways using a novel magnetic navigation system – a report of two cases. J Cardiovasc Electrophysiol 16:659–662

16. Ernst S, Ouyang F, Linder C, Hertting K, Stahl F, Chun J, Hachiya H, Bansch D, Antz M, Kuck KH (2004) Initial experience with remote catheter ablation using a novel magnetic navigation system: magnetic remote catheter ablation. Circulation 109:1472–1475

17. Ernst S, Schluter M, Ouyang F, Khanedani A, Cappato R, Hebe J, Volkmer M, Antz M, Kuck KH (1999) Modification of the substrate for maintenance of idiopathic human atrial fibrillation: efficacy of radiofrequency ablation using nonfluoroscopic catheter guidance. Circulation 100:2085–2092

18. Faddis MN, Blume W, Finney J, Hall A, Rauch J, Sell J, Bae KT, Talcott M, Lindsay B (2002) Novel, magnetically guided catheter for endocardial mapping and radiofrequency catheter ablation. Circulation 106:2980–2985

19. Faddis MN, Chen J, Osborn J, Talcott M, Cain ME, Lindsay BD (2003) Magnetic guidance system for cardiac electrophysiology: a prospective trial of safety and efficacy in humans. J Am Coll Cardiol 42:1952–1958

20. Fisher WG, Pelini MA, Bacon ME (1997) Adjunctive intracardiac echocardiography to guide slow pathway ablation in human atrioventricular nodal reentrant tachycardia: anatomic insights. Circulation 96:3021–3029

21. Friedman PA (2002) Novel mapping techniques for cardiac electrophysiology. Heart 87:575–582

22. Friedman PA, Asirvatham SJ, Grice S, Glikson M, Munger TM, Rea RF, Shen WK, Jahanghir A, Packer DL, Hammill SC (2002) Noncontact mapping to guide ablation of right ventricular outflow tract tachycardia. J Am Coll Cardiol 39:1808–1812

23. Gepstein L, Evans SJ (1998) Electroanatomical mapping of the heart: basic concepts and implications for the treatment of cardiac arrhythmias. Pacing Clin Electrophysiol 21:1268–1278

24. Gepstein L, Hayam G, Ben-Haim SA (1997) A novel method for nonfluoroscopic catheter-based electroanatomical mapping of the heart. In vitro and in vivo accuracy results. Circulation 95:1611–1622

25. Gornick CC, Adler SW, Pederson B, Hauck J, Budd J, Schweitzer J (1999) Validation of a new noncontact catheter system for electroanatomic mapping of left ventricular endocardium. Circulation 99:829–835

26. Haissaguerre M, Shah DC, Jais P, Hocini M, Yamane T, Deisenhofer I, Chauvin M, Garrigue S, Clementy J (2000) Electrophysiological breakthroughs from the left atrium to the pulmonary veins. Circulation 102:2463–2465

27. Hindricks G, Kottkamp H (2001) Simultaneous noncontact mapping of left atrium in patients with paroxysmal atrial fibrillation. Circulation 104:297–303

28. Hoffmann E, Reithmann C, Nimmermann P, Elser F, Dorwarth U, Remp T, Steinbeck G (2002) Clinical experience with electroanatomic mapping of ectopic atrial tachycardia. Pacing Clin Electrophysiol 25:49–56

29. Jais P, Shah DC, Haissaguerre M, Hocini M, Peng JT, Takahashi A, Garrigue S, Le Metayer P, Clementy J (2000) Mapping and ablation of left atrial flutters. Circulation 101:2928–2934

30. Jongbloed MR, Bax JJ, van der Burg AE, Van der Wall EE, Schalij MJ (2004) Radiofrequency catheter ablation of ventricular tachycardia guided by intracardiac echocardiography. Eur J Echocardiogr 5:34–40

31. Jongbloed MR, Schalij MJ, Zeppenfeld K, Oemrawsingh PV, van der Wall EE, Bax JJ (2005) Clinical applications of intracardiac echocardiography in interventional procedures. Heart 91:981–990

32. Kall JG, Rubenstein DS, Kopp DE, Burke MC, Verdino RJ, Lin AC, Johnson CT, Cooke PA, Wang ZG, Fumo M, Wilber DJ (2000) Atypical atrial flutter originating in the right atrial free wall. Circulation 101:270–279

33. Kalman JM, Olgin JE, Karch MR, Hamdan M, Lee RJ, Lesh MD (1998) "Cristal tachycardias": origin of right atrial tachycardias from the crista terminalis identified by intracardiac echocardiography. J Am Coll Cardiol 31:451–459

34. Kammeraad J, ten Cate FU, Simmers T, Emmel M, Wittkampf FH, Sreeram N (2004) Radiofrequency catheter ablation of atrioventricular nodal reentrant tachycardia in children aided by the LocaLisa mapping system. Europace 6:209–214

35. Khoury DS, Taccardi B, Lux RL, Ershler PR, Rudy Y (1995) Reconstruction of endocardial potentials and activation sequences from intracavitary probe measurements. Localization of pacing sites and effects of myocardial structure. Circulation 91:845–863

36. Kirchhof P, Loh P, Eckardt L, Ribbing M, Rolf S, Eick O, Wittkampf F, Borggrefe M, Breithardt GG, Haverkamp W (2002) A novel nonfluoroscopic catheter visualization system (LocaLisa) to reduce radiation exposure during catheter ablation of supraventricular tachycardias. Am J Cardiol 90:340–343

37. Kottkamp H, Hindricks G, Breithardt G, Borggrefe M (1997) Three-dimensional electromagnetic catheter technology: electroanatomical mapping of the right atrium and ablation of ectopic atrial tachycardia. J Cardiovasc Electrophysiol 8:1332–1337

38. Krum D, Goel A, Hauck J, Schweitzer J, Hare J, Attari M, Dhala A, Cooley R, Akhtar M, Sra J (2005) Catheter location, tracking, cardiac chamber geometry creation, and ablation using cutaneous patches. J Interv Card Electrophysiol 12:17–22

39. Kumagai K, Ogawa M, Noguchi H, Yasuda T, Nakashima H, Saku K (2004) Electrophysiologic properties of pulmonary veins assessed using a multielectrode basket catheter. J Am Coll Cardiol 43:2281–2289

40. Lamberti F, Calo L, Pandozi C, Castro A, Loricchio ML, Boggi A, Toscano S, Ricci R, Drago F, Santini M (2001) Radiofrequency catheter ablation of idiopathic left ventricular outflow tract tachycardia: utility of intracardiac echocardiography. J Cardiovasc Electrophysiol 12:529–535

41. Lee RJ, Kalman JM, Fitzpatrick AP, Epstein LM, Fisher WG, Olgin JE, Lesh MD, Scheinman MM (1995) Radiofrequency catheter modification of the sinus node for "inappropriate" sinus tachycardia. Circulation 92:2919–2928

42. Lesh MD, Van Hare GF, Epstein LM, Fitzpatrick AP, Scheinman MM, Lee RJ, Kwasman MA, Grogin HR, Griffin JC (1994) Radiofrequency catheter ablation of atrial arrhythmias. Results and mechanisms. Circulation 89:1074–1089

43. Love BA, Collins KK, Walsh EP, Triedman JK (2001) Electroanatomic characterization of conduction barriers in sinus/atrially paced rhythm and association with intra-atrial reentrant tachycardia circuits following congenital heart disease surgery. J Cardiovasc Electrophysiol 12:17–25

44. Macle L, Jais P, Scavee C, Weerasooriya R, Hocini M, Shah DC, Raybaud F, Choi KJ, Clementy J, Haissaguerre M (2003) Pulmonary vein disconnection using the LocaLisa three-dimensional nonfluoroscopic catheter imaging system. J Cardiovasc Electrophysiol 14:693–697

45. Marchlinski FE, Callans DJ, Gottlieb CD, Zado E (2000) Linear ablation lesions for control of unmappable ventricular tachycardia in patients with ischemic and nonischemic cardiomyopathy. Circulation 101:1288–1296

46. Marrouche NF, Martin DO, Wazni O, Gillinov AM, Klein A, Bhargava M, Saad E, Bash D, Yamada H, Jaber W, Schweikert R, Tchou P, Abdul-Karim A, Saliba W, Natale A (2003) Phased-array intracardiac echocardiography monitoring during pulmonary vein isolation in patients with atrial fibrillation: impact on outcome and complications. Circulation 107:2710–2716

47. Mitchel JF, Gillam LD, Sanzobrino BW, Hirst JA, McKay RG (1995) Intracardiac ultrasound imaging during transseptal catheterization. Chest 108:104–108

48. Molenschot M, Ramanna H, Hoorntje T, Wittkampf F, Hauer R, Derksen R, Sreeram N (2001) Catheter ablation of incisional atrial tachycardia using a novel mapping system: LocaLisa. Pacing Clin Electrophysiol 24:1616–1622

49. Nademanee K, Kosar EM (1998) A nonfluoroscopic catheter-based mapping technique to ablate focal ventricular tachycardia. Pacing Clin Electrophysiol 21:1442–1447

50. Nakagawa H, Shah N, Matsudaira K, Overholt E, Chandrasekaran K, Beckman KJ, Spector P, Calame JD, Rao A, Hasdemir C, Otomo K, Wang Z, Lazzara R, Jackman WM (2001) Characterization of reentrant circuit in macroreentrant right atrial tachycardia after surgical repair of congenital heart disease: isolated channels between scars allow "focal" ablation. Circulation 103:699–709

51. Olgin JE, Kalman JM, Chin M, Stillson C, Maguire M, Ursel P, Lesh MD (1997) Electrophysiological effects of long, linear atrial lesions placed under intracardiac ultrasound guidance. Circulation 96:2715–2721

52. Packer DL (2005) Three-dimensional mapping in interventional electrophysiology: techniques and technology. J Cardiovasc Electrophysiol 16:1110–1116

53. Pappone C, Rosanio S, Oreto G, Tocchi M, Gugliotta F, Vicedomini G, Salvati A, Dicandia C, Mazzone P, Santinelli V, Gulletta S, Chierchia S (2000) Circumferential radiofrequency ablation of pulmonary vein ostia: A new anatomic approach for curing atrial fibrillation. Circulation 102:2619–2628

54. Paul T, Windhagen-Mahnert B, Kriebel T, Bertram H, Kaulitz R, Korte T, Niehaus M, Tebbenjohanns J (2001) Atrial reentrant tachycardia after surgery for congenital heart disease: endocardial mapping and radiofrequency catheter ablation using a novel, noncontact mapping system. Circulation 103:2266–2271

55. Poty H, Saoudi N, Nair M, Anselme F, Letac B (1996) Radiofrequency catheter ablation of atrial flutter. Further insights into the various types of isthmus block: application to ablation during sinus rhythm. Circulation 94:3204–3213

56. Rostock T, Willems S, Ventura R, Weiss C, Risius T, Meinertz T (2004) Radiofrequency catheter ablation of a macroreentrant ventricular tachycardia late after surgical repair of tetralogy of Fallot using the electroanatomic mapping (CARTO). Pacing Clin Electrophysiol 27:801–804

57. Rotter M, Takahashi Y, Sanders P, Haissaguerre M, Jais P, Hsu LF, Sacher F, Pasquie JL, Clementy J, Hocini M (2005) Reduction of fluoroscopy exposure and procedure duration during ablation of atrial fibrillation using a novel anatomical navigation system. Eur Heart J 26:1415–1421

58. Schalij MJ, van Rugge FP, Siezenga M, van der Velde ET (1998) Endocardial activation mapping of ventricular tachycardia in patients : first application of a 32-site bipolar mapping electrode catheter. Circulation 98:2168–2179

59. Schilling RJ, Peters NS, Davies DW (1999) Feasibility of a noncontact catheter for endocardial mapping of human ventricular tachycardia. Circulation 99:2543–2552

60. Schilling RJ, Peters NS, Davies DW (1998) Simultaneous endocardial mapping in the human left ventricle using a noncontact catheter: comparison of contact and reconstructed electrograms during sinus rhythm. Circulation 98:887–898

61. Schmitt C, Ndrepepa G, Weber S, Schmieder S, Weyerbrock S, Schneider M, Karch MR, Deisenhofer I, Schreieck J, Zrenner B, Schomig A (2002) Biatrial multisite mapping of atrial premature complexes triggering onset of atrial fibrillation. Am J Cardiol 89:1381–1387

62. Schmitt C, Zrenner B, Schneider M, Karch M, Ndrepepa G, Deisenhofer I, Weyerbrock S, Schreieck J, Schomig A (1999) Clinical experience with a novel multielectrode basket catheter in right atrial tachycardias. Circulation 99:2414–2422

63. Schmitt H, Weber S, Tillmanns H, Waldecker B (2000) Diagnosis and ablation of atrial flutter using a high resolution, noncontact mapping system. Pacing Clin Electrophysiol 23:2057–2064

64. Schneider MA, Ndrepepa G, Dobran I, Schreieck J, Weber S, Plewan A, Deisenhofer I, Karch MR, Schomig A, Schmitt C (2003) LocaLisa catheter navigation reduces fluoroscopy time and dosage in ablation of atrial flutter: a prospective randomized study. J Cardiovasc Electrophysiol 14:587–590

65. Schneider MA, Ndrepepa G, Weber S, Deisenhofer I, Schomig A, Schmitt C (2004) Influence of high-pass filtering on noncontact mapping and ablation of atrial tachycardias. Pacing Clin Electrophysiol 27:38–46

66. Schneider MA, Ndrepepa G, Zrenner B, Karch MR, Schmieder S, Deisenhofer I, Schreieck J, Schomig A, Schmitt C (2001) Noncontact mapping-guided ablation of atrial flutter and enhanced-density mapping of the inferior vena caval-tricuspid annulus isthmus. Pacing Clin Electrophysiol 24:1755–1764

67. Schneider MA, Ndrepepa G, Zrenner B, Karch MR, Schreieck J, Deisenhofer I, Schmitt C (2000) Noncontact mapping-guided catheter ablation of atrial fibrillation associated with left atrial ectopy. J Cardiovasc Electrophysiol 11:475–479

68. Schreieck J, Ndrepepa G, Zrenner B, Schneider MA, Weyerbrock S, Dong J, Schmitt C (2002) Radiofrequency ablation of cardiac arrhythmias using a three-dimensional real-time position management and mapping system. Pacing Clin Electrophysiol 25:1699–1707

69. Seidl K, Schwacke H, Rameken M, Drogemuller A, Beatty G, Senges J (2003) Noncontact mapping of ectopic atrial tachycardias: different characteristics of isopotential maps and unipolar electrogram. Pacing Clin Electrophysiol 26:16–25

70. Seidl K, Schwacke H, Zahn R, Rameken M, Drogemuller A, Senges J (2003) Catheter ablation of chronic atrial fibrillation with noncontact mapping: are continuous linear lesions associated with ablation success? Pacing Clin Electrophysiol 26:534–543

71. Shah D, Jais P, Takahashi A, Hocini M, Peng JT, Clementy J, Haissaguerre M (2000) Dual-loop intra-atrial reentry in humans. Circulation 101:631–639

72. Shah DC, Haissaguerre M, Jais P, Fischer B, Takahashi A, Hocini M, Clementy J (1997) Simplified electrophysiologically directed catheter ablation of recurrent common atrial flutter. Circulation 96:2505–2508

73. Simmers TA, Sreeram N, Wittkampf FH, Derksen R (2003) Radiofrequency catheter ablation of junctional ectopic tachycardia with preservation of atrioventricular conduction. Pacing Clin Electrophysiol 26:1284–1288

74. Sra J, Thomas JM (2001) New techniques for mapping cardiac arrhythmias. Indian Heart J 53:423–444

75. Stabile G, Turco P, La Rocca V, Nocerino P, Stabile E, De Simone A (2003) Is pulmonary vein isolation necessary for curing atrial fibrillation? Circulation 108:657–660

76. Stevenson WG, Delacretaz E (2000) Radiofrequency catheter ablation of ventricular tachycardia. Heart 84:553–559

77. Strickberger SA, Knight BP, Michaud GF, Pelosi F, Morady F (2000) Mapping and ablation of ventricular tachycardia guided by virtual electrograms using a noncontact, computerized mapping system. J Am Coll Cardiol 35:414–421

78. Tai CT, Huang JL, Lin YK, Hsieh MH, Lee PC, Ding YA, Chang MS, Chen SA (2002) Noncon-

tact three-dimensional mapping and ablation of upper loop re-entry originating in the right atrium. J Am Coll Cardiol 40:746–753

79. Thiagalingam A, Wallace EM, Campbell CR, Boyd AC, Eipper VE, Byth K, Ross DL, Kovoor P (2004) Value of noncontact mapping for identifying left ventricular scar in an ovine model. Circulation 110:3175–3180

80. Ventura R, Rostock T, Klemm HU, Lutomsky B, Demir C, Weiss C, Meinertz T, Willems S (2004) Catheter ablation of common-type atrial flutter guided by three-dimensional right atrial geometry reconstruction and catheter tracking using cutaneous patches: a randomized prospective study. J Cardiovasc Electrophysiol 15:1157–1161

81. Verma A, Kilicaslan F, Schweikert RA, Tomassoni G, Rossillo A, Marrouche NF, Ozduran V, Wazni OM, Elayi SC, Saenz LC, Minor S, Cummings JE, Burkhardt JD, Hao S, Beheiry S, Tchou PJ, Natale A (2005) Short- and long-term success of substrate-based mapping and ablation of ventricular tachycardia in arrhythmogenic right ventricular dysplasia. Circulation 111:3209–3216

82. Walsh EP, Saul JP, Hulse JE, Rhodes LA, Hordof AJ, Mayer JE, Lock JE (1992) Transcatheter ablation of ectopic atrial tachycardia in young patients using radiofrequency current. Circulation 86:1138–1146

83. Wittkampf FH, Wever EF, Derksen R, Wilde AA, Ramanna H, Hauer RN, Robles de Medina EO (1999) LocaLisa: new technique for real-time 3-dimensional localization of regular intracardiac electrodes. Circulation 99:1312–1317

84. Zrenner B, Dong J, Schreieck J, Ndrepepa G, Meisner H, Kaemmerer H, Schomig A, Hess J, Schmitt C (2003) Delineation of intra-atrial re-entrant tachycardia circuits after mustard operation for transposition of the great arteries using biatrial electroanatomic mapping and entrainment mapping. J Cardiovasc Electrophysiol 14:1302–1310

85. Zrenner B, Ndrepepa G, Schmitt C (2000) Use of multielectrode basket catheters for mapping of cardiac arrhythmias. Herzschr Electrophys 11: 4–10

86. Zrenner B, Ndrepepa G, Schneider M, Karch M, Deisenhofer I, Schreieck J, Schomig A, Schmitt C (2000) Basket catheter-guided three-dimensional activation patterns construction and ablation of common type atrial flutter. Pacing Clin Electrophysiol 23:1350–1358

87. Zrenner B, Ndrepepa G, Schneider M, Karch M, Hofmann F, Schomig A, Schmitt C (1999) Computer-assisted animation of atrial tachyarrhythmias recorded with a 64-electrode basket catheter. J Am Coll Cardiol 34:2051–2060

88. Zrenner B, Ndrepepa G, Schneider MA, Karch MR, Brodherr-Heberlein S, Kaemmerer H, Hess J, Schomig A, Schmitt C (2001) Mapping and ablation of atrial arrhythmias after surgical correction of congenital heart disease guided by a 64-electrode basket catheter. Am J Cardiol 88:573–578

4 Accessory pathways

GABRIELE HESSLING, MICHAEL SCHNEIDER,
ALEXANDER PUSTOWOIT, CLAUS SCHMITT

4.1 Introduction

Over a century has passed since Stanley Kent reported in 1893 on the pathohistologic finding of myocardial fibers crossing the lateral aspect of the sulcus atrioventricularis which he thought were part of the normal "nodal" connection between the atrium and ventricle [23]. Although the interpretation of his findings was wrong, he was the first to describe an accessory connection between atrial and ventricular myocardium and these pathways are still referred to as "Kent fibers". In 1930, Wolff, Parkinson und White described a "syndrome" that consisted of a short PQ interval with bundle branch block on the surface ECG together with the clinical picture of paroxysmal tachycardia [46]. The authors did not recognize the anatomic and electrophysiological correlate of their findings but their report led to more investigation. Holzmann and Scherf [21] are thought to be the first to describe our current understanding of the pathogenesis of WPW syndrome in terms of a reentrant circuit involving the AV node and an extranodal accessory pathway.

From a developmental aspect, accessory pathways are the result of an incomplete regression of the embryonic muscular continuity between atrial and ventricular myocardium and can occur at different locations around the tricuspid and mitral annulus [33, 36]. The prevalence of WPW syndrome is approximately 0.15–0.25% but varies with patient population, age and gender [1, 11]. A "loss" of preexcitation during the first year of life and during mid-term adult life has been reported [25]. The genetic basis of preexcitation is still not completely understood. While preexcitation of the WPW type is seen mostly sporadic, familial forms and an association with hypertrophic cardiomyopathy and congenital heart defects like Ebstein's anomaly of the tricuspid valve or congenitally "corrected" transposition of the great arteries have been described [3].

4.1.1 Electrophysiological characteristics of accessory pathways

Accessory pathways (APs) vary in anatomic location and may be capable of conducting only antegrade from the atria to the ventricles, only retrograde from the ventricles to the atria or may have bidirectional conduction properties as seen in the classical WPW syndrome. Patients with antegrade conducting APs have a risk of sudden death from a rapid ventricular response to fast conduction over the AP if atrial fibrillation or fast atrial flutter occurs. The incidence of sudden death in the WPW population is reported to be 0.1–0.6% per year [36]. Attempts have been made to identify asymptomatic high-risk patients with WPW syndrome by invasive EP testing [37]. The presence of multiple APs or the combination of inducible atrioventricular tachycardia and a shortest preexcited RR interval of < 250 ms during atrial fibrillation seem to provide the strongest indications for catheter ablation in the adult population [37, 43].

APs showing only retrograde conduction properties are termed "concealed" as they are not detectable during normal sinus rhythm.

The classic tachycardia involving an AP is orthodromic reentrant tachycardia (ORT) with antegrade conduction over the AV node and retrograde conduction via the AP. For this type of tachycardia only retrograde conduction properties of the AP are required and it occurs in patients with overt preexcitation as well as with concealed APs. With overt preexcitation, antidromic reentrant tachycardia (ART) with antegrade conduction over the AP and retrograde conduction over the AV node is also possible. This type of tachycardia is rare as it requires a longer antegrade refractory period of the AV

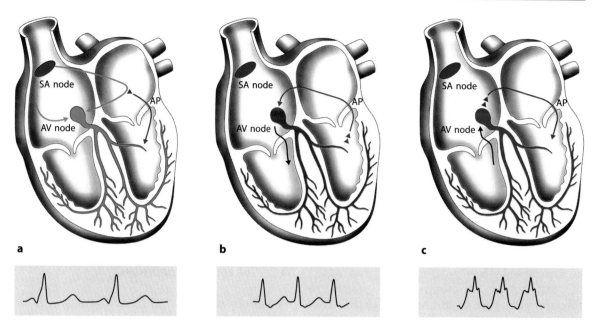

Fig. 4.1. a *Sinus rhythm with preexcitation of the WPW type*: Antegrade conduction (from the atria to the ventricles) occurs via the AV node (green) *and* the accessory pathway (red). Due to faster conduction over the AP, a part of ventricular myocardium is depolarized earlier than the rest which correlates to the surface delta wave. **b** *Orthodromic reentrant tachycardia*: Antegrade conduction over the AP is blocked due to its longer refractoriness. Conduction to the ventricles during tachycardia occurs *only* via the AV node (black) and reaches the AP when it is able to conduct back to the atria (blue). **c** *Antidromic reentrant tachycardia*: In this case, the AV node reaches refractoriness before the AP. Antegrade conduction occurs *only* via the AP (red) and reaches the AV node when it is able to conduct back to the atria (black)

node compared to the AP (which is usually the other way). Both antidromic and orthodromic tachycardia are also referred to as atrioventricular reentrant tachycardia (AVRT) with the AV node and the accessory pathway as necessary parts of the reentrant circuit (Figure 4.1).

"Decremental" conduction (cycle length-dependent prolongation of conduction) is a classic electrophysiological feature of the AV node, whereas the majority of APs (with overt preexcitation or concealed) show "nondecremental" conduction. APs with decremental conduction properties lead to specific clinical entities. Mahaim fibers (right-sided pathways often crossing the tricuspid annulus on the free wall) only have unidirectional conduction properties from the atria to ventricles [35]. APs in the permanent form of junctional reciprocating tachycardia only show retrograde decremental conduction properties and are often located posteroseptally on the right or left side [42].

To summarize, accessory pathways may occur singly or multiply, are found in almost every location around the AV groove, may exhibit uni-directional or bidirectional conduction properties and may show decremental or nondecremental conduction.

4.2 Basic approach to the ablation of accessory pathways

Catheter ablation has become the primary therapy for elimination of accessory pathways over the past decade. With current catheters and techniques precise localization of atrial and ventricular insertions of APs followed by temperature controlled heating of a small region of myocardium by radiofrequency energy is possible. In a survey reported in 1995 by Scheinman, success rates of radiofrequency (RF) ablation of accessory pathways were already over 90% [40]. In this chapter our standard approach with practical advices to ablation of accessory pathways is shown and highlighted by several case reports.

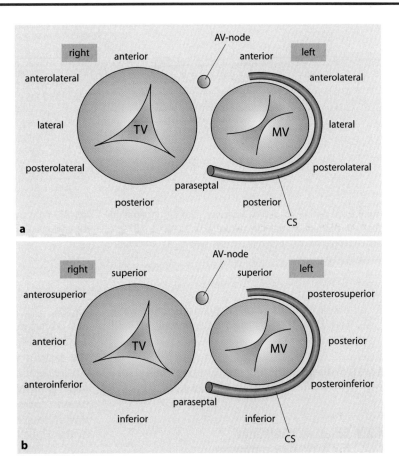

Fig. 4.2. Old (**a**) and New (**b**) nomenclature for the localization of accessory pathways around the atrioventricular junctions

4.2.1 Anatomic locations of accessory pathways

To describe the anatomy of the AV junctions, a new nomenclature was proposed in 1999 by an expert consensus conference [8]. This nomenclature is shown together with the old nomenclature in Figure 4.2. In this chapter, the "old" nomenclature will be used because of its widespread acceptance in describing the anatomic location of accessory pathways.

4.2.2 Localization of accessory pathways from the surface ECG

Before starting the electrophysiological procedure and ablation, the standard 12-lead surface ECG is assessed in patients with overt preexcitation. Various algorithms have been developed to predict the anatomic location of an accessory pathway from the surface delta wave polarity, QRS duration and axis or R/S ratio [4, 9, 14].

Visualization of premature ventricular contraction using ultrasound has also been used to predict AP localization [44]. All proposed algorithms for AP localization from the surface ECG have limited accuracy and should be regarded as an orientation rather than a precise localization tool. Nevertheless, some basic rules for AP localization can almost always be applied:

1. Left-sided free wall pathways are characterized by a positive delta wave in all precordial leads and a negative delta wave in lead I and aVL. Note that preexcitation in left free wall APs is sometimes discrete
2. Right-sided free wall pathways are characterized by a negative delta wave in leads V1-V2/V3 and a positive delta wave in lead I and aVL
3. If V1 is deeply negative and V2 is positive ("septal pattern"), this is suggestive for a septal pathway and subsequent rules 4–5 should be considered
4. A posteroseptal position is characterized by negative delta wave in the inferior leads (lead II, III, aVF)

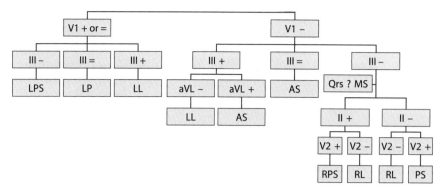

Fig. 4.3. Algorithm to detect accessory pathway localization from the QRS polarity on the surface ECG in adults (*LPS* left posteroseptal, *LP* left posterior, *LL* left lateral, *AS* anterosep- tal, *RPS* right posteroseptal, *RL* right lateral, *PS* posteroseptal, *MS* midseptal). From d'Avila et al. [9] with permission

5. Anteroseptal APs show a positive delta wave in lead I, II, III, aVL and aVF as well as lead V4–V6

An algorithm predicting AP location using surface ECG leads is shown in Figure 4.3.

4.2.3 Ablation guidelines for accessory pathways

Guidelines for the ablation of accessory pathways including personnel, policy, procedures and therapeutic recommendations were proposed in 2003 by the North American Society of Pacing and Electrophysiology and should be taken into consideration before taking a patient to the EP lab [39]. While in the adult population these guidelines aim at a curative treatment by catheter ablation in symptomatic patients, asymptomatic athletes or active younger people, more consideration regarding indications and natural history must be taken in children and young adults. The indications for RF ablation are discussed more extensively in Chapter 11 of this book.

4.2.4 General considerations regarding the ablation procedure

Usually, a single procedure is performed to diagnose the arrhythmia mechanism and to ablate the AP. Before AP mapping, standard electrophysiological techniques are used to evaluate the properties of the AP and tachycardia mech- anism. The general principles of the EP study and ablation are discussed in detail in Chapter 1 of this book. The procedure is performed in the fasting state and usually without sedation. Antiarrhythmic medication has been discontin- ued. Noninvasive or invasive (arterial sheath) blood pressure monitoring is mandatory throughout the procedure. After local anesthesia of the right (and if necessary the left) groin and right (left) femoral venous puncture, 2–3 stan- dard sheaths (6 F, 1×8 F) are introduced and heparin 5000 I.U. i.v. is administered. If a left- sided pathway is presumed from the surface ECG preexcitation pattern, an arterial 8 F sheath might be introduced instead of the 8 F venous sheath before EP testing. Catheter placement is usually possible from the femoral approach. If the surface ECG pattern points to an anterosep- tal or midseptal AP, a venous approach via the jugular or subclavian vein may be considered to facilitate catheter positioning at the septum (see below). Monoplane fluoroscopy is often suffi- cient to localize catheters (usually in the 45° or 60° left anterior oblique view), whereas biplane fluoroscopy (with an additional 30° right ante- rior oblique view) is helpful in difficult cases. A standard EP protocol with programmed ventri- cular and atrial stimulation using 2 to 3 6 F catheters (RV apex, coronary sinus and His po- sition) is routinely performed before mapping the AP.

The positioning of an octa- or decapolar 6 F catheter in the coronary sinus is helpful to dis- tinguish between right- and left-sided APs (especially in concealed APs during ventricular pacing or orthodromic tachycardia). In most

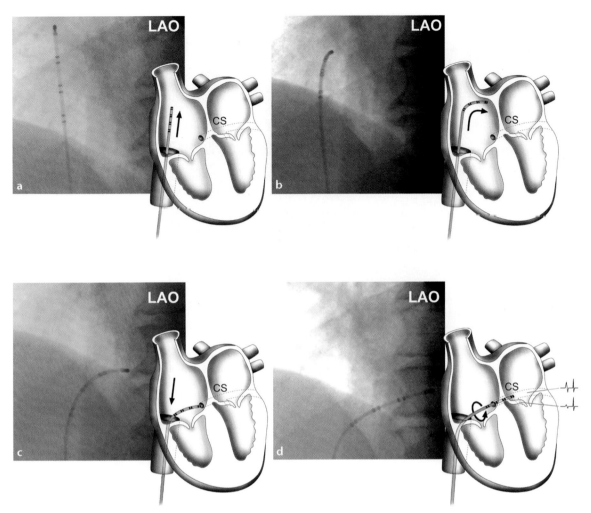

Fig. 4.4. Catheter placement in the coronary sinus using the femoral approach. **a** A steerable octapolar catheter is introduced via the femoral vein and advanced through the inferior caval vein into the right atrium. Fluoroscopy is then changed to a LAO 45° view. LAO angulation enables a frontal view of the atrioventricular valves. **b** The catheter tip is brought to a posteroseptal direction. **c** If necessary, the catheter is pulled back a little. When entering the ostium of coronary sinus, the tip starts nodding against the systolic heart movement. **d** Entering the coronary sinus, an atrial and ventricular electrogram will be recorded. The catheter should be advanced carefully without any force (danger of perforation!) while making a clockwise movement. From a lateral to anterior aspect, the epicardial tissue around the coronary sinus is thin. If a small atrial and larger ventricular signal is recorded, the catheter is caught in a ventricular vein and should be very carefully pulled back a bit and then advanced again

cases the coronary sinus can be cannulated using the femoral approach (Figure 4.4). In many EP labs, a superior approach (via right internal jugular or left subclavian vein) is still used. Rarely the coronary sinus is atretic and cannot be cannulated [31]. An angiography of the coronary sinus should be performed if cannulation is not easiliy achievable or a posteroseptal (epicardial) AP (see Section 4.3.2) is suspected.

As shown in Figure 4.5 (p. 82), once the catheter is introduced, the intracardiac CS signals can be helpful to differentiate a left- from a right-sided accessory pathway.

For mapping and ablation, a deflectable 7 F mapping/ablation catheter (4 mm tip) is used [19]. Especially with right and left free-wall APs, long sheaths might be introduced for better catheter stabilization. Recently developed nonfluoroscopic imaging tools like the LocaLisa

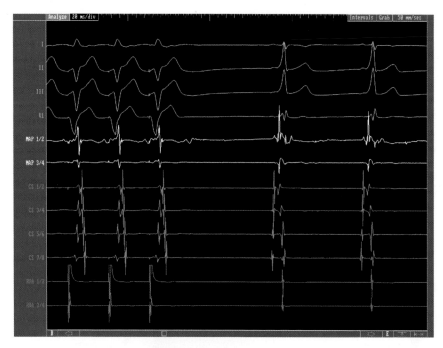

Fig. 4.5. Surface ECG and intracardiac ECG recordings from a patient with a left-sided AP during right ventricular pacing (left) and sinus rhythm (right). During right ventricular pacing (retrograde conduction over the AP), the earliest atrial CS activation (green) is seen on the distal CS poles (CS 1/2) with a distal to proximal (CS 7/8) sequence. During sinus rhythm (antegrade conduction over the AP), the activation sequence of the ventricular component has to be assessed and shows the earliest ventricular activation with the closest AV relation on the distal CS poles (CS 1/2). These findings are concordant with a left-sided pathway

or NavX system might be helpful in guiding the ablation catheter along the mitral annulus by visualizing the coronary sinus catheter (Figure 4.6). These systems are also particularly useful for relocating the ablation catheter in case of dislocation (as with termination of tachycardia during ablation of a concealed bypass tract).

Mapping of the AP depends on whether overt preexcitation is visible during sinus rhythm or the AP is concealed. It aims at

∎ the shortest atrioventricular (AV) time in preexcited sinus rhythm or paced atrial rhythm (only with overt preexcitation) or
∎ the shortest ventriculoatrial (VA) time during orthodromic reciprocating tachycardia or ventricular paced rhythm

A sharp AP potential can be recorded during preexcited sinus rhythm (Figure 4.7).

For ablation, RF energy is delivered using a generator that controls temperature of the catheter tip through power modulation between 0 and 50 W aiming at a target temperature over 50 °C up to 65 °C. Ablation using cryoenergy might be an alternative in pathways close to the AV node or in younger patients (see Chapter 11). In posteroseptal epicardial APs (see Section 4.3.2) the use of an irrigated tip catheter should be considered to avoid local edema and stenosis when ablating in the coronary sinus. Ablation can be performed during sinus rhythm, orthodromic tachycardia or right atrial or ventricular pacing to observe antegrade or retrograde conduction. If catheter stabilization is difficult, ablation during tachycardia is not advisable as the catheter might move with tachycardia termination.

Criteria for a successful AP ablation site have been described [13, 19]. They include maximal fusion of the atrial and ventricular signal and a stable A/V ratio at the ablation site as well as direct recording of a sharp AP potential. Permanent success is associated with early disappearance of the AP [29, 45]. Therefore, RF application is usually stopped after 10 seconds if there is no success. If the delta wave disappears or tachycardia terminates within this time, RF application should be continued for 60 seconds. During RF application, temperature, energy and impedance behavior as well as pain development [29] should be observed carefully. Following a successful RF attempt, patients should be monitored for at least 30 minutes in the EP lab and EP testing performed during/after this time to prove success of the procedure. Isoproterenol or the administration of adenosine might be helpful to unmask residual AP function. It should be kept in mind that approximately 5–10% of patients will show multiple accessory pathways, and in patients with congenital heart disease this number is even higher [30].

After the procedure an echocardiogram is performed routinely to rule out pericardial effusion. Patients are monitored for 12 hours and discharged the day after the procedure. Low-dose antithrombotic therapy with aspirine for 3 months is administered after ablation of a left-sided pathway.

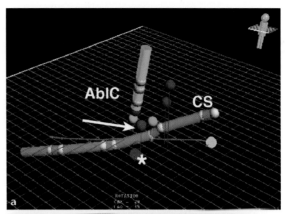
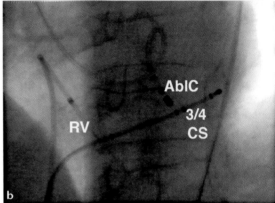

Fig. 4.6. Nonfluoroscopic catheter imaging (**a**) by using the LocaLisa system compared to the standard radiographic view (below) (**b**) CS coronary sinus catheter, AblC ablation catheter, RV right ventricular catheter; red dots= ablation sites

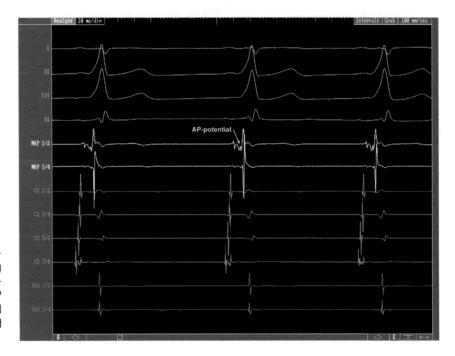

Fig. 4.7. Surface ECG and intracardiac recordings during sinus rhythm (left-sided accessory pathway). The MAP catheter (white) is positioned at the ablation site and shows a typical AP potential

4.3 Specific considerations in the ablation of accessory pathways

4.3.1 Left-sided free-wall accessory pathways

Left-sided APs are more prevalent (59%) and in most cases easier to ablate than right-sided APs [35]. The mitral annulus is generally smaller in diameter than the tricuspid annulus and forms a continuous ring of fibrous tissue between the left atrium and ventricle. APs mostly consist of small strands of tissue relatively close to the annulus. To localize left free-wall and left postero-septal APs, an octa- or decapolar 6 F catheter in the coronary sinus is helpful in guiding the mapping catheter (Figure 4.4). For the mapping and ablation of left-sided APs, the retrograde transaortal (Figure 4.8.) or the antegrade trans-septal approach (Figure 10.4) can be used.

Depending on the experience of the operator, success rates between 90–100% and recurrence rates <5% can be achieved by either approach for left-sided pathways [10, 35]. Unless a persistent Foramen ovale allows fast access to the left atrium (Figure 4.8), the transaortic approach (Figure 4.6) is routinely used at our institution. The curved catheter is pushed gently over the aortic valve into the left ventricle. The catheter tip is deflected and positioned under the mitral valve leaflet. Pathways on the anterior or antero-lateral aspect of the mitral valve might be reached easier with the retrograde approach than more posteroseptal located APs [35].

Complications of left-sided AP ablation are rare. The risk of myocardial perforation with cardiac tamponade or thromboembolic events with stroke or systemic emboli is 1–2%. Air embolism with the transseptal approach is also rare. Coronary artery thrombosis from delivery of RF current in the left main stem or left circumflex artery has been reported while AV block is also very rare with the retrograde approach [35].

∎ Left lateral accessory pathway – a tough case

This case highlights most of the features accessory connections can exhibit during an electrophysiological study and will therefore be reviewed extensively.

A 28-year old man was brought to the EP lab. He had a history of tachycardia as well as syncope; his standard 12-lead ECG was suggestive of a left lateral AP (Figure 4.9).

During the routine EP study, programmed atrial pacing showed maximal preexcitation (Figure 4.10).

With programmed atrial pacing, orthodromic reentrant tachycardia (ORT) was induced (Figure 4.11, p. 86).

After termination of ORT, also with programmed atrial stimulation, antidromic reentrant (ART) tachycardia was induced (Figures 4.12, p. 86 and 4.13, p. 87).

Shortly afterwards, atrial fibrillation occurred. (Figures 4.14, p. 87 and 4.15, p. 88).

After completing the mapping procedure, the AP could be successfully ablated at this position (Figure 4.16, p. 88).

4.3.2 (Epicardial) posteroseptal and left posterior accessory pathways

Epicardial APs are found most commonly in the posteroseptal and left posterior region. It is hypothesized that epicardial APs connect the myocardial coat of the coronary sinus to the ventricle [22]. These APs are associated with CS anomalies like diverticula (highly variable in size) or a trumpet-like enlargement of the ostium of the coronary sinus in approximately 20% of patients [22, 41]. In rare cases, epicardial APs encircle the mid cardiac vein. This rather small vein is difficult to cannulate and

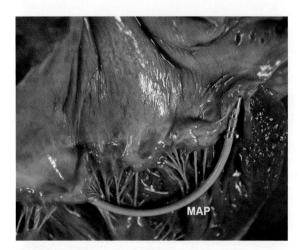

Fig. 4.8. Positioning of an ablation catheter (MAP) through the aortic valve towards the lateral mitral valve annulus. The corresponding fluoroscopic image is shown in Figure 4.16

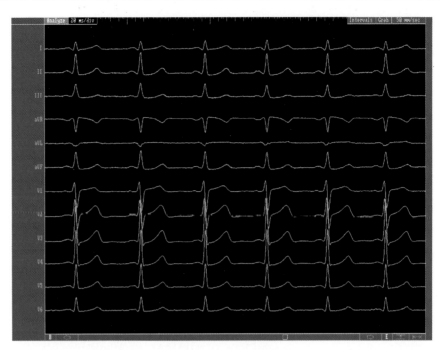

Fig. 4.9. Standard 12-lead ECG of the patient before ablation. During sinus rhythm, discrete preexcitation is present. The delta wave is positive in the precordial leads, negative in I and aVL

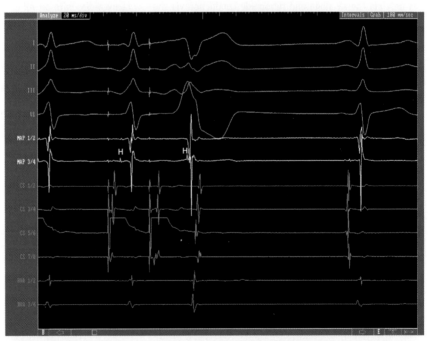

Fig. 4.10. Programmed atrial stimulation (from the CS) with one extrastimulus showing maximal preexcitation. Note the merging of the His potential (H) with the ventricular component on the MAP catheter which is positioned at the His bundle site. Due to dual AV nodal physiology, an AV nodal echo is observed on the CS leads (green) after the ventricular signal on the MAP catheter (white)

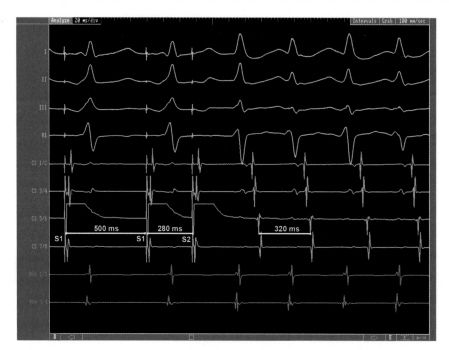

Fig. 4.11. Induction of orthodromic reentrant tachycardia (ORT) with decremental shortening of the coupling interval of the atrial extrastimulus. When the refractory period of the AP (narrow QRS complex) is reached, antegrade conduction occurs only via the AV node and retrograde conduction via the AP resulting in ORT. Of note is the distal to proximal activation sequence during tachycardia in the CS leads (green) corresponding to a left-sided AP. During tachycardia, an alternans of the QRS complex is observed (which is commonly seen in tachycardias with an AP as part of the reentrant circuit)

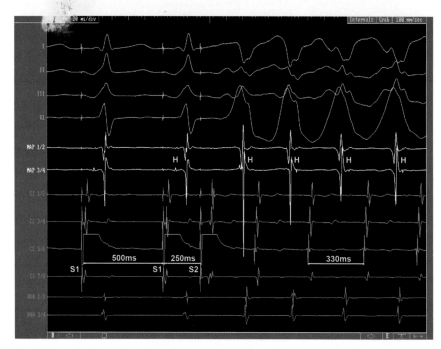

Fig. 4.12. Induction of antidromic reentrant tachycardia (ART) by programmed atrial stimulation from the CS (green). Of note is the retrograde His activation recorded on the MAP catheter (white). The activation sequence on the CS leads during tachycardia is now proximal (7/8) to distal (1/2) concordant with retrograde conduction via the AV node. (Proximal CS leads 7/8 are outside the coronary sinus os)

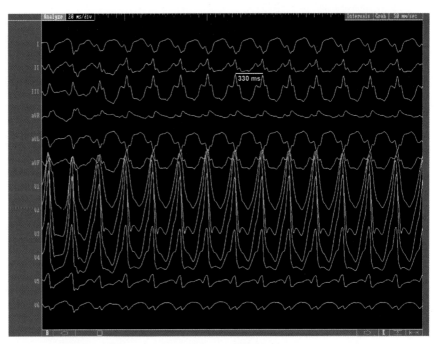

Fig. 4.13. Surface 12-lead ECG during antidromic reentrant tachycardia (cycle length 330 ms). Note the maximal preexcitation (and compare it to the standard 12-lead ECG in Figure 4.9 during sinus rhythm)

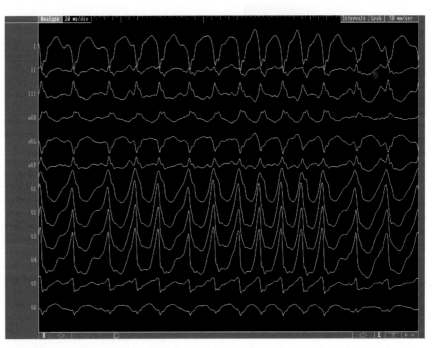

Fig. 4.14. Surface 12-lead ECG during atrial fibrillation with variable degree of antegrade conduction over the AP (minimal RR interval 255 ms)

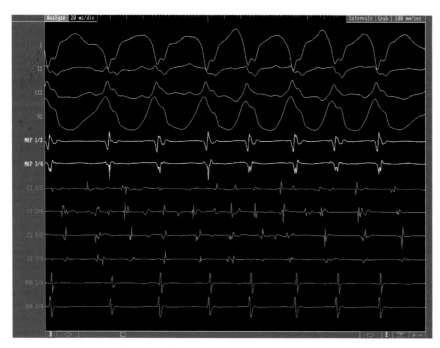

Fig. 4.15. Surface and intracardiac recordings during atrial fibrillation. Atrial fibrillation can be clearly detected on the CS leads (green)

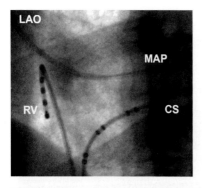

Fig. 4.16. Fluoroscopic view (LAO 45° projection) of the successful ablation site. The ablation catheter (MAP) is positioned via the aortic valve into the left ventricle and beneath the mitral valve in a left lateral position (guided by the CS catheter)

sometimes a superior approach via the jugular or subclavian vein has advantages to the transfemoral route.

In patients with a CS diverticulum, an AP potential is often recorded from the neck of the diverticulum. Mapping often reveals a distinct AP potential and earliest ventricular activation from the middle cardiac or posterior vein or within a CS diverticulum (Figure 4.17). Right and left ventricular mapping often show local endocardial activation 15–40 ms later than in

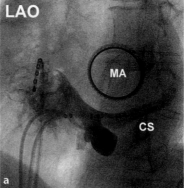

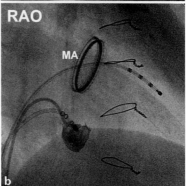

Fig. 4.17. CS angiography from a patient with a CS diverticulum. The ablation catheter is positioned at the neck of the diverticulum. The mitral annulus (MA) is shown (patient with a mitral valve prosthesis)

the vein. The delta wave in lead II is usually broad and deeply negative. Before starting ablation, a CS angiography from a transfemoral or right jugular venous approach should be performed to delineate coronary venous anatomy. Ablation along the mitral and tricuspid annulus is often ineffective. The most successful locations are in the mid cardiac vein, posterior coronary vein or CS diverticulum at the site of the largest, sharpest unipolar signal. As the distal right coronary artery is in close proximity, it is also advisable to perform a coronary angiography before starting ablation with reduced RF energy (5–15 W). Ablation of these APs is often only possible using irrigated tip catheters to avoid local edema and stenosis of the coronary sinus and its branches.

In the following, ECG tracings and ablation sites of a left and right posteroseptal pathway are shown.

∎ Left posteroseptal accessory pathway

Figures 4.18 and 4.19 (p. 90) show the ECG tracings and the ablation site of a patient with a left posteroseptal AP. For this location, which is often difficult to approach, going transseptally may sometimes be necessary for successful ablation.

∎ Right posteroseptal epicardial accessory pathway

This case shows the above mentioned features of a right posteroseptal epicardial AP (Figures 4.20–4.22, pp. 91, 92).

4.3.3 Permanent form of junctional reciprocating tachycardia (PJRT)

Accessory pathways in the permanent form of junctional reciprocating tachycardia may be located in many places around the AV groove but are most often found in the posteroseptal region [42]. PJRT accounts for 1–6% of SVT in childhood (see also Chapter 11) but is rare after adolescence [30, 41]. Catheter ablation should be first line treatment for patients with this entity especially if ventricular dysfunction is present. Tachycardia is orthodromic reciprocating involving a concealed AP with only retrograde decremental conduction properties (see Figure 11.6). PJRT can be distinguished from focal atrial tachycardia or atypical AVNRT during ventricular pacing if tachycardia termination happens when the His bundle is refractory. Ablation is often successful in or around the

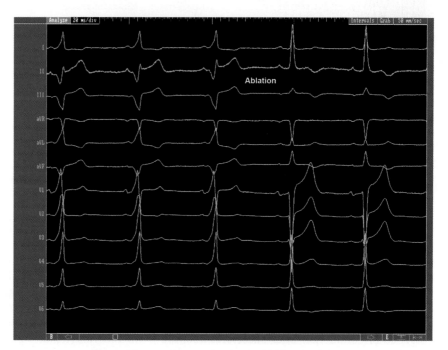

Fig. 4.18. Surface ECG of a patient with a left posteroseptal AP (positive delta wave in V1, I and aVL, negative delta wave in II, III and aVF). Preexcitation disappears during ablation. Note that after ablation the T waves are negative in lead II, III, aVF and V6, a feature that can persist for weeks ("cardiac memory")

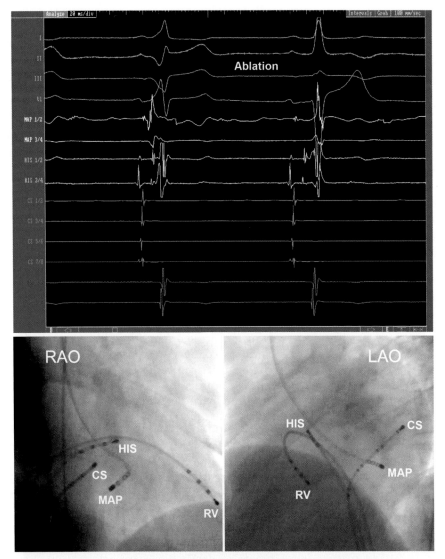

Fig. 4.19. Intracardiac recordings and fluoroscopic views of the successful ablation site in the same patient (transaortic approach). Again note that the CS catheter can be used as a guiding structure (MAP between CS 3/4 and CS 5/6)

mouth of the coronary sinus and the majority if not all of these APs are ablated without a risk of AV block (Figure 4.23, p. 92).

4.3.4 Right-sided free-wall accessory pathways

Success rates for RF ablation of right-sided APs are lower than elsewhere (88 vs. 96%) and recurrence of conduction after successful ablation is more common [7, 35]. There are several reasons for those findings. The tricuspid annulus is larger, thinner and less complete than the mi-

tral annulus which allows broad APs to bridge these gaps. Some of the right-sided APs also tend to take a more epicardial course. Mapping of right-sided APs is demanding as there is no guiding structure like the coronary sinus on the left. It is usually performed along the tricuspid annulus via the transfemoral approach. The catheter tip is most likely on or near the tricuspid annulus if the atrial signal at the catheter tip is approximately one-third of the amplitude of the ventricular signal. In difficult cases as in Ebstein's anomaly of the tricuspid valve (see Section 4.3.5), the tricuspid annulus can be defined by an angiogram of the right coronary

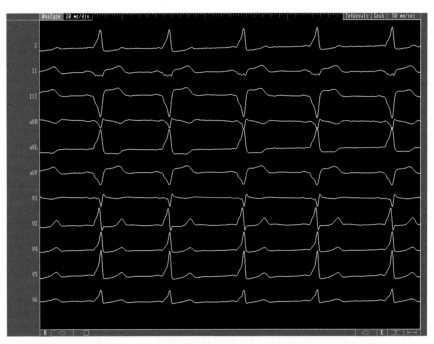

Fig. 4.20. Surface 12-lead ECG from a patient with a right posteroseptal epicardial AP. Note the broad negative delta wave in lead II (also negative in III and avF)

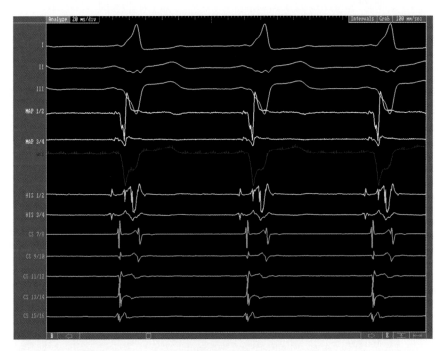

Fig. 4.21. Surface ECG and intracardiac recordings of the same patient. On the MAP catheter a discrete AP potential is visible. The red unipolar recording (UNI) shows a sharp negative deflection without any "R" wave. Typically the onset of the ventricular signal on the unipolar lead is just prior to the delta wave and slightly later than the ventricular signal on the MAP catheter

artery (or in rare instances by inserting a small catheter into the right coronary artery). Unipolar electrograms at the ablation site are different from the left side as they show a sharper QS downstroke than on the left side.

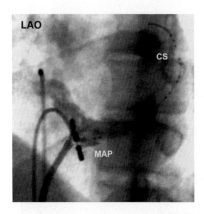

Fig. 4.22. Fluoroscopic view with the ablation catheter (MAP) positioned in the mid cardiac vein. A small multielectrode catheter (CS) is positioned in the coronary sinus (CS). An angiography of the CS was performed shortly before ablation to confirm catheter placement. Same patient as in Figures 4.20 and 4.21

Maintaining stable catheter contact is also more challenging than in other positions. While right posterior APs can usually be ablated with an IVC approach, for anterior APs an approach via the superior vena cava might be useful to place the catheter tip in the right ventricle under the tricuspid valve. In right lateral APs, a long sheath to stabilize the catheter position is often required. It should be kept in mind that temperatures at the catheter tip are often lower (45–55°C) than on the left side due to greater electrode cooling and less consistent tissue contact. The risk of complications is low [5]; damage to the AV node should not occur with right free-wall APs. Occlusion of the right coronary artery during RF ablation has been reported in a child [24].

▌ Right anterolateral pathway

This patient is a 9-year old girl with a right anterolateral pathway. Due to the young age of the patient, 2 F diagnostic catheters (3 catheters over one 7.5 sheath) were used (Figures 4.24–4.27, pp. 93–95).

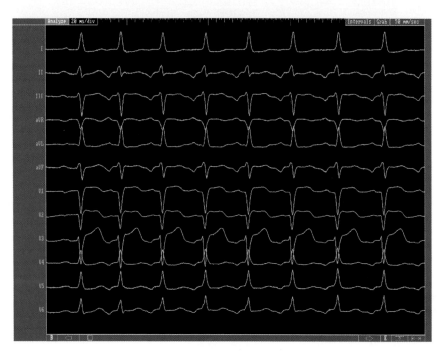

Fig. 4.23. Surface 12-lead ECG from a patient with PJRT. Due to the slow and decremental conduction properties of the AP, tachycardia shows a long RP interval with a superior P wave axis (neg. in II, III, aVF; posteroseptal pathway location). Intracardiac recordings are shown in Figure 11.6 (Chapter 11)

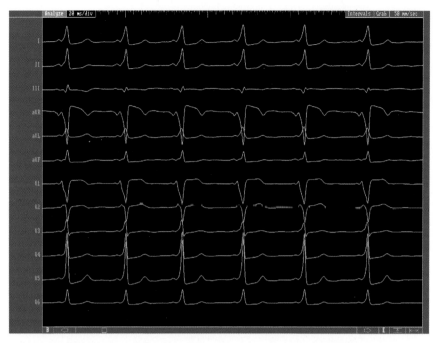

Fig. 4.24. Surface 12-lead ECG of the patient with a right anterolateral AP. The delta wave is negative in leads V1 and V2, positive in leads I, II and avL

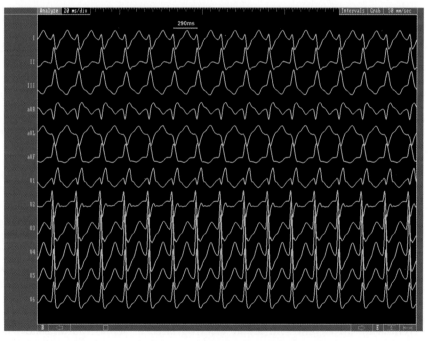

Fig. 4.25. Surface 12-lead ECG tracings (50 mm/s) during orthodromic reentrant tachycardia (CL 290 ms) with right bundle branch block (RBBB) in the same patient

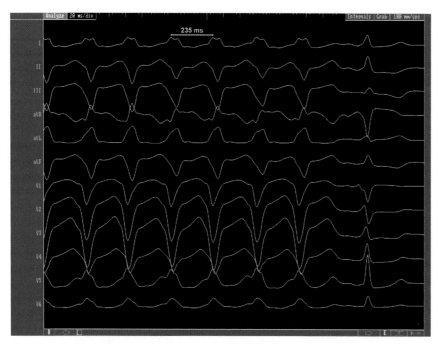

Fig. 4.26. In this patient, orthodromic reentrant tachycardia with left bundle branch block (LBBB) was also induced (12-lead surface ECG; paper speed 100 mm/s). Tachycardia cycle length with LBBB is 235 ms and therefore 55 ms shorter than with RBBB (see Figure 4.25). Conduction time of the reentrant circuit involving a right sided accessory pathway is prolonged if there is RBBB

4.3.5 Ebstein's anomaly of the tricuspid valve

Patients with Ebstein's anomaly of the tricuspid valve show a higher incidence of accessory pathways (30%) compared to other individuals [6, 20]. Multiple APs might be present in up to 50% of cases and decremental APs (Mahaim fibers) are also found. Ablation of these pathways can be a demanding and time consuming task. The success rate of the ablation is around 75% with recurrence rates up to 25% [6, 20]. Localization of the AV groove, differentiation of atrial and ventricular signals and defining the optimal ablation site are difficult due to the large size of the right atrium and low amplitude, fragmented "pseudo" AP potentials often found near the AV groove [20, 35].

Atrial extrastimuli have been helpful in differentiating atrial and ventricular electrograms. Atrial pacing during tachycardia is also useful to differentiate atrial and ventricular components of the fragmented electrograms. It should be kept in mind that the APs connect the atrium to ventricle at the site of the tricuspid annulus although the leaflets of the valve are displaced downward to the right ventricle. The use of long sheaths is often necessary to improve catheter stabilization. For ablation, the ventricular side of the tricuspid valve should be approached which is often quite difficult [38].

▌ Ebstein's anomaly and right posterolateral pathway

This case shows the findings of a patient with Ebstein's anomaly of the tricuspid valve and a right posterolateral AP (Figures 4.28 and 4.29, pp. 96, 97).

4.3.6 Anteroseptal (parahissian) and midseptal accessory pathways

Accessory pathways in the midseptal or anteroseptal (parahissian) location require specific attention due to the proximity of the AV node and His bundle. Anatomically, APs in the midseptal region are related to the atrial and ventricular septum. "Anteroseptal" APs are usually located anteriorly along the central fibrous body at the right anterior free wall [26]. Mapping of anteroseptal APs in the His area shows a simul-

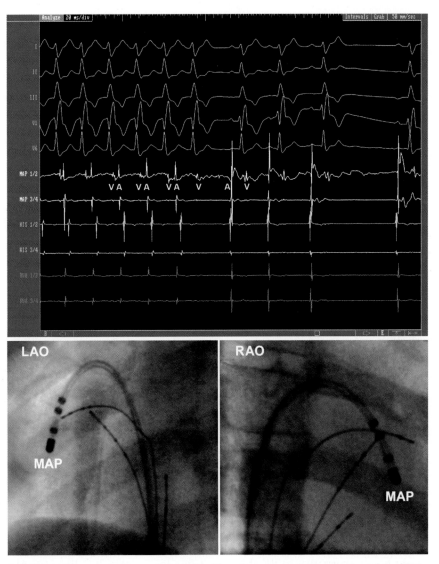

Fig. 4.27. Surface and intracardial ECG tracings and the radiographic views of the successful ablation site from the same patient. Ablation was performed during orthodromic tachycardia. There is a progressive lengthening of the VA interval on the MAP catheter during ablation before tachycardia terminates. During sinus rhythm, RBBB is again visible

taneous recording of an AP potential as well as a His bundle potential in over 90% of cases [27]. His activity might be superimposed by the early ventricular pathway activation; therefore, atrial or ventricular stimulation with premature beats should be performed to differentiate local His activity (Figure 4.30). If the catheter locates an AP signal in an area bound anterior by a His signal and posterior by the CS ositum, it is in the midseptal region.

Ablation of anteroseptal APs via a cranial approach over the right internal jugular vein is an alternative to the standard transfemoral approach as catheter position is often more stable with the approach via the SVC. The catheter is positioned at the atrial aspect of the tricuspid annulus or advanced to the right ventricle and curved to ablate the AP from the ventricular aspect of the tricuspid annulus. Radiographically the catheter is anterior and superior to the His bundle catheter (Figure 4.31). Midseptal pathways are ablated by the transfemoral approach and the catheter is positioned more to the ventricular aspect of the tricuspid annulus. The catheter is located posterior and inferior to the His bundle catheter. Midseptal APs are

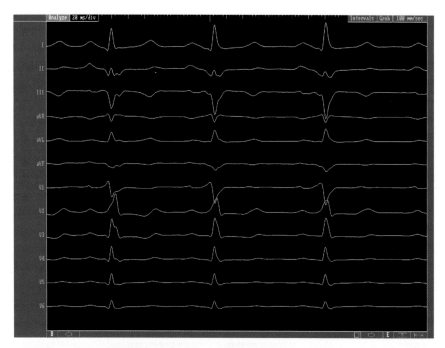

Fig. 4.28. Surface ECG from the patient with Ebstein's anomaly and a right posterolateral pathway. The delta wave is positive in leads V1 and V2 (which is rather unusual for this location) and negative in leads II, III and aVF

usually ablated from the rightside; left-sided midseptal APs might be approached transseptally or by a transaortic approach and the catheter placed as decribed. Power settings should start with low energy (15–25 W). Ablation success in anteroseptal or midseptal APs is reported to be 95–98% with a very low risk of transient or permanent AV block [26, 27]. Cryoablation, especially in younger patients, might be an alternative to RF ablation at this location as the risk of permanent AV block is further reduced [15].

4.3.7 Mahaim fibers

Mahaim fibers were originally described as connections between the AV node and the bundle branches or ventricular myocardium and termed as "nodofascicular" or "nodoventricular" [16, 32]. With mapping and catheter ablation studies it has become obvious that these pathways are usually right-sided crossing the tricuspid annulus preferentially on the free wall. Mahaim fibers show some features of the AV node ("nodal-like tissue") like antegrade decremetal conduction with relatively long baseline conduction times, transient conduction block

after adenosine injection [12] and conduction only in the antegrade direction [28]. Anatomically, Mahaim fibers occurring along the atrial margin of the tricuspid annulus connect directly to ventricular muscle either at the annulus or more distally (atrioventricular) or (in the majority of cases) connect to a long fiber that crosses the annulus and inserts into the right bundle branch [18]. On the ECG, preexcitation may be discrete. Although the PR interval increases with atrial pacing, the QRS complex widens due to ventricular preexcitation. Tachycardia shows a typical LBBB pattern with a superior frontal axis (Figures 4.32 and 4.33, p. 99).

For mapping and ablation, it must be remembered that most of these APs cannot be mapped in the usual way looking for the point of earliest ventricular activation. Conduction of these fibers is often sensitive to mechanical stimulation which can intermittently eliminate conduction [2]. Mapping for the pathway potential around the tricuspid annulus during atrial pacing or SVT is most commonly used (looking for a His-like potential; Figure 4.34, p. 100). Finding a site along the tricuspid annulus at which the catheter tip produces transient AP conduction block is also used. Ablation aims at

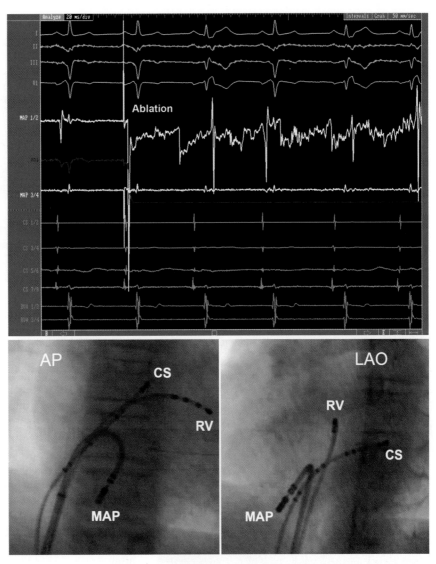

Fig. 4.29. Intracardiac recordings and fluoroscopic view from the same patient. The ablation catheter (MAP) is positioned in a posterior to posterolateral position. When ablation starts, the second beat shows right bundle branch block without preexcitation on the surface ECG (and a ventricular spike on the MAP catheter after the surface QRS); on the third beat preexcitation is back (early ventricular spike on the MAP catheter), but from the fourth beat on preexcitation is gone and right bundle branch block is visible

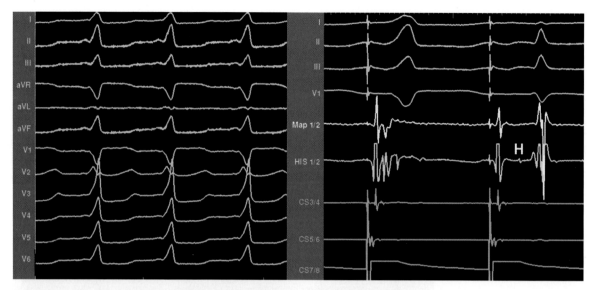

Fig. 4.30. (Left) Surface 12-lead ECG from a patient with a parahissian accessory pathway. The delta wave is negative in V1, positive in V2 ("septal pattern") and positive in leads II, III and aVF. (Right) Surface ECG and intracardiac recordings during atrial pacing from the CS. The first beat still shows pre-excitation, but on the second beat there is no preexcitation, and a His deflection (H) is now clearly detectable on the His catheter (HIS 1/2), but not on the ablation catheter (Map 1/2)

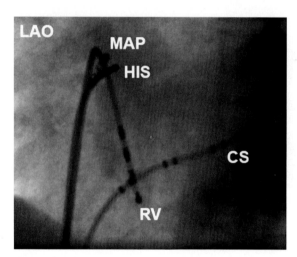

Fig. 4.31. Fluoroscopic view of the ablation site in the same patient as in Figure 4.30 with a parahissian AP. The ablation catheter (MAP) is just slightly anterior and superior to the His catheter

the atrial insertion of the AP but sometimes is only successful at the ventricular side of the tricuspid annulus or the ventricular insertion of the fiber along the right bundle branch [17, 34]. The majority of Mahaim fibers have been successfully ablated in the lateral or anterolateral aspect of the tricuspid valve with success rates over 90%. Electroanatomical mapping might be useful in difficult cases as the catheter can be moved around and relocated if it produces mechanical block of the AP and was moved thereafter.

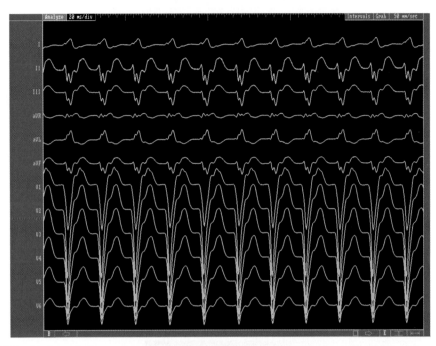

Fig. 4.32. The 12-lead surface ECG of tachycardia in a patient with a Mahaim fiber. Tachycardia shows a typical LBBB pattern with a superior frontal axis (neg. in II, III, aVF)

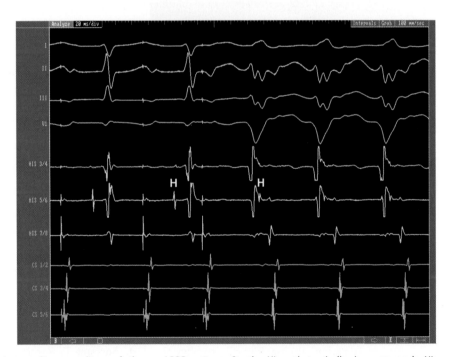

Fig. 4.33. Surface ECG and intracardiac recordings of the same patient. Antidromic tachycardia is induced by atrial pacing via the coronary sinus and shows a superior axis and LBBB pattern. On the His catheter (yellow), a retrograde His potential is seen shortly after the QRS complex during tachycardia (retrograde conduction via the AV node)

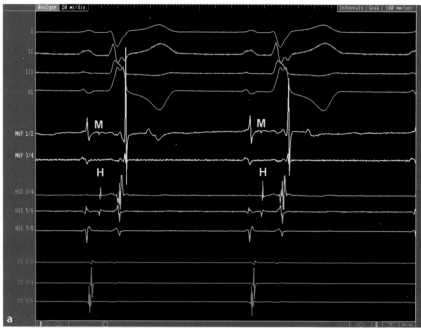

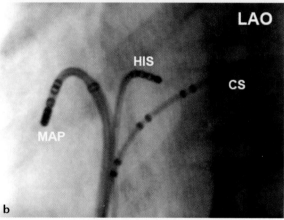

Fig. 4.34. a Surface ECG and intracardiac recordings during mapping of a Mahaim (M) fiber. On the distal poles (MAP 1/2) of the MAP catheter a sharp Mahaim potential is recorded (see text). The right bundle branch pattern in V1 is the result of a previous ablation attempt close to the right bundle. **b** Fluoroscopic view of the successful ablation site in the same patient. The MAP catheter is positioned at the lateral aspect of the tricuspid ring

▮ References

1. Anderson RH, Ho SY (1997) Anatomy of the atrioventricular junctions with regard to ventricular preexcitation. Pacing Clin Electrophysiol 20:2072–2076
2. Belhassen B, Viskin S, Fish R, Glick A, Glikson M, Eldar M (1999) Catheter-induced mechanical trauma to accessory pathways during radiofrequency ablation: incidence, predictors and clinical implications. J Am Coll Cardiol 33:767–774
3. Benson DW Jr (2001) Genetic basis of disturbances of cardiac rhythm and conduction. In: Walsh EP, Saul JP, Triedman JK (eds) Cardiac arrhythmias in children and young adults with congenital heart disease. Lippincott Williams & Wilkins, Baltimore, pp 23–33
4. Boersma L, Garcia-Moran E, Mont L, Brugada J (2002) Accessory pathway localization by QRS polarity in children with Wolff-Parkinson-White syndrome. J Cardiovasc Electrophysiol 13:1222–1226
5. Calkins H, Yong P, Miller JM, Olshansky B, Carlson M, Saul JP, Huang SK, Liem LB, Klein LS, Moser SA, Bloch DA, Gillette P, Prystowsky E (1999) Catheter ablation of accessory path-

ways, atrioventricular nodal reentrant tachycardia, and the atrioventricular junction: final results of a prospective, multicenter clinical trial. The Atakr Multicenter Investigators Group. Circulation 99:262–270

6. Cappato R, Schluter M, Weiss C, Antz M, Koschyk DH, Hofmann T, Kuck KH (1996) Radiofrequency current catheter ablation of accessory atrioventricular pathways in Ebstein's anomaly. Circulation 94:376–383

7. Chen SA, Chiang CE, Tsang WP, Hsia CP, Wang DC, Yeh HI, Ting CT, Chiou CW, Yang CJ, Kong CW et al (1993) Recurrent conduction in accessory pathway and possible new arrhythmias after radiofrequency catheter ablation. Am Heart J 125:381–387

8. Cosio FG, Anderson RH, Kuck KH, Becker A, Benditt DG, Bharati S, Borggrefe M, Campbell RW, Gaita F, Guiraudon GM, Haissaguerre M, Klein G, Langberg J, Marchlinski F, Rufilanchas JJ, Saksena S, Thiene G, Wellens HJ (1999) ESCWGA/NASPE/P experts consensus statement: living anatomy of the atrioventricular junctions. A guide to electrophysiologic mapping. Working Group of Arrhythmias of the European Society of Cardiology. North American Society of Pacing and Electrophysiology. J Cardiovasc Electrophysiol 10:1162–1170

9. d'Avila A, Brugada J, Skeberis V, Andries E, Sosa E, Brugada P (1995) A fast and reliable algorithm to localize accessory pathways based on the polarity of the QRS complex on the surface ECG during sinus rhythm. Pacing Clin Electrophysiol 18:1615–1627

10. Deshpande SS, Bremner S, Sra JS, Dhala AA, Blanck Z, Bajwa TK, al-Bitar I, Gal R, Sarnoski JS, Akhtar M et al (1994) Ablation of left freewall accessory pathways using radiofrequency energy at the atrial insertion site: transseptal versus transaortic approach. J Cardiovasc Electrophysiol 5:219–231

11. Dunnigan A (1986) Developmental aspects and natural history of preexitation syndromes. In: Benditt DG, Benson DW Jr (eds) Cardiac preexitation syndromes: origins, evaluation and treatment. Martinus Nijhoff Publishing, Boston, pp 21–29

12. Ellenbogen KA, Rogers R, Old W (1989) Pharmacological characterization of conduction over a Mahaim fiber: evidence for adenosine sensitive conduction. Pacing Clin Electrophysiol 12:1396–1404

13. Ernst S, Ouyang F, Antz M (2004) Catheter ablation of atrioventricular reentry. In: Zipes DP, Jalife J (eds) Cardiac electrophysiology. From cell to bedside. WP Saunders, Philadelphia, pp 1078–1086

14. Fitzpatrick AP, Gonzales RP, Lesh MD, Modin GW, Lee RJ, Scheinman MM (1994) New algorithm for the localization of accessory atrioventricular connections using a baseline electrocardiogram. J Am Coll Cardiol 23:107–116

15. Gaita F, Haissaguerre M, Giustetto C, Grossi S, Caruzzo E, Bianchi F, Richiardi E, Riccardi R, Hocini M, Jais P (2003) Safety and efficacy of cryoablation of accessory pathways adjacent to the normal conduction system. J Cardiovasc Electrophysiol 14:825–829

16. Gallagher JJ, Smith WM, Kasell JH, Benson DW Jr, Sterba R, Grant AO (1981) Role of Mahaim fibers in cardiac arrhythmias in man. Circulation 64:176–189

17. Grogin HR, Lee RJ, Kwasman M, Epstein LM, Schamp DJ, Lesh MD, Scheinman MM (1994) Radiofrequency catheter ablation of atriofascicular and nodoventricular Mahaim tracts. Circulation 90:272–281

18. Haissaguerre M, Cauchemez B, Marcus F, Le Metayer P, Lauribe P, Poquet F, Gencel L, Clementy J (1995) Characteristics of the ventricular insertion sites of accessory pathways with anterograde decremental conduction properties. Circulation 91:1077–1085

19. Haissaguerre M, Sha DC, Takahashi A (1998) A conceptual approach to radiofrequency catheter ablation of accessory pathways focusing on electrocardiogram criteria. In: Singer I, Barold SS, Camm AJ (eds) Nonpharmacological therapy of arrhythmias for the 21st century: the state of the art. Futura Publishing Co, Inc, Armonk, NY, pp 57–71

20. Hebe J (2000) Ebstein's anomaly in adults. Arrhythmias: diagnosis and therapeutic approach. Thorac Cardiovasc Surg 48:214–219

21. Holzmann M, Scherf D (1932) Über Elektrokardiogramme mit verkürzter Vorhof-Kammer Distanz und positiven P-Zacken. Z Klin Med 121:404–410

22. Jackman WM, Sun Y, Beckman KJ (2002) Proposed anatomy and catheter ablation of epicardial posteroseptal and left posterior accessory AV pathways. In: Zipes DP, Haissaguerre M (eds) Catheter ablation of arrhythmias. Futura Publishing Co, Inc, Armonk, NY, pp 321–343

23. Kent AFS (1893) Researches on the structure and function of the mammalian heart. J Physiol 14:233

24. Khanal S, Ribeiro PA, Platt M, Kuhn MA (1999) Right coronary artery occlusion as a complication of accessory pathway ablation in a 12-year-old treated with stenting. Catheter Cardiovasc Interv 46:59–61

25. Klein GJ, Yee R, Sharma AD (1989) Longitudinal electrophysiologic assessment of asymptomatic patients with the Wolff-Parkinson-White electrocardiographic pattern. N Engl J Med 320:1229–1233

26. Kuck KH, Ouyang F, Goya M, Boczor S (2002) Ablation of anteroseptal and midseptal accessory pathways. In: Zipes DP, Haissaguerre M (eds) Catheter ablation of arrhythmias. Futura Publishing Co, Inc, Armonk, NY, pp 305–320

27. Kuck KH, Schluter M, Gursoy S (1992) Preservation of atrioventricular nodal conduction during radiofrequency current catheter ablation of midseptal accessory pathways. Circulation 86: 1743–1752

28. Kuck KH, Siebels J, Braun E (1997) Mahaim fibers – a second atrioventricular conduction system. Pacing Clin Electrophysiol 20:1201

29. Laohaprasitiporn D, Walsh EP, Saul JP, Triedman JK (1997) Predictors of permanence of successful radiofrequency lesions created with controlled catheter tip temperature. Pacing Clin Electrophysiol 20:1283–1291

30. Lesh MD, Van Hare GF, Schamp DJ, Chien W, Lee MA, Griffin JC, Langberg JJ, Cohen TJ, Lurie KG, Scheinman MM (1992) Curative percutaneous catheter ablation using radiofrequency energy for accessory pathways in all locations: results in 100 consecutive patients. J Am Coll Cardiol 19:1303–1309

31. Luik A, Deisenhofer I, Estner H, Ndrepepa G, Pflaumer A, Zrenner B, Schmitt C (2006) Atresia of the Coronary Sinus in Patients with Supraventricular Tachycardia. Pacing Clin Electrophysiol 29(2):171–174

32. Mahaim I, Benatt A (1938) Nouvelle recherches sur les connexions superieures de la branch gauche du faisceau de His-Tawara avec cloison interventriculaire. Cardiologia 1:61–76

33. Mantakas ME, McCue CM, Miller WW (1978) Natural history of Wolff-Parkinson-White syndrome discovered in infancy. Am J Cardiol 41:1097–1103

34. McClelland JH, Wang X, Beckman KJ, Hazlitt HA, Prior MI, Nakagawa H, Lazzara R, Jackman WM (1994) Radiofrequency catheter ablation of right atriofascicular (Mahaim) accessory pathways guided by accessory pathway activation potentials. Circulation 89:2655–2666

35. Miller JM, Olgin JE (2002) Catheter ablation of free-wall accessory pathways and Mahaim fibres. In: Zipes DP, Haissaguerre M (eds) Catheter ablation of arrhythmias. Futura Publishing Co, Inc, New York, pp 277–303

36. Munger TM, Packer DL, Hammill SC, Feldman BJ, Bailey KR, Ballard DJ, Holmes DR Jr, Gersh BJ (1993) A population study of the natural history of Wolff-Parkinson-White syndrome in Olmsted County, Minnesota, 1953–1989. Circulation 87:866–873

37. Pappone C, Santinelli V, Rosanio S, Vicedomini G, Nardi S, Pappone A, Tortoriello V, Manguso F, Mazzone P, Gulletta S, Oreto G, Alfieri O (2003) Usefulness of invasive electrophysiologic testing to stratify the risk of arrhythmic events in asymptomatic patients with Wolff-Parkinson-White pattern: results from a large prospective long-term follow-up study. J Am Coll Cardiol 41:239–244

38. Saul JP (2001) Ablation of accessory pathways. In: Walsh EP, Saul JP, Triedman JK (eds) Cardiac arrhythmias in children and young adults with congenital heart disease. Lippincott Williams & Willkins, Baltimore, pp 393–425

39. Scheinman M, Calkins H, Gillette P, Klein R, Lerman BB, Morady F, Saksena S, Waldo A (2003) NASPE policy statement on catheter ablation: personnel, policy, procedures, and therapeutic recommendations. Pacing Clin Electrophysiol 26:789–799

40. Scheinman MM (1995) NASPE survey on catheter ablation. Pacing Clin Electrophysiol 18:1474–1478

41. Schneider MAE, Zrenner B, Karch MR (1998) Incidence of morphologic coronary sinus variations in 118 patients – impact on electrophysiologic study and catheter ablation. Pacing Clin Electrophysiol 21:944

42. Ticho BS, Saul JP, Hulse JE, De W, Lulu J, Walsh EP (1992) Variable location of accessory pathways associated with the permanent form of junctional reciprocating tachycardia and confirmation with radiofrequency ablation. Am J Cardiol 70:1559–1564

43. Todd DM, Klein GJ, Krahn AD, Skanes AC, Yee R (2003) Asymptomatic Wolff-Parkinson-White syndrome: is it time to revisit guidelines? J Am Coll Cardiol 41:245–248

44. Tuchnitz A, Schmitt C, von Bibra H, Schneider MA, Plewan A, Schomig A (1999) Noninvasive localization of accessory pathways in patients with Wolff-Parkinson-White syndrome with the use of myocardial Doppler imaging. J Am Soc Echocardiogr 12:32–40

45. Willems S, Chen X, Kottkamp H, Hindricks G, Haverkamp W, Rotman B, Shenasa M, Breithardt G, Borggrefe M (1996) Temperature-controlled radiofrequency catheter ablation of manifest accessory pathways. Eur Heart J 17: 445–452

46. Wolff L, Parkinson J, White P (1930) Bundle branch block with short PR interval in healthy young people prone to paroxysmal tachycardia. Am Heart J 5:585–704

5 Atrioventricular nodal reentrant tachycardia

Heidi Estner, Isabel Deisenhofer

Atrioventricular nodal reentrant tachycardia (AVNRT) is the most frequent paroxysmal supraventricular tachycardia (SVT) with an incidence in the general population of approximately 5/1000. AVNRT is regarded as a benign arrhythmia although hemodynamic compromise (e.g., dizziness or syncope) can occur. It is usually not associated with structural heart disease. AVNRT can be more frequent in women (~60%) with a peak incidence in our patient population at a mean age of 50 years [9], but AVNRT can be encountered at any age, even in children. AVNRT may cause a significant worsening of the quality of life especially with frequent recurrence. The development of catheter ablation has provided the possibility to definitely cure this arrhythmia.

5.1 Mechanism

AVNRT has traditionally been thought to be due to a reentrant mechanism. The AV node in affected patients is characterized by a so-called longitudinal dissociation due to the existence of fibers with differences in conduction velocity and refractory periods. The part of the AV node called the "fast pathway" has a faster conduction time and a longer refractory period, while the "slow pathway" has a long conduction time and a shorter refractory period. Initially, dual AV nodal physiology was thought to be exclusively present in patients with AVNRT and rare in patients without this arrhythmia. However, studies demonstrated that this pattern can be found in up to 10% of normal subjects who have never suffered from an AVNRT [5]. Subsequent observations suggested that fast and slow pathway represent conduction over different atrionodal connections. Sung et al. [4] first demonstrated that the two pathways actually have two anatomically distinct atrial insertions. During ventricular pacing in patients with dual ventriculoatrial conduction, these authors were able to demonstrate a different retrograde atrial activation sequence depending on whether conduction utilizes the fast or the slow pathway. The retrograde atrial exit of the fast pathway was localized in the anterior part of the septum near the His bundle recording site, while the retrograde atrial exit of the slow pathway was located in the posterior part of the septum near the coronary sinus ostium (CS os), i.e., inferior and posterior to the exit of the fast pathway.

During sinus rhythm, an atrial impulse traverses the fast AV nodal conduction pathway and activates the ventricles via the His bundle. The impulse simultaneously conducts down the slow AV pathway, reaching the His bundle shortly after it has been depolarized via the fast pathway and therefore is refractory (Figure 5.1a).

When an atrial premature depolarization occurs, the impulse may not conduct over the fast AV pathway due to its longer refractory period, and proceeds slowly down the slow AV pathway. This leads to a sudden prolongation of the AH interval and to a corresponding prolonged PR interval. A beat-to-beat change of the AH interval during programmed atrial pacing is a marker for dual pathway physiology. The phenomenon of a sudden prolongation (≥ 50 ms) of the AH interval (see also Chapter 1, Figure 1.14) during decremental programmed stimulation (with a 10 ms decrement in coupling interval) is called a "jump" (Figure 5.1b).

If conduction down the slow pathway is sufficiently delayed to allow the fast pathway to recover from refractoriness, retrograde conduction over the fast pathway leads to an early retrograde atrial activation. This early retrograde atrial activation is referred to as an "AV nodal echo beat" (Figure 5.1b).

Both phenomena, "jump" and "echo" are often associated and can initiate AVNRT. Some-

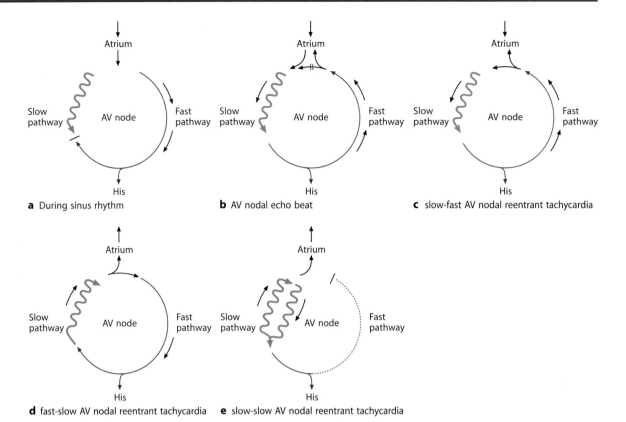

a During sinus rhythm   **b** AV nodal echo beat   **c** slow-fast AV nodal reentrant tachycardia

d fast-slow AV nodal reentrant tachycardia   **e** slow-slow AV nodal reentrant tachycardia

Fig. 5.1. The mechanism of AVNRT. (**a**) During sinus rhythm an atrial impulse antegradely penetrates both the fast and slow pathways simultaneously. Because the impulse reaches the His bundle via the fast pathway, the PR interval is normal. (**b**) The effective refractory period of the fast pathway is longer than that of the slow pathway. Conduction over the fast pathway is blocked by an atrial premature beat and conducts down the slow pathway to activate the His bundle. Therefore the PR interval is prolonged. Because the antegrade conduction via the slow pathway is slow, the fast pathway has enough time to regain its excitability. The impulse that was conducted down the slow pathway may therefore reexcite the fast pathway retrogradely, resulting in an AV nodal echo beat. (**c**) Conduction over the fast path-way is blocked by a short coupling atrial premature beat and conducts down the slow pathway very slowly. This provides time for the fast pathway to recover to allow retrograde conduction. The slow pathway now also has had time to recover to allow repetitive antegrade reentrance. The continuation of this process leads to the development of typical slow-fast AVNRT. (**d**) Fast-slow AVNRT: In this uncommon type of AVNRT, antegrade conduction occurs over the fast pathway while the retrograde conduction is over the slow pathway with a short AH interval and a long HA interval. (**e**) Slow-slow ANVRT: In this type of tachycardia, the slow pathway is used for antegrade conduction and retrograde conduction is over a different slow pathway. It is characterized by relatively long and similar HA and AH intervals

times the following phenomenon is observed with programmed atrial stimulation: Decreasing the coupling interval in 10 ms steps, a jump and an echo can be observed, but only after further decremental pacing tachycardia is initiated. An explanation for this phenomenon might be that retrograde fast pathway excitation is only possible if an earlier atrial premature beat (blocked in the fast pathway) conducts more slowly down the slow pathway and arrives later at the fast pathway, when the latter is again excitable. Because of the longer overall conduction time

from the first atrial premature beat until atrial reexcitation via the retrograde fast pathway, the slow pathway has had more time to recover excitability and sustained tachycardia results (Figure 5.1 c).

Individuals may demonstrate "dual AV nodal physiology" but will not have spontaneous or inducible AVNRT. It is important to distinguish patients with dual AV nodal physiology but no inducible AVNRT from those with inducible AVNRT. Isoproterenol infusion may be required for initiation of the tachycardia and should be titrated to increase the sinus rate by 20-35%. Reproducible and reliable mode(s) of initiation should be assessed before ablation since the endpoint of successful ablation is the noninducibility of AVNRT.

▮ Stimulation protocol in AVNRT – characterization of AV node conduction properties and induction of tachycardia

As explained above, the ante- and retrograde conduction velocity and the effective refractory period (ERP) of the (dual) AV nodal pathway(s) are the determining factors in AVNRT initiation and maintenance. To test these, a standardized stimulation protocol should be performed (details are given in Chapter 1).

First, ventricular stimulation is performed at a basic cycle length of 600–400 ms (S1) with one shorter coupled extrastimulus (S2). S2 is decreased in 10 ms steps until the ERP of the ventricle is reached. The focus of interest lies on the retrograde conduction to the atria. Afterwards stimulation to test the retrograde Wenckebach interval is performed.

The following questions should be answered:

- Is a retrograde conduction demonstrable and does it occur via the AV node (watch the CS sequence)
- Is the retrograde conduction decremental (which would be a marker of AV-nodal retrograde conduction) and
- Is there a dual retrograde VA conduction ("retrograde jump")?

Similarly, atrial stimulation (programmed and Wenckebach) is performed with two different basic cycle lengths (e.g., 500 ms and 400 ms). If initiation of AVNRT is not possible with these stimulation settings, a second extrastimulus (S3), isoproterenol perfusion and/or atrial burst pacing at the antegrade Wenckebach interval are performed.

5.2 Different types of AVNRT

In some cases, more than one slow pathway is present. The presence of two slow pathways and one fast pathway may sustain various types of tachycardias with different cycle lengths or the finding of an alternating cycle length during AVNRT. Considering the reentrant circuit, three different types of AVNRT may be present.

5.2.1 Slow-fast AVNRT

The typical (common) form of AVNRT, representing about 90% of cases, consists of a reentrant circuit with conduction over the slow pathway in antegrade direction and over the fast pathway in retrograde direction (slow-fast; Figure 5.1 c). Endocardial recordings typically show simultaneous atrial and ventricular depolarization (Figures 5.2 and 5.3). The tachycardia P wave is usually obscured by the QRS complex, because the retrograde (fast pathway) activation of the atria occurs almost simultaneously with the (antegrade) ventricular activation (QRS complex) via the His bundle. Less frequently, the atrial electrogram may be recorded just before (very fast retrograde atrial activation or delayed antegrade ventricular activation via the His bundle) or immediately after the ventricular electrogram (delayed retrograde atrial activation via the fast pathway or very early antegrade ventricular activation). If the P wave is placed at the end of the QRS complex, it may lead to a characteristic late positive component in electrocardiogram lead V1 (pseudo-r') and a pseudo-S wave in the inferior leads (Figure 5.4).

The spontaneous initiation of typical AVNRT almost always occurs with an atrial premature beat that is associated with long PR and AH intervals (Figure 5.2). It is logical to assume that if spontaneous atrial premature beats are the most frequent method of AVNRT initiation, then programmed atrial extrastimuli could simulate the spontaneous situation and induce tachycardia (Figure 5.3). If no dual nodal conduction properties (i.e., the increase in AH interval = "jump") can be documented, then ANVRT is unlikely. As mentioned above, by definition, a sudden increase of at least 50 ms in AH (or PR) interval with a small (i.e., 10 ms) decrease in the coupling interval of an atrial premature extrastimulus must be observed to diagnose dual nodal pathway conduction (Figure 5.3.). This sudden increase in PR or AH interval representing change of antegrade activation from fast to slow pathway conduction is sometimes also observed during sinus rhythm or at fixed pacing rates (see Figure 1.15).

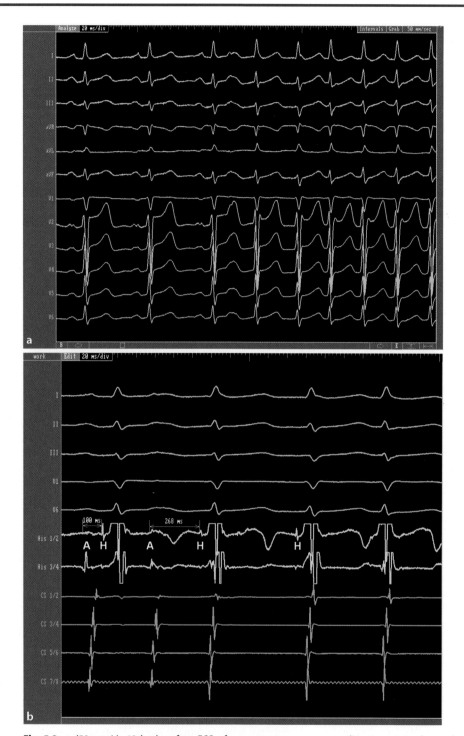

Fig. 5.2. a (50 mm/s): 12-lead surface ECG of a spontaneous initiation of AVNRT. Following three sinus complexes, a spontaneous atrial premature beat initiates SVT. **b** (100 mm/s): The initiating atrial premature beat (second beat) is associated with a markedly prolonged AH interval (268 ms), corresponding to antegrade conduction over the slow pathway. During SVT, atrial depolarization occurs simultaneously with the QRS complex representing retrograde conduction over the fast pathway

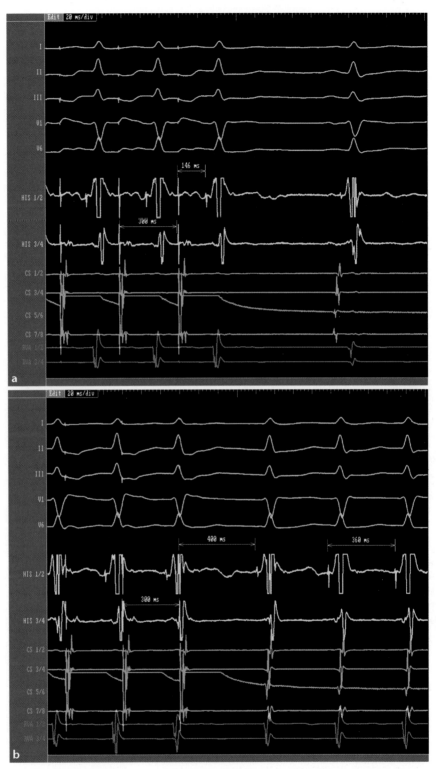

Fig. 5.3. SVT induction with atrial programmed stimulation. **a** An atrial premature extrastimulus delivered at a coupling interval of 310 ms is conducted with an AH interval of 146 ms without inducing SVT. **b** An atrial premature extrastimulus delivered at a slightly shorter coupling interval of 300 ms is conducted with a much longer AH interval of 400 ms and initiates the SVT. The sudden prolongation of the AH interval is characteristic for a shift from fast to slow AV nodal pathway conduction ("jump"). Speed in both panels 100 mm/s

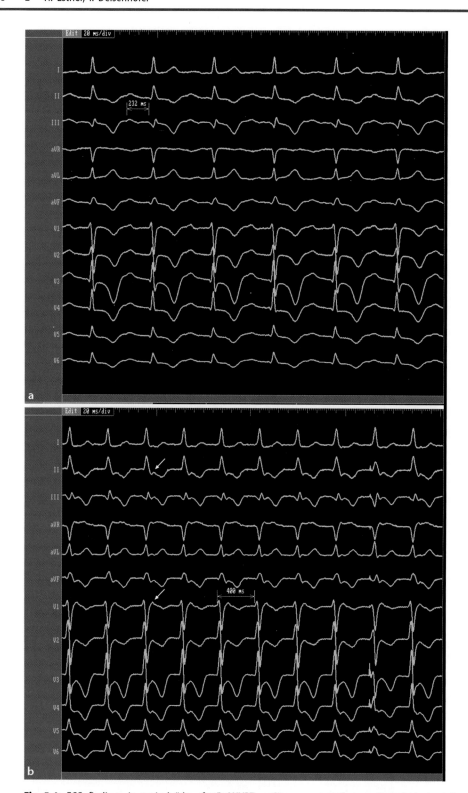

Fig. 5.4. ECG findings in typical "slow-fast" ANVRT. **a** Sinus rhythm with AV block I°. **b** During typical AVNRT retrograde P waves are observed at the terminal portion of the QRS complex, particularly in lead II or aVF (pseudo S) mimicking terminal delay and as a pseudo r′ wave (arrows) in lead V1. The negative T waves are probably tachycardia related

5.2.2 Fast-slow AVNRT

This less frequently observed (uncommon) form of AVNRT is characterized by antegrade conduction over the fast pathway and retrograde conduction over the slow pathway ("fast-slow" AVNRT). Consequently, during fast-slow AVNRT, the AH interval is shorter than the HA interval and the RP interval is longer than the PR interval (Figures 5.1d and 5.5). The deeply negative P waves, which are hidden in the QRS complex in typical slow-fast AVNRT, now precede the (next) QRS complex and can easily be distinguished in leads II, III and aVF. The earliest retrograde atrial activation occurs late after the ventricular electrogram and is recorded in the posterior part of the triangle of Koch close to the CS os, i.e., the classical slow pathway location. Atrial activation is preceded by a distinct slow-pathway potential, best recorded along the posteroseptal right atrium between the coronary sinus and the tricuspid annulus. During the EP study, fast-slow AVNRT is mostly induced by programmed ventricular stimulation (burst or by ventricular premature programmed stimulation). After a premature ventricular stimulus, retrograde VA conduction over the still refractory fast pathway is impossible. Therefore, VA conduction occurs over the slow pathway. When the delayed activation wave front reaches the atrial insertion of the slow pathway, antegrade conduction via the fast pathway (which is not refractory anymore) is possible again. Fast-slow AVNRT is rarely induced by programmed atrial stimulation. The initiation may occur with or without a significant increase in AH interval, suggesting that the antegrade AV conduction delay is not relevant for tachycardia onset.

5.2.3 Slow-slow AVNRT

In slow-slow AVNRT, the bidirectional limbs of the reentrant circuit consist of two distinct slow AV pathways. Therefore, retrograde conduction is also located close to the CS ostium. As both

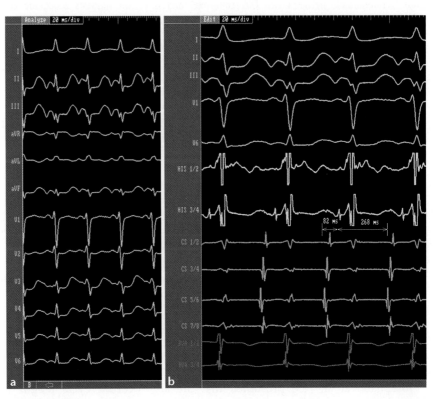

Fig. 5.5. Fast-slow AVNRT. **a** Surface ECG (50 mm/s). The P wave is recognizable before the QRS complex and is deeply negative in leads II, III and aVF. **b** Intracardiac recordings (100 mm/s). The AH interval is shorter than the HA interval, and consequently, the RP interval is longer than the PR interval

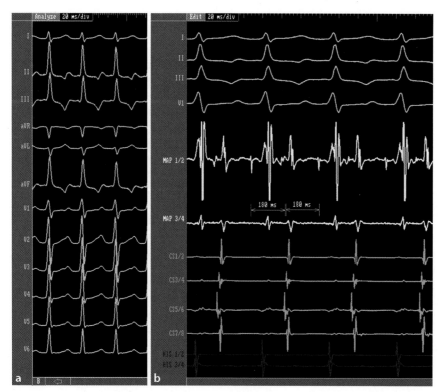

Fig. 5.6. Slow-slow AVNRT. **a** Surface ECG 50 mm/s. The P wave is recognizable between two QRS complexes and is negative in leads II, III and aVF. **b** Surface and intracardiac recordings (100 mm/s): Map catheter in His position. His catheter (in red) placed in the RVA. The AH interval and HA interval are both long and almost similar. The long AH interval suggests antegrade conduction over a slow AV nodal pathway and the long HA interval points to a slow pathway retrograde conduction as well

the antegrade and retrograde limb are characterized by slow conduction, the resulting tachycardia cycle length might be long and the AH interval is often similar to the HA interval (Figures 5.1e and 5.6).

5.2.4 Concept of upper and lower common pathway block

AVNRT is associated with 2:1 AV conduction block in approximately 10% of patients [22]. The AV block in this setting is probably a functional infranodal block within the bundle of His ("lower common pathway" block) (Figure 5.7). Similarly, an "upper common pathway" block with 2:1 conduction to the atria can be present (Figure 5.8). This is due to a supranodal block (between the AV node and atrium).

Josephson et al. [15] presumed that the atrium is not a necessary component of the AVNRT reentry circuit. Many other observations also suggest that supra- or infranodal structures are not necessarily required to maintain AVNRT. There are reported examples of tachycardia persistence in the presence of AV block [12, 22, 28]. The site of block most commonly occurs infrahisian in either a 2:1 or Wenckebach fashion. Block above the bundle of His is rarely observed [25]. Although AV block has most commonly been observed during typical AVNRT, atypical AVNRT with infrahisian block might also be observed.

5.2.5 AVNRT with right or left bundle branch block

Bundle branch block is produced by alterations in His-Purkinje conduction and refractoriness and should therefore have no influence on a reentrant process confined to the AV node. Tachycardia cycle length is not affected, neither if bundle branch block develops during ongoing AVNRT nor if the bundle branch block is observed during different tachycardia episodes. A

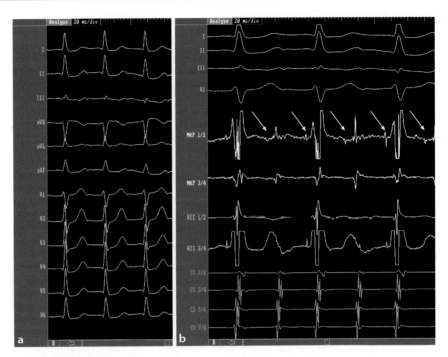

Fig. 5.7. 2:1 lower common pathway block during AVNRT. Surface ECG (50 mm/s) and intracardiac recordings (100 mm/s) demonstrate a typical slow-fast AVNRT with 2:1 block. The Map catheter is placed in an optimal His recording position. An infrahisian block can be seen: only every second re-corded His potential (arrows) conducts to the ventricle. This results in an "isolated" (negative) P wave exactly between the two conducted cycles (visible at the end of the T wave) (right panel 100 mm/s)

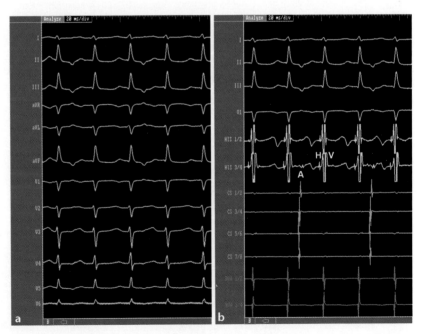

Fig. 5.8. Upper common pathway block in an atypical slow-slow AVNRT. (**a**) Surface ECG 50 mm/s. AVNRT with a 2:1 retrograde conduction block is present. Negative P waves in II, III and aVF are present only after every second QRS complex. (**b**) Atrial depolarization as recorded on the CS catheter is not required for the maintenance of tachycardia (right panel 50mm/s)

right bundle branch block is most commonly observed, rarely a left bundle branch block. The lack of influence of bundle branch block on AVNRT is in contrast to AV reentrant tachycardia involving an (extra-nodal) ipsilateral accessory pathway (see Figure 4.26).

5.2.6 Excluding other arrhythmia mechanisms

It has to be emphasized that before the diagnosis of any form of AVNRT can be made, other arrhythmia mechanisms have to be excluded.

5.3 Differential diagnosis in typical slow-fast AVNRT

A typical AVNRT should be differentiated from an AV reentrant tachycardia in patients with an accessory pathway. Slow-fast AVNRT can be distinguished from orthodromic AV reentrant tachycardia by the following maneuvers.

∎ Differentiating an accessory pathway

∎ Timing of retrograde atrial activation:
In AV reentrant tachycardia with a right anteroseptal accessory pathway, the reentrant wave front activates the ventricles through the His-Purkinje system. The impulse then propagates to the base of the ventricles before activating the accessory pathway in the retrograde direction. This results in a ventriculoatrial (VA) conduction time of at least 50 ms (usually 65–85 ms), corresponding to an HA interval of 100–140 ms [2]. The retrograde P wave begins near the end of the QRS complex or within the ST segment. In AVNRT, the ventricles are not a part of the reentrant circuit. Retrograde conduction over the fast pathway begins close in time to the onset of His bundle activation. VA intervals of less than 50 ms are common in AVNRT and exclude orthodromic AV reentrant tachycardia.

∎ Atypical retrograde activation sequence:
In typical slow-fast AVNRT, the retrograde (VA) conduction sequence should be compatible with a retrograde conduction via the AV

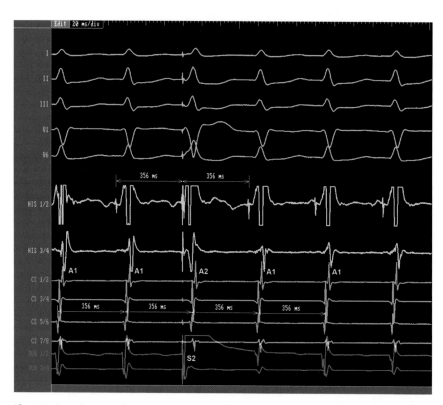

Fig. 5.9. Negative preceding maneuver: A premature ventricular extrastimulus (S2) during typical AVNRT with surface electrogram (I,II, III, V1) and intracardiac recordings. The ventricular extrastimulus is delivered at a time when the His bundle is refractory (H1S2=H1H1). The premature ventricular stimulus does not precede the atrium (A1A2=A1A1) (100 mm/s)

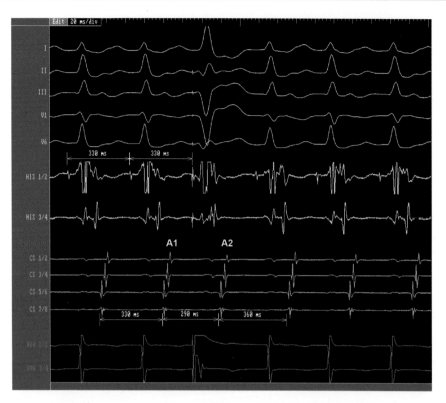

Fig. 5.10. Positive preceding maneuver: A ventricular extra-stimulus delivered during the refractory period of the His bundle advances atrial activation (A2). This indicates the presence of retrograde conduction over an accessory path-way. The atrial activation sequence of A2 is identical to that during tachycardia (A1), indicating that retrograde conduc-tion occurs over the accessory pathway during tachycardia. This is an example of an orthodromic AV reentrant tachycar-dia in a patient with a concealed anteroseptal accessory pathway. Of note, the VA interval during tachycardia is con-siderably longer than in Figure 5.9 showing a slow-fast AVNRT (100 mm/s)

node. If the earliest retrograde atrial activa-tion is not located in the antero-septal part of the tricuspid annulus, close to the His-poten-tial location, an AV reentrant tachycardia in-volving an accessory pathway inserting some-where else is very probable.

▮ Ventricular extrastimulus – "preceding man-euver" (Figures 5.9 and 5.10): Decrementally coupled single ventricular extrastimuli are delivered during tachycardia, at or slightly prior to His bundle activation and, thus, dur-ing refractoriness of the His bundle. Ventri-cular stimulation at the timing of His with ventricular capture results in a slightly de-formed QRS complex. The timing of atrial activation immediately after the ventricular extrastimulus is observed along with the at-rial activation sequence. An advancement in the timing of atrial activation, when retro-grade conduction could not have occurred over the refractory His bundle, establishes the presence of an accessory pathway. An ac-cessory pathway can be considered absent if retrograde atrial activation is unchanged by the ventricular extrastimulus. The most reli-able results are obtained when the ventricular extrastimulus is delivered at the time of the His bundle depolarization.

▮ Parahisian pacing:
If tachycardia does not sustain long enough to deliver ventricular extrastimuli, the ab-sence of a septal accessory pathway can be verified by "parahisian pacing" [13] during sinus rhythm. The parahisian pacing tech-nique can be used to differentiate retrograde conduction over the fast AV nodal pathway from retrograde conduction over a concealed anteroseptal accessory pathway. During sinus rhythm, pacing is performed at the anteroba-sal right ventricular septum adjacent to the

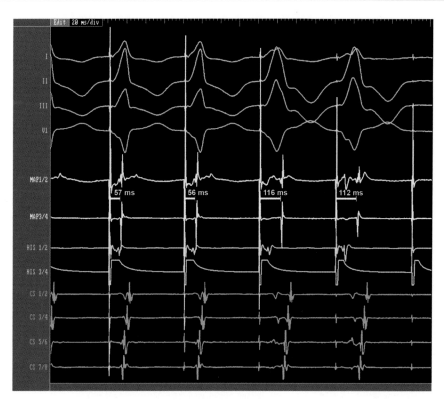

Fig. 5.11. Negative parahisian pacing: Ventricular pacing is performed adjacent to the His bundle/proximal right bundle branch; Map is placed in His localization. At high output pacing, the pacing stimulus captures both the local ventricular myocardium and the proximal right bundle branch. This results in an early retrograde activation of the His bundle and in a stimulus-atrial (SA) interval of 56 ms. A reduction in pacing current results in loss of direct capture of the proximal right bundle branch while capture of the ventricular myocardium is maintained. This is associated with an increase in the width of the QRS complex and a late timing of the His bundle potential. The delay in timing of the His bundle activation resulted in prolongation of the SA interval to 112 ms. This indicates retrograde conduction over the AV node. Further decrease of pacing output leads to loss of ventricular capture following the last stimulus (Speed 100 mm/s)

His bundle. Pacing is initiated with high output and the pacing catheter is maneuvered progressively closer to the His bundle until simultaneous capture of the His bundle and right ventricle occurs, reflected in an abrupt narrowing of the QRS complex. The pacing output is then decreased until direct capture of the His bundle is lost while maintaining right ventricular capture. A delay in the timing of atrial activation, equal to the delay in the timing of His bundle activation, identifies retrograde conduction over the AV node. Retrograde conduction over an accessory pathway is identified either by an absence of change in the timing of atrial activation with loss of His bundle capture or by delay in atrial activation that is less than the delay in the timing of His bundle activation (Figures 5.11 and 5.12).

▌ Differentiating atrial tachycardia

Typical slow-fast AVNRT can be differentiated from atrial tachycardia by administration of intravenous adenosine (Figure 5.13). An atrial tachycardia is present when tachycardia continues in the atrium and is completely dissociated from the ventricle. In case of adenosine-sensitive atrial tachycardia, an AVNRT can be assumed when the features of a typical AVNRT are observed:

▌ Dual AV nodal physiology is present and induction of tachycardia is achieved with a simultaneous prolongation of the A2H2 interval (jump)

▌ The earliest retrograde activation during tachycardia is recorded at the His bundle site because the retrograde AV conduction is through the fast pathway

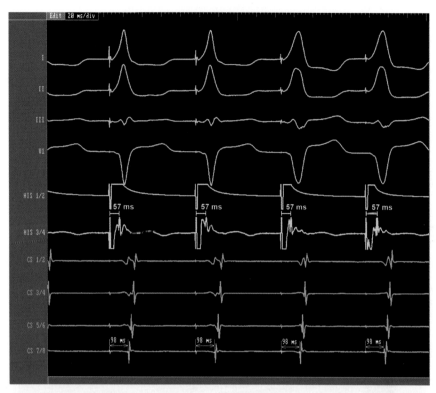

Fig. 5.12. Positive parahisian pacing: The pacing principle is the same as that in Figure 5.11. In the two left complexes, the pacing stimulus captures the ventricular myocardium and the His bundle with a short SA interval and relatively narrow QRS complexes. In the two right complexes, the pacing stim- ulus captured only the ventricular myocardium, as evidenced by the late timing of the His potential and by the increase in width of the QRS complex. The SA interval remains constant, indicating that retrograde conduction occurs over an accessory pathway (100 mm/s)

5.3.1 Differential diagnosis in atypical fast-slow or slow-slow AVNRT

∎ **Differentiating an posteroseptal accessory pathway**

1. Ventricular extrastimuli: as described for slow-fast AVNRT
2. Parahisian pacing: as described for slow-fast AVNRT

∎ **Differentiating an atrial tachycardia**

Differentiation of fast-slow AVNRT from atrial tachycardia may be more difficult. The following observations or maneuvers can be consulted for differential criteria:

∎ Initiation of tachycardia by ventricular stimulation with evidence of a retrograde jump accounts for an atypical AVNRT (Figure 5.14)

∎ Administration of adenosine: Atrial tachycardia is suggested in the presence of complete AV dissociation. This can be achieved by administering intravenous adenosine
∎ Carotis sinus massage: In atypical AVNRT, termination is in the retrograde slow pathway
∎ Atrial tachycardia can be ruled out by ventricular pacing at a cycle length 10 ms shorter than the tachycardia cycle length which is able to entrain tachycardia (with the identical atrial activation sequence). This means that after discontinuation of ventricular pacing, the first return cycle of atypical AVNRT (atrial activation measured in CS or His catheter) is identical to the stimulation cycle length
∎ When tachycardia termination occurs by ventricular extrastimuli that do not conduct to the atrium, atrial tachycardia can be ruled out

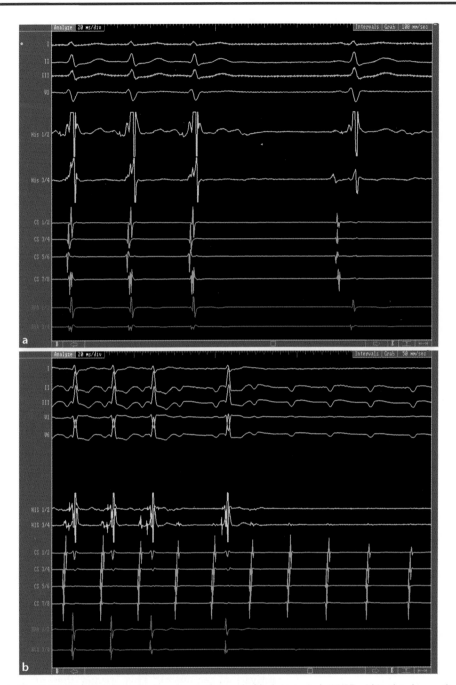

Fig. 5.13. Administration of adenosine. **a** Antegrade block in typical AVNRT within the slow pathway followed by sinus rhythm. **b** AV dissociation in atrial tachycardia

5.4 Catheter ablation of typical AVNRT

5.4.1 Fast pathway

Considering the fact that in the common form of AVNRT retrograde conduction is through the fast pathway, the first attempts of catheter ablation were performed at this location [8, 11]. Se-lective catheter ablation of the fast pathway was effective in about 80–90% of patients. Unfortu-nately, due to the proximity of the fast pathway to the compact AV node and the His bundle, the risk of complete AV block ranged from 0-22% [3, 18, 21].

To perform fast pathway modification, the ab-lation catheter is first positioned in the His

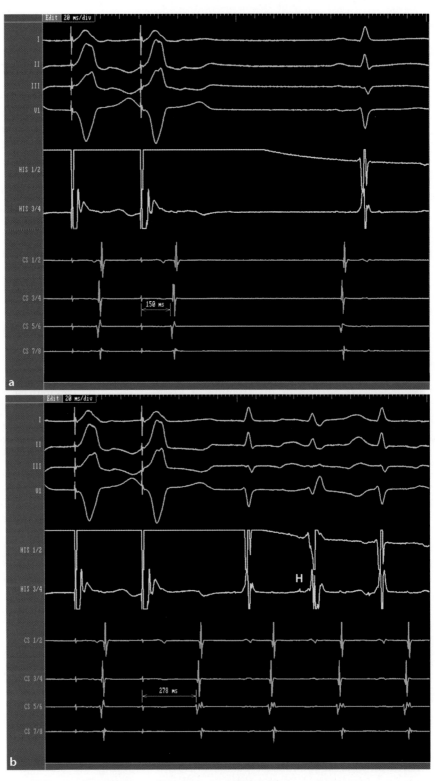

Fig. 5.14. Initiation of a slow-slow AVNRT with a retrograde jump by ventricular pacing. **a** His catheter is advanced into the RV: Ventricular stimulation is performed at a cycle length of 500 ms (S1) and a decreasing coupling interval for S2 is used. A premature ventricular stimulus (S2) at 380 ms results in a fast retrograde atrial activation (S2-A2 = 150 ms). **b** Same drive cycle length with a premature beat (S2) of 370 ms results in a sudden prolongation of retrograde VA interval to 270 ms ("retrograde jump") and induction of an atypical slow-slow AVNRT (100 mm/s)

bundle region to record the maximum amplitude of the bipolar His bundle potential. The catheter is then carefully withdrawn until the His bundle potential becomes smaller or barely visible or disappears while the atrial amplitude becomes larger than the ventricular amplitude. At the optimal site, the earliest atrial activation via the retrograde conduction (i.e., fast pathway) is visible here during typical AVNRT and vice versa the earliest ventricular activation during atypical AVNRT. However, the risk of complete AV block is too high a price to pay for a generally well-tolerated and not life-threatening arrhythmia. AVNRT fast pathway ablation had only been performed before a technique for slow pathway ablation was developed. Currently, fast pathway ablation has been widely abandoned.

5.4.2 Slow pathway

Jackman et al. [14] showed in 1990 that during atypical (fast-slow) AVNRT, the earliest retrograde atrial activation was recorded in the inferoposterior portion of the triangle of Koch close to the CS os, confirming what Sung et al. had previously observed. Based on this finding, selective ablation of the slow pathway in the posteroseptal region, far from the His bundle, was possible using retrograde mapping during atypical AVNRT. Subsequently, ablation approaches of the slow pathway for all types of AVNRT have been investigated.

5.4.3 Anatomical approach

The anatomical approach was proposed by Jazayeri et al. [3] and is performed using only anatomical landmarks to guide slow pathway ablation. The triangle of Koch, i.e., the area of the right atrium that is bounded by the base of the septal leaflet of the tricuspid valve inferiorly, the anterior margin of the coronary sinus orifice and the tendon of Todaro anterosuperiorly (Figure 1.2), is identified in the RAO fluoroscopic view: catheters placed at the His location and in the coronary sinus determine these two structures, whereas the inferior border of Koch's triangle is demarcated by the ablation catheter placed at the most inferior septal position possiblly on the tricuspid annulus.

The ventricular border of Koch's triangle is then divided into three regions: anterior (closest

to the His localization), mid and posterior regions (closest to the base of the tricuspid annulus). The ablation catheter is sequentially moved along the tricuspid septal annulus down to the most posteroinferior aspect of the interatrial septum adjacent to the CS ostium obtaining an A:V electrogram ratio of 1:10 to 1:2. At the end of each RF delivery, inducibility of AVNRT is tested and, if AVNRT is still inducible, another RF application is delivered at an adjacent site with a higher AV ratio. In case of further unsuccessful RF applications, the catheter is moved towards a more mid and anterior position. Using this approach, the success rate varies between 95 and 99% with a mean of six RF pulses. Inadvertent fast pathway ablation occurs in 0.8–0.9% of cases and AV block incidence ranges from 0.6–0.9% [3, 24].

5.4.4 Electrophysiological guided approach

Endocardial potentials and anatomical markers to guide application of RF energy were proposed by Jackman et al. [14] and later by Haissaguerre and Gaita [10]. They describe two specific potentials that are different not only morphologically but also for the site where they are recorded and in their electrophysiological behavior and importance.

Jackman et al. described a potential that is sharp and is the latest atrial electrogram following a low amplitude atrial electrogram during sinus rhythm. During atypical AVNRT the sequence is inverted and the sharp potential precedes the atrial electrogram. The location of this potential varies among patients and the region in which it is usually recorded is very small. It can be recorded near the CS os, sometimes anterior to the CS os or even inside. The authors suggest that this potential represents the activation of the atrial connection of the slow pathway in the posteroanterior direction.

5.4.5 The integrated approach

In daily practice, an integrated approach combining the electrogram-guided and anatomical approach is used for slow pathway ablation (Figure 5.15). As described above, the "triangle of Koch" is divided into posteroseptal, midseptal and anteroseptal zones. The electrogram-guided approach is used initially to identify the

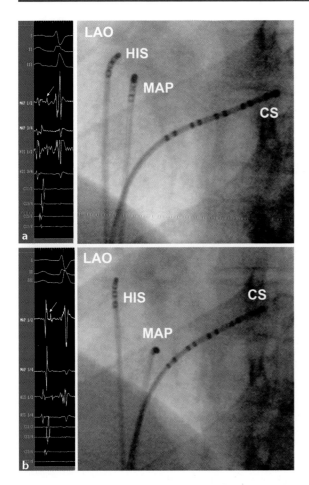

Fig. 5.15. Integrated ablation approach. **a** After crossing the tricuspid valve, the ablation catheter is placed at the maximum His bundle potential recording site (arrow) and this position is documented in the upper fluoroscopic LAO view. **b** From this position, the ablation catheter is deflected inferoposteriorly and slowly withdrawn so that the tip of the catheter is positioned along the tricuspid annulus near the coronary sinus. This area is carefully mapped. In our example, a possible slow pathway potential has been identified: A sharp discrete potential following the atrial potential (arrow). Note: The simultaneously recorded His potential (on His catheter recordings) occurs shortly after the described slow pathway potential (100 mm/s)

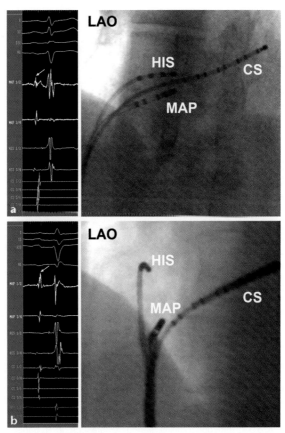

Fig. 5.16. Variability of slow pathway localizations (both successful ablation sites). **a** The recorded slow pathway potential shows a multicomponent atrial electrogram, the Map catheter is positioned beneath the coronary sinus (catheter) and inferior to the distal His catheter. Note: The His bundle potential is also recorded relatively low, at the roof of the CS os. **b** The recorded slow pathway potential also showing a multicomponent atrial electrogram is found at the bottom of the coronary sinus. To achieve better stability for the MAP catheter, a long sheath is inserted (100 mm/s)

target sites where an atrial to ventricular electrogram ratio is 1:2 to 1:10 and a possible slow-pathway potential is present. Mapping is started at the posteroseptal zone and proceeds to the midseptal zones. Rarely, the anteroseptal zone has to be targeted. If the characteristic atrial electrogram is not identified in a more cranial region, the area posterior to or at the os of the coronary sinus ostium should be mapped (Figure 5.16).

5.4.6 Ablation catheter and settings

The ablation catheter should have a distal electrode that is at most 4 mm in length and a deflectable distal segment. The fluoroscopic view that is used for mapping and ablation is usually the left anterior oblique view (LAO) at 40–60° or the right anterior oblique view (RAO) at 20–30°. Usually, monoplane fluoroscopy is adequate, but before ablation, the catheter position

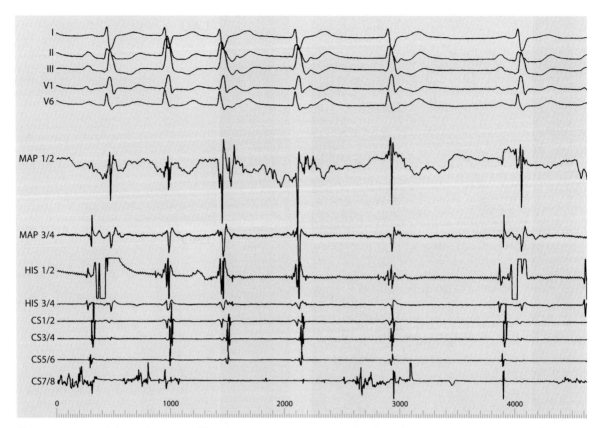

Fig. 5.17. Junctional beats during RF ablation in a patient with a typical AVNRT. Note: The retrograde activation of the atrium (atrial potentials simultaneous to QRS complex in the CS recordings) is always present

should be checked in both of the above mentioned projections. When an appropriate target site for slow pathway ablation is identified, RF energy is usually delivered at power output of 20–30 Watts for up to 60 seconds. A temperature of more than 50 °C should be reached. The RF energy is delivered during sinus rhythm under continuous electrocardiographic monitoring. Accelerated junctional rhythm (Figure 5.17) during RF energy application occurs in nearly 100% of effective sites. However, this is not a specific finding of successful selective ablation, as it also occurs in up to 65% of ineffective applications. On the other hand, the absence of junctional rhythm usually predicts inefficacy of the lesion and the RF energy delivery should not be continued for more than 15 seconds at this site. If accelerated junctional rhythm is absent, the ablation catheter may be withdrawn carefully 2–3 mm from its initial position while the energy delivery is continued. Bursts of accelerated junctional rhythm may develop and then subside after several seconds. Guided by the electrogram, an additional lesion ("safety burn") may be applied within Koch's triangle to support the ablation effect on slow pathway conduction. Since a location of the catheter tip in the anterior third of the distance between the His potential recording site and the coronary sinus ostium increases the risk of fast pathway and/or the His bundle lesion, "safety burns" should not be applied if these sites were targeted with (successful) ablation.

In our daily practice, we mostly use the integrated approach combining the electrogram-guided and anatomical approach. However, if no adequate slow pathway potential is detectable, we perform the anatomical approach. The majority of successful ablation sites are near or superior to the coronary sinus ostium. Occasionally, target sites posterior or within the coronary sinus ostium can be found (Figure 5.16).

∎ Pitfalls

During the accelerated junctional rhythm that accompanies slow pathway ablation, intact VA

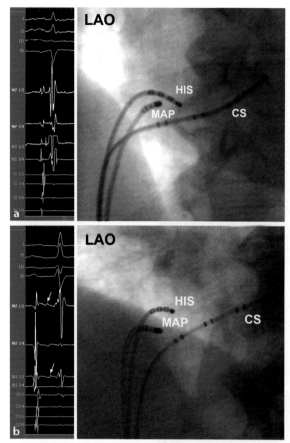

Fig. 5.18. Ablation sites from two patients with AV block III° after ablation. **a** The recorded atrial potential is multifractionated, representing a split atrium but no slow pathway potential. Fluoroscopically, the maximal recorded His bundle potential on the His catheter and the misinterpreted slow pathway potential on the Map catheter are very close together. **b** The Map catheter is positioned fluoroscopically below the His catheter. However, Map 1/2 shows a small His potential (simultaneous to the His potential recorded in the His catheter tracing) and no slow pathway potential (arrow) (Speed 100 mm/s)

conduction has to be present (Figure 5.17). The occurrence of VA block during ablation-induced accelerated junctional rhythm may herald the onset of an AV block. In junctional beats occurring during slow pathway ablation, atrial and ventricular activation is simultaneous and atrial activation is due to retrograde fast pathway conduction. Therefore, junctional beats showing VA block indicate alteration of the fast pathway and therefore herald AV block (Figure 5.21). Energy application must be discontinued immediately as VA block occurs to reduce the risk of AV block. Correct interpretation of the recorded electrogram in the ablation position and thor-

oughly mapping of the slow pathway region are extremely important to avoid undesirable fast pathway alterations (Figure 5.18).

5.4.7 Endpoints and results

The endpoint for slow pathway ablation is the inability to induce AVNRT with a previously reliable induction maneuver. In general, this will be atrial programmed stimulation (with or without isoproterenol perfusion). This can be achieved by either *complete ablation* of slow pathway conduction or by *modification* of slow pathway conduction properties, meaning that the ERP of antegrade slow pathway and retrograde fast pathway conduction do not "fit" together anymore to allow reentry.

The major electrophysiological effects of complete slow pathway ablation are as follows (Figure 5.19):
∎ Loss of a previously demonstrable critical prolongation of the AH interval (= antegrade jump) during atrial extrastimulation that resulted in the initiation of AVNRT (and loss of retrograde jump during ventricular extrastimulation)
∎ Prolongation of the 1:1 AV conduction cycle length

Electrophysiological effects of slow pathway modification are (Figure 5.20):
∎ A demonstrable jump after RF application (at the same programmed stimulation interval as before ablation)
∎ **But:** Maximum of one atrial echo beat, but no inducibility of the arrhythmia

5.4.8 Endpoint, short-term success and complications in AVNRT ablation

The persistence of dual AV nodal physiology with or without a single AV nodal reentrant echo beat is generally considered acceptable and usually is not an indication for continuing ablation attempts. When residual slow pathway conduction is present after successful ablation in terms of noninducibility of AVNRT, the patient may not have changes in the Wenckebach cycle length or AV nodal effective refractory period.

Other complications of slow pathway ablation are rare and are similar to the complications that are associated with any invasive electro-

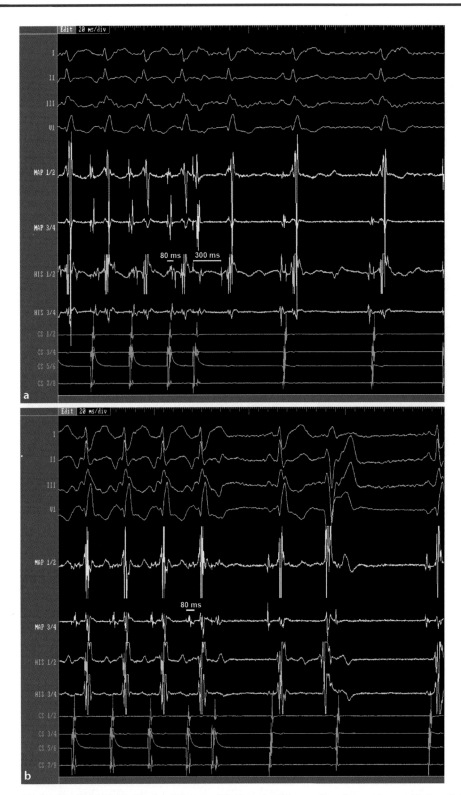

Fig. 5.19. a (100 mm/s): Slow pathway modification. A typical AVNRT had been induced with programmed atrial stimulation with an antegrade jump. After successful slow pathway modification, there is still a sudden AH prolongation, but AVNRT induction is no longer possible. **b** (100 mm/s): Complete slow pathway ablation: Before RF ablation, initiation of AVNRT was observed after a jump when stimulating with the same coupling intervals. After successful slow pathway ablation, there was no antegrade slow pathway conduction (no jump) or inducible AVNRT

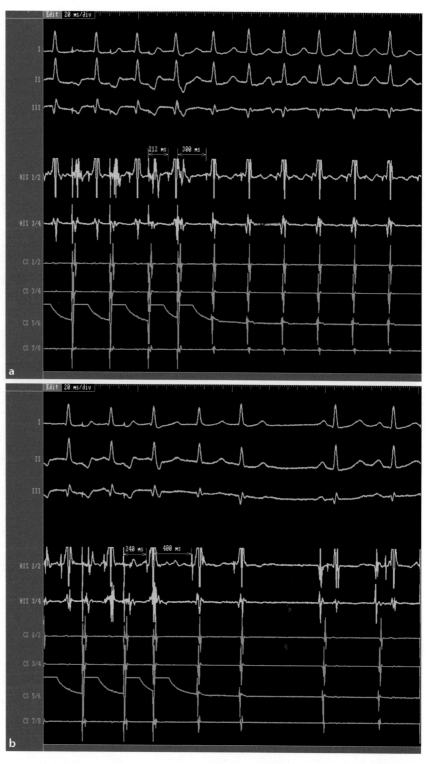

Fig. 5.20. a (50 mm/s): Induction of AVNRT with a typical jump. **b** (100 mm/s): After slow pathway modification with RF current, an antegrade jump with *two* echo beats is still inducible. The endpoint of slow pathway ablation is the elimination of the AVNRT. Although it remains controversial whether the risk of recurrence is higher with residual slow pathway function, the persistence of dual AV nodal physiology with a *single* AV nodal reentrant beat is generally accepted. However, two AV nodal echo beats as in the presented example are an indication for continuing RF ablation attempts

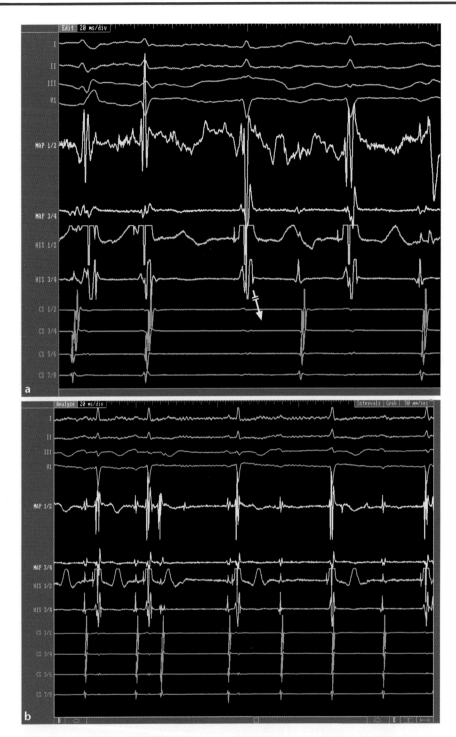

Fig. 5.21. Accelerated junctional rhythm develops shortly after the onset of RF energy application. **a** (100 mm/s): VA dissociation occurs during accelerated junctional rhythm (arrow). The next atrial activation is conducted with AV block I° with an AV interval of 234 ms. This indicates injury of the fast pathway. RF energy delivery should be stopped immediately. **b** (50 mm/s): Continued RF application causes AV block III°

physiological study including vascular damage, deep venous thrombosis, pulmonary emboli and cardiac tamponade.

5.4.9 Recurrence

Overall, primary success rates range from 96–100% no matter whether a complete slow pathway ablation or a modification was achieved. Late recurrence rates range from 1–6% and the incidence of inadvertent complete AV block is reported to be less than 3% [7, 10, 14, 17, 21, 31].

The predictors of AVNRT recurrence after successful slow pathway modification have been discussed controversially. Several studies found that the recurrence rate was higher in patients with residual slow pathway conduction [1, 23, 26]. In contrast, other studies showed that after successful elimination of AVNRT, residual slow pathway conduction does not correlate with clinical tachycardia recurrence [19, 20, 30].

In a study from our group with 506 patients after slow pathway ablation, the risk of recurrence was not higher when residual slow pathway function persisted after successful elimination of AVNRT [9]. Residual slow pathway conduction may be present in approximately 40% of patients after successful elimination of sustained AVNRT. However, the risk of complete AV block may increase substantially by continuing ablation attempts to eliminate the residual slow pathway. Thus, the persistence of residual dual AV nodal physiology and an inducible single AV nodal reentrant echo beat should not be considered an indication for continuing ablation attempts as long as AVNRT is no longer inducible.

5.4.10 AV Block related to slow pathway ablation

Atrioventricular block generally occurs during RF energy delivery and only rarely in the first 24 hours following ablation. A few parameters have been proposed as predictors of this complication:

▮ *The anatomical ablation site:* The anatomical site is crucial since it is important not to deliver RF energy close to the compact AV node or His bundle to avoid damaging these structures. This is generally checked before and during RF delivery, using the fluoroscopic projection and the catheters in the CS and His bundle regions as landmarks for the septal area (Figure 5.18).

▮ *Occurrence of junctional rhythm either rapid or with ventriculoatrial block during RF delivery:* The occurrence of junctional ectopy during RF ablation of the slow pathway is common and it has been suggested to be a response to thermal injury of the AV node or the perinodal tissue comprising the input of fast and slow pathways. Its presence is a highly sensitive finding, occurring in over 90% of effective sites [16]. However, the presence of faster junctional tachycardia or VA block during junctional rhythm is generally considered predictive for complete permanent AV block [29]. This parameter also seems to be relevant in predicting late AV block [6].

▮ *Worsening of AV antegrade conduction:* The importance of monitoring antegrade AV conduction (PR or AH interval) during RF energy is obvious since a progressive or abrupt lengthening may be a sign of more extensive damage involving the compact AV node or proximal His bundle.

▮ *Number of RF applications related to the amount of the tissue damage:* It is very important to limit the extent of tissue damage by minimizing the number of RF energy applications, because in some cases the actual lesion size could progress beyond the border of the pathological lesion explaining acute and late complications (see Section 2.14).

5.4.11 Slow pathway ablation with cryoenergy

AV block is a severe complication considering the generally young patient age and the benign nature of the arrhythmia. To further reduce the risk of AV block, the use of catheter cryoablation has been recently proposed [27]. The main advantages using cryoenergy are the possibility to create lesions that are initially reversible and the stability of the catheter once an iceball has formed. It is possible to induce a reversible lesion after several seconds of freezing at –30 °C. This allows testing of the functional effect of any prospective lesion before the formation of permanent tissue damage. In contrast to cryoenergy, ablation using RF energy allows the evaluation of the lesion only after the lesion is (permanently) created.

During RF energy delivery, the appearance of junctional rhythm with 1:1 VA conduction is a reliable sign of thermal injury to the slow pathway and a probably effective ablation site. During cryoablation of the slow pathway, no junctional rhythm is observed, but antegrade conduction properties of the AV node can be tested. This is generally performed using various pacing protocols during the ice-mapping at –30°C. Stimulation of the atrium at the planned ablation site to test the modification or disappearance of conduction through the slow pathway is constantly feasible. At this temperature, the lesion is reversible and the catheter is "adhesive" to the atrial endocardium by the formation of an iceball around the tip electrode (Figure 2.6). Some criteria predict the effect of slow pathway ablation or modification, such as disappearance of dual AV node physiology, noninducibility of AVNRT, interruption of ongoing AVNRT due to the slowing down and then block of conduction over the slow pathway, or modification of the fast pathway effective refractory period. If one or more of these criteria are present, then the temperature is lowered to –75°C for 4 min, creating an irreversible lesion. The adhesion of the catheter tip to the atrial endocardium during cryomapping as well as ablation prevents catheter dislocation, resulting in a reduction of fluoroscopy time [32].

In case of AV conduction lengthening or appearance of AV block during ice mapping at –30°C, the interruption of cryoenergy delivery allows a prompt rewarming of the tissue, reversibility of the lesion and the restoration of normal AV conduction.

The possibility to test a potential lesion may be particularly important in case of patients with abnormal AV nodal anatomy, such as a posterior displacement of the fast pathway or AV node, a small space in the triangle of Koch between the His bundle region, the compact AV node and the CS, or if ablation has to be performed in the midseptum. In these subgroups of patients, the risk of AV block, in fact, is higher when using RF energy since the ablation site is close to the compact AV node.

In our experience, although slow pathway ablation using RF energy is currently a routine procedure, the use of cryoenergy may increase the safety of the procedure, especially in patients with a higher risk of AV block [32].

∎ References

1. Baker JH, 2nd, Plumb VJ, Epstein AE, Kay GN (1994) Predictors of recurrent atrioventricular nodal reentry after selective slow pathway ablation. Am J Cardiol 73:765–769
2. Benditt DG, Pritchett EL, Smith WM, Gallagher JJ (1979) Ventriculoatrial intervals: diagnostic use in paroxysmal supraventricular tachycardia. Ann Intern Med 91:161–166
3. Blanck Z, Dhala A, Deshpande S, Sra J, Jazayeri M, Akhtar M (1993) Bundle branch reentrant ventricular tachycardia: cumulative experience in 48 patients. J Cardiovasc Electrophysiol 4:253–262
4. Sung RJ, Styperek JL, Myerburg RJ, Castellanos A (1978) Initiation of two distinct forms of atrioventricular nodal reentrant tachycardia during programmed ventricular stimulation in man. Am J Cardiol 42(3):404–415
5. Denes P, Wu D, Amat-y-Leon F, Dhingra R, Wyndham CR, Rosen KM (1977) The determinants of atrioventricular nodal reentrance with premature atrial stimulation in patients with dual A-V nodal pathways. Circulation 56:253-259
6. Elhag O, Miller HC (1998) Atrioventricular block occurring several months after radiofrequency ablation for the treatment of atrioventricular nodal reentrant tachycardia. Heart 79:616-618
7. Epstein LM, Lesh MD, Griffin JC, Lee RJ, Scheinman MM (1995) A direct midseptal approach to slow atrioventricular nodal pathway ablation. Pacing Clin Electrophysiol 18:57–64
8. Epstein LM, Scheinman MM, Langberg JJ, Chilson D, Goldberg HR, Griffin JC (1989) Percutaneous catheter modification of the atrioventricular node. A potential cure for atrioventricular nodal reentrant tachycardia. Circulation 80:757–768
9. Estner HL, Ndrepepa G, Dong J, Deisenhofer I, Schreieck J, Schneider M, Plewan A, Karch M, Weyerbrock S, Wade D, Zrenner B, Schmitt C (2005) Acute and long-term results of slow pathway ablation in patients with atrioventricular nodal reentrant tachycardia – an analysis of the predictive factors for arrhythmia recurrence. Pacing Clin Electrophysiol 28:102–110
10. Haissaguerre M, Gaita F, Fischer B, Commenges D, Montserrat P, d'Ivernois C, Lemetayer P, Warin JF (1992) Elimination of atrioventricular nodal reentrant tachycardia using discrete slow potentials to guide application of radiofrequency energy. Circulation 85:2162–2175
11. Haissaguerre M, Warin JF, Lemetayer P, Saoudi N, Guillem JP, Blanchot P (1989) Closed-chest ablation of retrograde conduction in patients

with atrioventricular nodal reentrant tachycardia. N Engl J Med 320:426–433

12. Hamdan MH, Page RL, Scheinman MM (1997) Diagnostic approach to narrow complex tachycardia with VA block. Pacing Clin Electrophysiol 20:2984–2988

13. Hirao K, Otomo K, Wang X, Beckman KJ, McClelland JH, Widman L, Gonzalez MD, Arruda M, Nakagawa H, Lazzara R, Jackman WM (1996) Para-Hisian pacing. A new method for differentiating retrograde conduction over an accessory AV pathway from conduction over the AV node. Circulation 94:1027–1035

14. Jackman WM, Beckman KJ, McClelland JH, Wang X, Friday KJ, Roman CA, Moulton KP, Twidale N, Hazlitt HA, Prior MI et al (1992) Treatment of supraventricular tachycardia due to atrioventricular nodal reentry, by radiofrequency catheter ablation of slow-pathway conduction. N Engl J Med 327:313–318

15. Josephson ME, Kastor JA (1976) Paroxysmal supraventricular tachycardia: is the atrium a necessary link? Circulation 54:430–435

16. Kalbfleisch SJ, Strickberger SA, Williamson B, Vorperian VR, Man C, Hummel JD, Langberg JJ, Morady F (1994) Randomized comparison of anatomic and electrogram mapping approaches to ablation of the slow pathway of atrioventricular node reentrant tachycardia. J Am Coll Cardiol 23:716–723

17. Kay GN, Epstein AE, Dailey SM, Plumb VJ (1992) Selective radiofrequency ablation of the slow pathway for the treatment of atrioventricular nodal reentrant tachycardia. Evidence for involvement of perinodal myocardium within the reentrant circuit. Circulation 85:1675–1688

18. Kottkamp H, Hindricks G, Willems S, Chen X, Reinhardt L, Haverkamp W, Breithardt G, Borggrefe M (1995) An anatomically and electrogram-guided stepwise approach for effective and safe catheter ablation of the fast pathway for elimination of atrioventricular node reentrant tachycardia. J Am Coll Cardiol 25:974–981

19. Lindsay BD, Chung MK, Gamache MC, Luke RA, Schechtman KB, Osborn JL, Cain ME (1993) Therapeutic end points for the treatment of atrioventricular node reentrant tachycardia by catheter-guided radiofrequency current. J Am Coll Cardiol 22:733–740

20. Manolis AS, Wang PJ, Estes NA, 3rd (1994) Radiofrequency ablation of slow pathway in patients with atrioventricular nodal reentrant tachycardia. Do arrhythmia recurrences correlate with persistent slow pathway conduction or site of successful ablation? Circulation 90:2815–2819

21. Mitrani RD, Klein LS, Hackett FK, Zipes DP, Miles WM (1993) Radiofrequency ablation for atrioventricular node reentrant tachycardia: comparison between fast (anterior) and slow (posterior) pathway ablation. J Am Coll Cardiol 21:432–441

22. Movsowitz C, Schwartzman D, Callans DJ, Preminger M, Zado E, Gottlieb CD, Marchlinski FE (1996) Idiopathic right ventricular outflow tract tachycardia: Narrowing the anatomical location for successful ablation. Am Heart J 131:930–936

23. Nakagawa H, Beckman KJ, McClelland JH, Wang X, Arruda M, Santoro I, Hazlitt HA, Abdalla I, Singh A, Gossinger H et al (1993) Radiofrequency catheter ablation of idiopathic left ventricular tachycardia guided by a Purkinje potential. Circulation 88:2607–2617

24. Scheinman MM, Huang S (2000) The 1998 NASPE prospective catheter ablation registry. Pacing Clin Electrophysiol 23:1020–1028

25. Schmitt C, Miller JM, Josephson ME (1988) Atrioventricular nodal supraventricular tachycardia with 2:1 block above the bundle of His. Pacing Clin Electrophysiol 11:1018–1023

26. Schwacke H, Brandt A, Rameken M, Vater M, Fischer F, Senges J, Seidl K (2002) [Long-term outcome of AV node modulation in 387 consecutive patients with AV nodal reentrant tachycardia]. Z Kardiol 91:389–395

27. Skanes AC, Dubuc M, Klein GJ, Thibault B, Krahn AD, Yee R, Roy D, Guerra P, Talajic M (2000) Cryothermal ablation of the slow pathway for the elimination of atrioventricular nodal reentrant tachycardia. Circulation 102:2856–2860

28. Strohmer B, Schernthaner C, Pichler M (2003) Paroxysmal supraventricular tachycardia with persistent ventriculoatrial block. J Cardiovasc Electrophysiol 14:90–93

29. Thakur RK, Klein GJ, Yee R, Stites HW (1993) Junctional tachycardia: a useful marker during radiofrequency ablation for atrioventricular node reentrant tachycardia. J Am Coll Cardiol 22:1706–1710

30. Wang CC, Yeh SJ, Wen MS, Hsieh IC, Lin FC, Wu D (1994) Late clinical and electrophysiologic outcome of radiofrequency ablation therapy by the inferior approach in atrioventricular node reentry tachycardia. Am Heart J 128:219–226

31. Wetzel U, Hindricks G, Dorszewski A, Schirdewahn P, Gerds-Li JH, Piorkowski C, Kobza R, Tanner H, Kottkamp H (2003) Electroanatomic mapping of the endocardium. Implication for catheter ablation of ventricular tachycardia. Herz 28:583–590

32. Zrenner B, Dong J, Schreieck J, Deisenhofer I, Estner H, Luani B, Karch M, Schmitt C (2004) Transvenous cryoablation versus radiofrequency ablation of the slow pathway for the treatment of atrioventricular nodal reentrant tachycardia: a prospective randomized pilot study. Eur Heart J 25:2226–2231

6 Cavotricuspid isthmus-dependent atrial flutter – common-type atrial flutter

Martin Karch

6.1 Introduction

Cavotricuspid isthmus (CTI)-dependent atrial flutter represents the most common type of macroreentrant atrial tachycardia in patients with and without structural heart disease. In this chapter the focus will be on common-type atrial flutter which represents the vast majority of CTI-dependent flutter cases. Due to historical reasons, lower loop reentrant atrial flutter as a rare subtype of CTI-dependent flutter will be addressed in Chapter 7 of this book (atypical atrial flutter).

Common-type atrial flutter is well known as a stable arrhythmia which can usually be terminated by overdrive stimulation or electrocardioversion. Drug treatment proved to be insufficient to maintain sinus rhythm and to control ventricular rate during ongoing flutter [4, 22]. With the introduction of radiofrequency catheter ablation, a curative treatment approach has become available for this arrhythmia.

6.2 Historical perspective

One of the first electrocardiographic descriptions of human atrial flutter was made by Jolly and Ritchie in 1911 [15] and later by Sir T. Lewis in 1913 [19]. He reported about restless electrical activity and a sawtooth-pattern with a negative deflection of the atrial activity on the surface ECG leads II and III. The exact mechanism of atrial flutter remained a matter of debate for many years. A rapidly firing atrial focus as well as macroreentry involving the right atrium were discussed as possible mechanisms [32]. Puech et al. concluded in 1970 that atrial flutter involves the whole right atrium [26]. Waldo et al. found in postoperative patients that

atrial flutter after atriotomy is based on atrial reentrant activation [40]. He demonstrated an excitable gap with the possibility to speed up the flutter rate and to terminate flutter by overdrive stimulation. However, the exact pathway of common-type flutter remained unclear. In the early 1990s, a protected, narrow isthmus of conduction was identified in the low right atrium between the tricuspid ring and the ostium of the inferior vena cava [6, 10, 24]. This area was characterized by a conduction slowing and it was shown that the typical atrial flutter reentry had to pass this area as a necessary part of the reentrant circuit. Two important findings clarified the exact course of the common-type flutter reentry within the right atrium. In 1995, using intracardiac ultrasound, Olgin et al. identified the crista terminalis (a muscular ridge assigning the border between the trabeculated lateral and the smooth posterior right atrium) and its posterior extension, the eustachian ridge, as an electrical obstacle during atrial flutter. One year later, the tricuspid annulus was defined as the anterior barrier of the typical atrial flutter circuit by Kalman et al. [16, 21]. Thus common-type atrial flutter was clearly defined as a reentrant tachycardia around the tricuspid annulus being protected from shortcut activation towards the posterior right atrium by the crista terminalis.

Attempts of terminating atrial flutter by direct current shocks [28] and the successful cryosurgical destruction of the CTI in the low right atrium [18] initiated the area of catheter ablation. Direct current ablation and focal ablation attempts in the CTI mostly resulted in termination of atrial flutter but showed high recurrence rates. This was mainly due to edema mimicking complete isthmus ablation and resulting in the inability of immediate flutter reinduction. However, the flutter substrate recovered in the majority of patients [37]. In the early 1990s groups led by Feld et al. [10] and Cosio et al.

[7, 8] developed a safe and practical approach for radiofrequency ablation of the CTI by the creation of a continuous ablation line across the isthmus. Pacing maneuvers for testing the completeness of isthmus conduction block – not requiring attempts for reinduction of atrial flutter – significantly increased the permanent success rates of this approach [1, 20, 36]. Further 3D mapping studies helped to differentiate the mechanism of CTI-dependent and atypical variants of atrial flutter [14, 42]. Different ablation concepts have been developed based on these findings. However, the high permanent success rate of isthmus ablation for curative treatment of CTI-dependent atrial flutter has not been reached for atypical flutter variants so far.

6.3 Definitions

Over the years, different classifications have been introduced to describe the various forms of atrial flutter. Most of these nomenclatures are ambiguous and have created some confusion. In 2001, the Joint Expert Group of the Working Group of Arrhythmias of the European Society of Cardiology and the North American Society of Pacing and Electrophysiology published an updated version of the current classification of atrial tachycardia and flutter [29]. Table 6.1

shows a modified version of this nomenclature provided by Scheinman et al. in 2004 which has found widespread acceptance [31].

6.3.1 Common-type atrial flutter

Common-type atrial flutter is characterized by two important features:

▮ The excitation wave has to pass through an isthmus confined by the entry of the inferior vena cava into the right atrium and the eustachian ridge on the posterolateral side and the tricuspid annulus at the anteroseptal side. This isthmus not only represents the narrowest part of the flutter circuit but also a region of significant conduction slowing. Several different notations have been given to this area in the literature, e.g., inferior isthmus, flutter isthmus or the subeustachian isthmus. In this chapter it will be called the "cavotricuspid isthmus (CTI)".

▮ The macroreentrant circuit of common-type atrial flutter is characterized by a defined course around the tricuspid annulus. This reentrant circuit is bounded toward the posterior wall by the crista terminalis with its inferoseptal extension into the eustachian ridge. The crista terminalis possesses fixed or functional properties in a transverse direction, which protect the flutter circuit from shortcut activation (Figure 6.2). The macro-

Table 6.1. Classification of atrial flutter

Right atrial CTI-dependent flutter	Common-type atrial flutter: – **Counterclockwise flutter** – **Clockwise flutter** – **Lower loop reentrant flutter**
▮ Right atrial non-CTI-dependent flutter	– Scar-related flutter – Upper loop flutter
▮ Left atrial flutter	– Perimitral flutter – Scar- and pulmonary vein related flutter – Left septal flutter and others

CTI Cavotricuspid-isthmus; flutter variants described in this article are displayed in bold letters, other flutter forms are described in Chapter 7

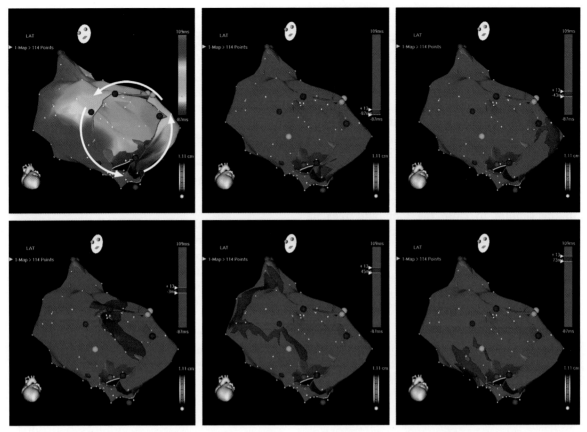

Fig. 6.1. Electroanatomical map (CARTO) of a typical flutter circuit. The use of a CARTO map is not necessary for isthmus ablation but nicely demonstrates the flutter circuit and might help to find a gap in the ablation line. The upper left panel shows an activation map, the other figures show propagation maps of the circuit around the tricuspid valve

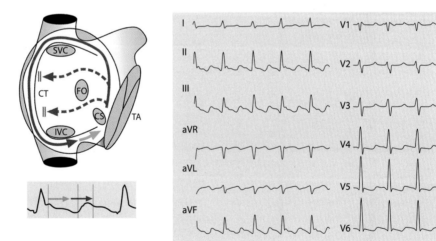

Fig. 6.2. ECG showing common-type counterclockwise atrial flutter with the typical sawtooth pattern in the inferior leads. The intraatrial activation is demonstrated by a schematic drawing of a right atrial cut open view. The red arrows shows the course of the flutter circuitry through the right atrium. Activation across the crista terminalis (CT) is blocked protecting the flutter wavefront from shortcut activation. Conduction through the flutter isthmus (green arrow) is re-presented by the first slightly negative sloping part of the P wave (plateau phase) in the surface ECG; the activation of the interatrial septum is reproduced by the second part of the downsloping P wave, the following steep upstroke of the P wave in the inferior leads is caused by the craniocaudal activation of the lateral right atrial wall. *CS* coronary sinus ostium, *FO* fossa ovalis, *IVC* inferior vena cava, *SVC* superior vena cava, *TA* tricuspid annulus

reentrant circuit involves the complete right atrium, the left atrium being activated only as a bystander via right-to-left atrial connections like the coronary sinus, the Fossa ovalis and Bachmann's bundle.

6.3.2 Counterclockwise atrial flutter

In the most common form of atrial flutter (90% of clinical cases), the activation front moves down the anterolateral right atrium with a lateral-to-septal activation over the CTI to climb up the septum to close the loop and reexcite the anterolateral part of the circuit at its superior pivotal point anterior to the superior vena cava entry. This type of atrial flutter is called "counterclockwise" as the reentrant circuit moves in a counterclockwise direction around the tricuspid annulus in the LAO view.

6.3.3 Clockwise atrial flutter

Typical atrial flutter with an activation front rotating around the tricuspid annulus in a clockwise direction (LAO view) occurs in only 10% of clinical cases. This subtype is called "clockwise" atrial flutter.

6.4 ECG Diagnosis

Atrial flutter is primarily an ECG diagnosis implicating undulating atrial activity without a baseline. The most common form, counterclockwise atrial flutter, is characterized by a stereotypic surface ECG pattern showing negative sawtooth-like waves in the inferior leads II, III and aVF at a rate of 200–300 beats/minute (Figure 6.3).

These flutter waves comprise a segment which shows a slow downslope followed by a sharp upstroke with a positive overshoot that

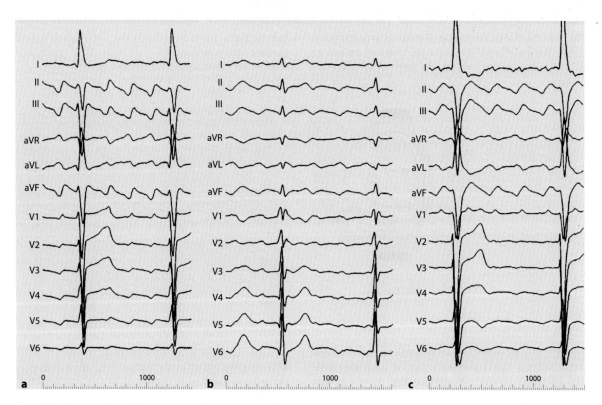

Fig. 6.3. Characteristic ECG appearance of counterclockwise AFl. Three different morphologies in lead I are shown. **a** Predominantly negative; **b** Predominantly positive; **c** Triphasic. Morphology in other leads is stereotypical. The plateau is clearly visible in the inferior leads. From Ndrepepa et al. [23] with permission

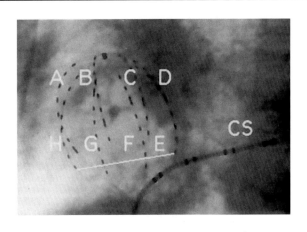

Fig. 6.4. Fluoroscopic appearance of a basket catheter and CS catheter in LAO 45° projection. Letters from A to H identify the basket splines. Splines A–H are located at the lateral wall, spline B at the posterior wall, spline C at the postero-septal wall, splines D–E at the septal wall and splines F–G across the tricuspid annulus. The thick white line represents the isthmus distance. Numbers represent arrangement of the electrode pairs in BC splines

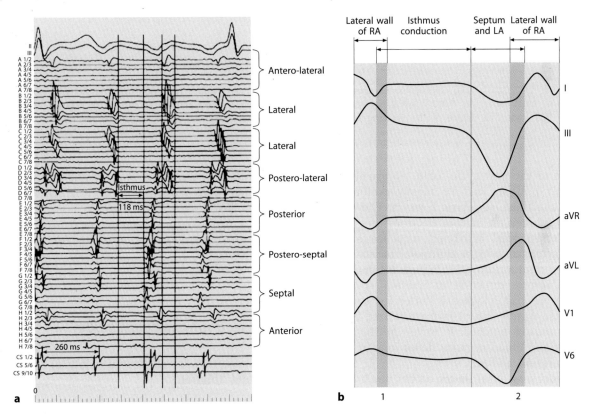

Fig. 6.5. Relationship between endocardial activation sequence and surface ECG morphology in counterclockwise atrial flutter. **a** Two inferior leads and 56 bipolar basket catheter electrograms are shown. Spline locations in relation to the RA wall are shown on the right side. The lateral wall (splines B and C) is activated in a craniocaudal sequence from electrode pairs 1/2 to 7/8. Double potentials are recorded in posterolateral region (spline D). The septal and posteroseptal walls (splines G and F) are activated in a caudocranial direction from electrode pair 7/8 to electrode pair 1/2. The posterior wall is activated in a simultaneous way from the horizontally emerging wavefronts of septal origin. **b** Schematic of the relation between endocardial activation and surface ECG. The morphology in lead I is triphasic. Lead III is selected as representative of inferior leads and leads V1 and V6 as representative of the precordial leads. Shaded areas 1 and 2 represent superimposition of the activation of the lateral wall of the RA over the isthmus conduction and the left atrium, respectively. (From Ndrepepa et al. with permission)

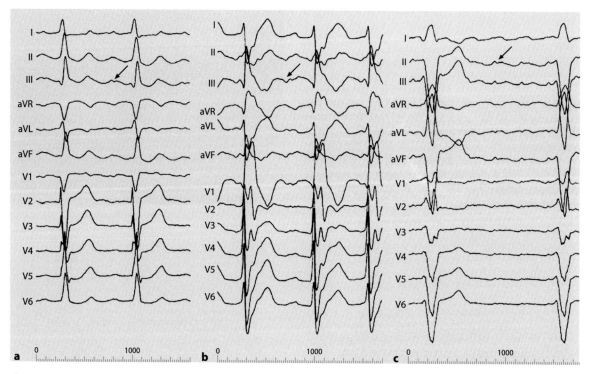

Fig. 6.6. Characteristic ECG appearance of CTI-dependent clockwise atrial flutter. The flutter wave is notched (arrows) in all ECG leads. The degree of the notching varies from slight (**a**) until almost two distinctive deflections (**c**).Typically the plateau is short and has a concave shape in the inferior leads. (From Ndrepepa et al. [23] with permission)

leads to the next cycle. Lead V1 usually shows clearly positive, lead V6 mostly exhibits negative or almost isoelectric P waves. The relationship between the surface electrocardiogram and the endocardial activation sequence has been characterized using a multipolar basket catheter in the right atrium [23] (Figures 6.4 and 6.5).

A reverse direction of rotation around the tricuspid ring, clockwise flutter (or sometimes reverse typical flutter) is characterized by broad and mostly notched P waves in the inferior leads and broad negative deflections in lead V1 (Figures 6.6 and 6.7).

Clockwise atrial flutter occurs much less frequently in the clinical setting (about 10% of cases). Interestingly, it turns out to be inducible in the majority of patients with counterclockwise flutter during an electrophysiological study. The reason for its lower incidence is unclear. Specific conduction properties of the CTI and the lateral right atrial wall as well as the predominantly left atrial origin of atrial premature complexes initiating atrial flutter episodes might play a role. It has been observed that during atrial fibrillation wavefronts spread much more frequently in a craniocaudal compared to a caudocranial direction along the anterolateral right atrium. This craniocaudal direction as existent during normal sinus rhythm might be the preferred direction of excitation along the lateral right atrium [17, 27].

6.5 Electrophysiological study

6.5.1 Indication for electrophysiological study and ablation

Recurrence of common-type atrial flutter after the initial presentation requiring cardioversion and/or drug treatment is extremely common [4]. Therefore, in our view, a single documentation of common-type atrial flutter already justifies the indication for an electrophysiological study and ablation. In a small study, Natale et al. investigated the outcome of patients with atrial flutter comparing two treatment strategies: radiofrequency ablation of the flutter isthmus

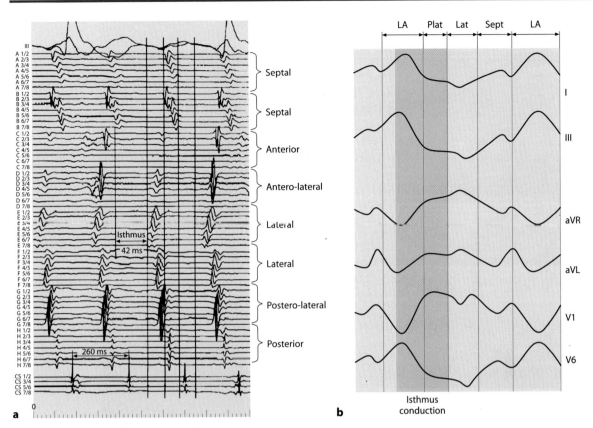

Fig. 6.7. a Relationship between endocardial activation sequence and surface ECG morphology in clockwise atrial flutter. Two inferior leads and 56 bipolar basket catheter (see Figure 6.4) electrograms are shown. Spline locations relative to the RA wall are shown on the right side. The lateral (splines E and F) and posterolateral (spline G) walls are activated in a caudocranial sequence from electrode pairs 7/8 to 1/2. The septal (splines **a** and **b**) wall is activated in a cra-

niocaudal direction from electrode pair 1/2 to electrode pair 7/8. Again, the posterior wall is activated in a simultaneous way from the horizontally emerging wave-fronts of septal origin. **b** Schematic of the relationship between the endocardial activation and the surface ECG. The shaded area represents the isthmus conduction. *LA* left atrium, *Lat* lateral wall, *Plat* plateau, *Sept* septal wall (From Ndrepepa et al. [23] with permission)

and the treatment with antiarrhythmic drugs. During a follow-up period of 21 months, they demonstrated that ablation was associated with a significant improvement in quality of life, a reduction of atrial fibrillation episodes and fewer hospital admissions [22]. Findings from our laboratory show that in patients with concurrent atrial fibrillation and atrial flutter a significant reduction of atrial fibrillation episodes could be achieved after successful flutter ablation [33].

6.5.2 Catheter placement

Different catheter setups can be chosen for an electrophysiological study in a patient with suspected common-type atrial flutter. From a pragmatic standpoint, testing of the CTI-dependency

of the flutter reentry from a septal and a low lateral pacing position appears to be sufficient. The use of a multipolar coronary sinus catheter has proven to be very helpful in providing information about the activation of the basal septum. In addition it offers a stable pacing position on the septal aspect of the flutter isthmus. A second multipolar catheter with at least four electrodes should be placed upside down along the lateral right atrial wall (Figure 6.8). Due to historical reasons, this catheter is often called a "Halo" catheter. At the beginning of the flutter ablation era, ring-shaped Halo catheters with 20 and more electrodes were used to cover the complete typical flutter circuit. Nowadays, this is no longer necessary in typical flutter cases. Attention must be paid to position the Halo catheter as anterior as possible along the lateral

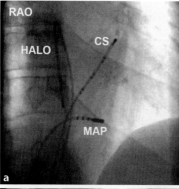

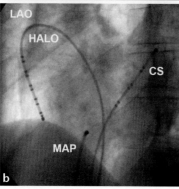

Fig. 6.8. Fluoroscopic images of catheter positions during ablation of CTI-dependent atrial flutter. A 30° right anterior oblique (**a**) and a 45° left anterior oblique (**b**) projection demonstrate the ablation catheter (MAP) in the 6 o'clock position at the flutter isthmus; a decapolar Halo catheter is placed at the tricuspid annulus along the anterolateral right atrium and an octapolar catheter is inserted into the coronary sinus (CS)

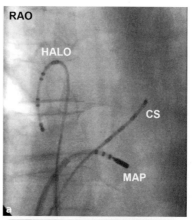

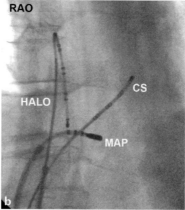

Fig. 6.9. Fluoroscopic 30° right anterior oblique projection to demonstrate a misplacement (**a**) of the Halo catheter posterior to the crista terminalis and its correct position (**b**) in an anterior position. The anterior position of the Halo catheter is crucial for the diagnosis of CTI-dependent flutter as well as for the detection of isthmus block. For abbreviations see Figure 6.8

right atrium to assure a position anterior of the crista terminalis (proven by right anterior oblique fluoroscopy). If the Halo catheter is misplaced posterior to the crista terminalis, it will show a caudocranial activation sequence during counterclockwise atrial flutter instead of the proper craniocaudal activation as expected. Second, the distal end of the catheter must be placed as caudally as possible close to the lateral entry of the flutter isthmus (Figure 6.9). This is of particular importance for testing of the completeness of the isthmus ablation line.

6.6 Catheter ablation

The mapping and ablation procedure for common-type atrial flutter can be performed during ongoing atrial flutter as well as during sinus rhythm.

6.6.1 Mapping during common-type atrial flutter

If atrial flutter is present at the beginning of the electrophysiological study the activation sequence can be recorded and evaluated. Two questions need to be answered:
1. Is the recorded intracardiac activation sequence compatible with CTI-dependent atrial flutter?
   - Depending on the direction of the flutter circuit, the activation along the right atrial lateral wall will be craniocaudal (counterclockwise) or caudocranial (clockwise) (Figures 6.10 und 6.12)
   - Activation of the coronary sinus from the proximal to the distal bipoles

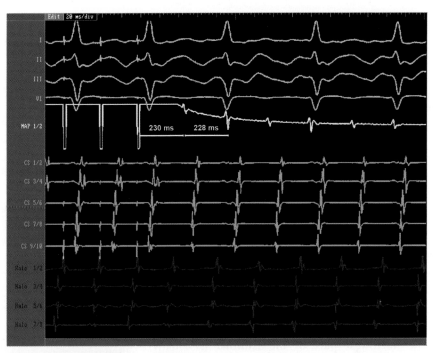

Fig. 6.10. Concealed entrainment from the ablation catheter (MAP) placed right at the flutter isthmus during ongoing counterclockwise atrial flutter. The postpacing interval is similar to the flutter cycle length and thus the isthmus is a necessary part of the flutter circuit. For abbreviations see Figure 6.7

– Sequential, not simultaneous activation of Halo and coronary sinus catheter. If a (ablation) catheter is already placed at the CTI, its activation occurs in the plateau phase (in counterclockwise atrial flutter) (Figure 6.2)
2. Can concealed entrainment be achieved inside the assumed flutter reentry, i.e. along the tricuspid annulus?
   – Preferentially, pacing should be performed from the distal part of the Halo catheter to prove the anterolateral right atrium being a necessary part of the flutter reentry (entrainment stimulation from the CS ostium is less helpful due to the possibility of septal or perimitral flutter reentry)

If both questions are answered with "yes", an ablation catheter should be inserted and placed to the CTI (Figure 6.8). Entrainment stimulation should be performed from here (Figure 6.10). In case of concealed entrainment the ongoing flutter must be CTI-dependent. The rare case of lower loop reentrant atrial flutter (Figure 7.1) shows isthmus dependency of the flutter reentry with fusion of activation along the lateral right atrial wall.

Concealed entrainment: During stimulation from inside the flutter circuitry during ongoing flutter with a rate faster than the flutter cycle length, the surface P wave should remain unchanged. After termination of stimulation, the first postpacing interval must be identical (up to 20–30 ms) to the flutter cycle length, to prove a location of the pacing site inside the circuit.

6.6.2 Pacing procedures during sinus rhythm

If sinus rhythm is present at the beginning of the electrophysiological study, conduction times from the proximal coronary sinus electrodes to the distal lateral wall electrodes and vice versa should be measured. These values can be compared with conduction times evaluated after ablation. Pacing from the low septum/coronary sinus ostium is more likely to induce counterclockwise atrial flutter. Clockwise flutter more likely results from lateral wall pacing. As soon as atrial flutter is induced, its isthmus dependency must be tested as described above. In our EP lab, we do not attempt the induction of atrial flutter if a 12-lead ECG is available which clearly shows typical atrial flutter. This is mainly due to the common problem of inducing atrial fibrillation or clinically irrelevant forms of atypical atrial flutter.

6.6.3 Location of the ablation line

For achieving permanent cure of typical atrial flutter, the ablation line across the CTI must provide a bidirectional, complete line of conduction block without gaps or residual slow conduction. To achieve this goal, the ablation line has to span from the tricuspid annulus to the inferior vena cava and/or the eustachian ridge. The CTI itself represents a complex 3D structure: The thickness of muscle in the CTI is variable showing "deep valleys and high mountains". The narrowest distance which has to be spanned by ablation also varies significantly from a few millimeters to more than 3 cm in width. In a 45° left anterior oblique projection, the narrowest part of the isthmus is usually found at the 6 o'clock position (Figure 6.8). A more septal position is frequently associated with a longer ablation line. If placed very septally it actually consists of two lines, one from the tricuspid annulus to the coronary sinus ostium and a second line from here to the orifice of the inferior caval vein (Figure 6.11).

Furthermore, in addition to a generally more painful ablation in a septal position a potential risk of AV block exists. An anterior and lateral position is also associated with a longer ablation line compared to the 6 o'clock position. In addition, the atrial myocardium appears to be thicker at this location. The optimal site of the ablation line is the location with the shortest distance at which an acceptable catheter contact can be achieved. Due to distinctive anatomical characteristics, it might be impossible in some cases to complete a lesion at a 6 o'clock position due to myocardial thickness or insufficient catheter-wall contact. A septal or lateral approach might then be justified.

6.6.4 Ablation: technical considerations

Isthmus ablation is usually performed with the catheter being advanced via the inferior vena cava to the right ventricle. The ablation should be started as soon as firm tissue contact is achieved with a ratio of the atrial to ventricular bipolar electrogram amplitude of less than 1:3.

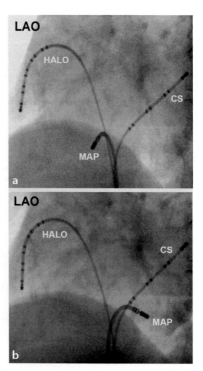

Fig. 6.11. Fluoroscopic 45° left anterior oblique projection depicting a lateral (**a**) and septal (**b**) ablation position of the ablation (MAP) catheter. For abbreviations see Figure 6.8

For successful ablation it is crucial to achieve firm tissue catheter contact during ablation. For this purpose, different ablation catheter curvatures and long vascular sheaths are available. Due to the size and shape of the flutter isthmus, a complete bidirectional conduction block can not be achieved with a single ablation lesion. Therefore, progressive drag lesions or sequential point-by-point lesions are necessary. Ablation should be stopped with the disappearance of atrial signals on the ablation catheter, signaling that the border of the right atrium to the inferior vena cava has been reached.

6.6.5 Ablation technology

Isthmus ablation might be achieved with 4 mm standard ablation catheters in the majority of cases. However, several studies demonstrated that radiofrequency ablation catheters with larger tips (8–10 mm) and 4 mm cooled tip catheters (closed loop or open irrigated, see Chapter 2) significantly shorten the procedure and fluoroscopy time without increasing ablation related risks [3, 13, 34]. These catheters allow the application of more energy and the achievement of larger and deeper lesions. In the presence of thick muscle bundles within the isthmus, this might be crucial for final ablation success [9, 12, 13, 30]. Ablation with large tip radiofrequency catheters and irrigated catheters seem to be of comparable value [34].

Duration, power and temperature settings of the ablation must be chosen considering that the location of the ablation line is a high flow area. Therefore, electrode temperature does not always exactly reflect tissue temperature due to significant convective blood cooling of the ablation catheter. Entrapment of a catheter tip while creating linear lesions on one of the above mentioned "deep valleys" might lead to excessive heating and subsequent power down-regulation. This limitation can be overcome by an open irrigated tip catheter system. In our laboratory, 8 mm radiofrequency catheters are usually used with a power of 50–60 W and a temperature limitation of 60 °C.

More recently, cryoablation for creation of ablation lesions within the heart has been introduced to clinical use. The main advantage of this new technology in the setting of flutter ablation seems to be the painless creation of deep transmural lesions in the subeustachian isthmus [39]. Cryoablation catheters are available with 8 or 10 mm ablation tips for application of the cooling energy. During the application of cryoenergy, the catheter sticks to the endocardium, and therefore, the application of a dragging technique is not possible.

6.6.6 Ablation endpoint

▌ Flutter termination during ablation

Isthmus ablation can be performed during atrial flutter or during sinus rhythm. Termination of flutter during ablation proves the isthmus dependency of the flutter circuit (Figure 6.12) but it is rarely equivalent to a complete bidirectional conduction block [35]. Other criteria need to be applied to confirm a complete ablation line.

▌ Reversion of activation along the lateral right atrium

If atrial flutter ablation is performed during sinus rhythm, a conduction block in the clock-

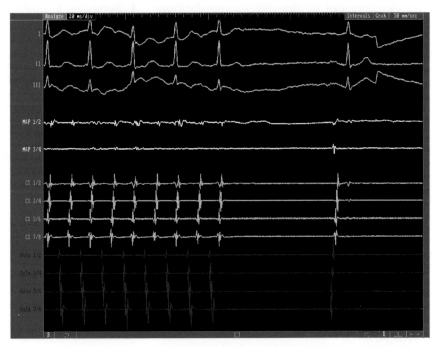

Fig. 6.12. Termination of common-type clockwise flutter during ablation in the CTI. The activation sequence of the Halo catheter depicts a caudocranial direction along the antero-lateral right atrium in accordance with a clockwise activation around the tricuspid ring. For abbreviations see Figure 6.7

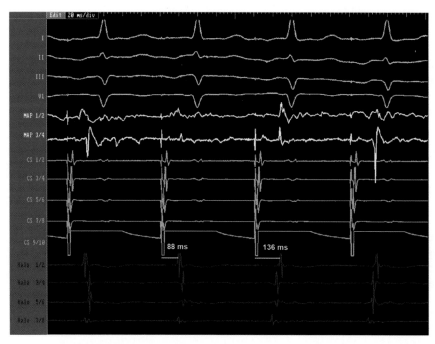

Fig. 6.13. Proximal coronary sinus (CS) pacing during ablation. As soon as complete isthmus block is achieved, the activation sequence of the Halo catheter changes to a complete craniocaudal activation. For the first two beats of this tracing, the distal electrodes (Halo 1/2) are activated before Halo 3/4 due to residual conduction through the isthmus. From the second to the third activation, complete isthmus block occurs with a sudden increase of activation time from the proximal CS to the distal Halo catheter. For catheter setup see Figure 6.8

wise direction can be detected during ablation by pacing from the coronary sinus. With clockwise isthmus conduction block, the activation front along the lateral right atrium during proximal coronary sinus pacing changes from a caudocranial to a complete craniocaudal direction (observed on the Halo catheter). For this pacing maneuver, it is crucial that the Halo catheter is placed as described above with the distal part positioned close to the lateral isthmus (Figure 6.13).

∎ Increase of isthmus conduction times

A significant prolongation of the conduction times from one to the other side of the isthmus (distal Halo to proximal coronary sinus and vice versa) can be used as a criterion for isthmus conduction block when compared to baseline values obtained in sinus rhythm. However, a specific cut off value has not been determined.

∎ Recording of double (split)-potentials along the ablation line

For this purpose, the ablation catheter is placed on the former ablation line. In sinus rhythm, a fractionated low amplitude potential is visible on the lesion site. During pacing from either side of the line, widely split double potentials can be recorded on the line, if the lesion is already complete. Note: The wider the separation of both potentials, the more complete the line is.

∎ Differential pacing: pacing from the Halo catheter distal and proximal

With this pacing maneuver a conduction block in the counter clockwise direction can be tested. If a block of the CTI in a counterclockwise direction is achieved the second split component of the ablation catheter (placed on the ablation line) occurs later with distal compared to proximal Halo pacing (Figures 6.14 and 6.15). Timing of the first split potential can be checked to prove the correctness of the pacing

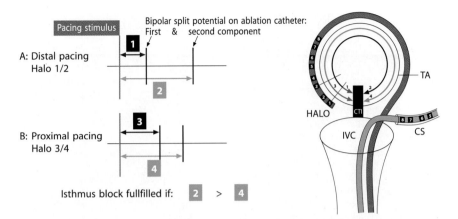

Fig. 6.14. Schematic depiction of the chronology of the two components of the split potential recorded from the ablation catheter placed along a complete linear ablation lesion in the flutter isthmus. Signals are recorded during distal (A) and proximal (B) Halo pacing. With pacing from the distal Halo catheter, an early potential (after interval 1) and a second late potential (after interval 2) can be recorded on the ablation line. During pacing from the proximal Halo catheter, the time to the second interval shortens (interval 4), while the first potential on the ablation line occurs later (interval 3) compared to distal Halo pacing. The corresponding electrogram recordings (with the MAP catheter placed on the ablation line) are shown in Figure 6.15

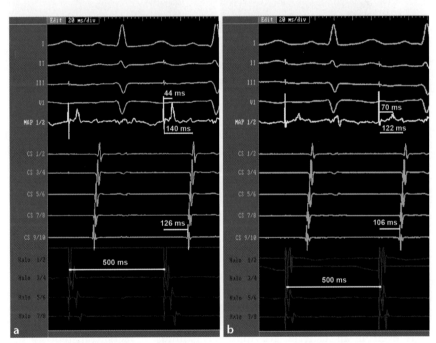

Fig. 6.15. Differential pacing: The ablation catheter (MAP) is placed across the ablation line in the flutter isthmus recording split potentials during pacing from the distal Halo bipole 1/2 (**a**) and the more proximal bipole Halo 3/4 (**a**). For further explanation see Figure 6.15. Abbreviations see Figure 6.7

locations. Pacing from the distal Halo catheter results in a shorter stimulus to the first split component interval compared to pacing from a more proximal bipole.

▌ Change of P wave morphology

With the achievement of complete isthmus block, the surface P waves in the inferior leads change their morphology from double negative

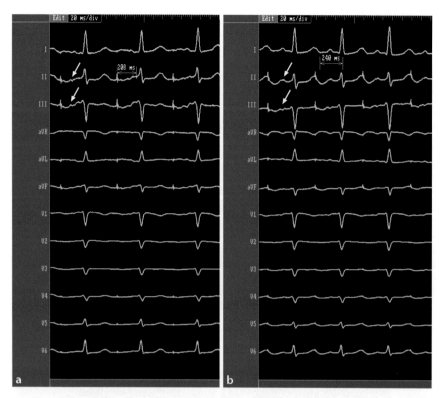

Fig. 6.16. Distal Halo pacing with double negative P waves at the inferior surface ECG leads as long as isthmus conduction is present (**a**). In contrast distal Halo pacing leads to negative-positive P waves in the inferior surface ECG leads as soon as isthmus block has been achieved (**b**)

to a biphasic (negative-positive) waveform with pacing from the low lateral wall. In addition, the stimulus to QRS interval will be prolonged due to a later activation of the AV node when the isthmus is blocked (Figure 6.16).

6.6.7 Short- and long-term success

Isthmus conduction tests must be repeated 20–30 minutes after the ablation as a high short-term recovery rate of isthmus conduction (20–30%) is reported [5]. It needs to be emphasized that even if all criteria are fulfilled, isthmus block might not be complete and only a marked delay of conduction might have been achieved. These patients might present with a relapse of atrial flutter with very long cycle lengths.

A complete interruption of isthmus conduction can be achieved in our EP lab in a high percentage of cases (over 90%) [33]. Recurrence of atrial flutter usually occurs within 6 months after ablation and only 25% of recurrences are observed later [11]. During the first year after the ablation, about 10% of patients with initial verification of complete bidirectional isthmus block experience a flutter recurrence and in 95% of these patients a second ablation proves to be successful [33].

6.6.8 Complications

The most frequently encountered epiphenomenon of flutter ablation is the perception of pain during radiofrequency energy application. Triggered by intense pain and caused by vagal effects, transient AV block may occur during ablation even far away from the septum. This type of AV block is reversible and can be prevented by the administration of atropine and/or analgetics during ablation. Permanent AV block might occur if the ablation line is located septally, close to the caudal part of the triangle of Koch [2, 33, 38]. Delivery of a high amount of energy via a small electrode without sufficient cooling might result in carbonization of blood at the catheter tip (Figure 2.4). This might especially happen if the catheter tip is trapped within trabeculae. A sudden heating of tissue might then cause a development of steam resulting in an explosion of tissue. This so-called "popping" phenomenon might cause a life-threatening complication due to disruption of cardiac tissue. Persistent sinuatrial block after flutter termination should not be mistaken for an ablation-associated complication. This problem is almost exclusively observed in patients with long lasting atrial flutter and/or a higher degree AV block during atrial flutter (with an atrial to ventricular conduction ratio of more than 3:1 as a hint towards binodal disease). Implantation of a dual chamber pacemaker is usually necessary to solve this problem. Despite close proximity, an acute obstruction of the right coronary artery during CTI ablation appears to be a rare complication [25].

∎ References

1. Anselme F, Saoudi N (2001) Assessment of complete isthmus block after ablation of typical atrial flutter: can we rely on a single criterion? J Cardiovasc Electrophysiol 12:400–401
2. Anselme F, Saoudi N, Poty H, Douillet R, Cribier A (1999) Radiofrequency catheter ablation of common atrial flutter: significance of palpitations and quality-of-life evaluation in patients with proven isthmus block. Circulation 99:534–540
3. Atiga WL, Worley SJ, Hummel J, Berger RD, Gohn DC, Mandalakas NJ, Kalbfleisch S, Halperin H, Donahue K, Tomaselli G, Calkins H, Daoud E (2002) Prospective randomized comparison of cooled radiofrequency versus standard radiofrequency energy for ablation of typical atrial flutter. Pacing Clin Electrophysiol 25: 1172–1178
4. Babaev A, Suma V, Tita C, Steinberg JS (2003) Recurrence rate of atrial flutter after initial presentation in patients on drug treatment. Am J Cardiol 92:1122–1124
5. Bru P, Duplantier C, Bourrat M, Valy Y, Lorillard R (2000) Resumption of right atrial isthmus conduction following atrial flutter radiofrequency ablation. Pacing Clin Electrophysiol 23: 1908–1910
6. Cosio FG, Lopez-Gil M, Goicolea A, Arribas F (1992) Electrophysiologic studies in atrial flutter. Clin Cardiol 15:667–673
7. Cosio FG, Lopez-Gil M, Goicolea A, Arribas F, Barroso JL (1993) Radiofrequency ablation of the inferior vena cava-tricuspid valve isthmus in common atrial flutter. Am J Cardiol 71:705–709
8. Cosio FG, Lopez Gil M, Arribas F, Goicolea A (1993) Radiofrequency catheter ablation for the

9. Feld GK (2004) Radiofrequency ablation of atrial flutter using large-tip electrode catheters. J Cardiovasc Electrophysiol 15:S18–S23
10. Feld GK, Fleck RP, Chen PS, Boyce K, Bahnson TD, Stein JB, Calisi CM, Ibarra M (1992) Radiofrequency catheter ablation for the treatment of human type 1 atrial flutter. Identification of a critical zone in the reentrant circuit by endocardial mapping techniques. Circulation 86:1233–1240
11. Gilligan DM, Zakaib JS, Fuller I, Shepard RK, Dan D, Wood MA, Clemo HF, Stambler BS, Ellenbogen KA (2003) Long-term outcome of patients after successful radiofrequency ablation for typical atrial flutter. Pacing Clin Electrophysiol 26:53–58
12. Jais P, Hocini M, Gillet T, Shah DC, Haissaguerre M, Yamane T, Deisenhofer I, Garrigue S, Le Metayer P, Roudaut R, Clementy J (2001) Effectiveness of irrigated tip catheter ablation of common atrial flutter. Am J Cardiol 88:433–435
13. Jais P, Shah DC, Haissaguerre M, Hocini M, Garrigue S, Le Metayer P, Clementy J (2000) Prospective randomized comparison of irrigated-tip versus conventional-tip catheters for ablation of common flutter. Circulation 101: 772–776
14. Jais P, Shah DC, Haissaguerre M, Hocini M, Peng JT, Takahashi A, Garrigue S, Le Metayer P, Clementy J (2000) Mapping and ablation of left atrial flutters. Circulation 101:2928–2934
15. Jolly WA, Ritchie TW (1911) Auricular flutter and fibrillation. Heart 3:177–221
16. Kalman JM, Olgin JE, Saxon LA, Fisher WG, Lee RJ, Lesh MD (1996) Activation and entrainment mapping defines the tricuspid annulus as the anterior barrier in typical atrial flutter. Circulation 94:398–406
17. Karch MR, Ndrepepa G, Zrenner B, Saur C, Schneider MA, Schomig A, Schmitt CS (2003) Simultaneous multisite endocardial mapping of sustained and non-sustained atrial fibrillation in humans. J Invasive Cardiol 15:257–262
18. Klein GJ, Guiraudon GM, Sharma AD, Milstein S (1986) Demonstration of macroreentry and feasibility of operative therapy in the common type of atrial flutter. Am J Cardiol 57:587–591
19. Lewis T (1913) Observations upon a curious and not uncommon form of extreme accelerations of the auricle: atrial flutter. Heart 7:171–178
20. Mangat I, Tschopp DR, Jr, Yang Y, Cheng J, Keung EC, Scheinman MM (2003) Optimizing the detection of bidirectional block across the flutter isthmus for patients with typical isthmus-dependent atrial flutter. Am J Cardiol 91: 559–564
21. Nakagawa H, Lazzara R, Khastgir T, Beckman KJ, McClelland JH, Imai S, Pitha JV, Becker AE, Arru-

da M, Gonzalez MD, Widman LE, Rome M, Neuhauser J, Wang X, Calame JD, Goudeau MD, Jackman WM (1996) Role of the tricuspid annulus and the eustachian valve/ridge on atrial flutter. Relevance to catheter ablation of the septal isthmus and a new technique for rapid identification of ablation success. Circulation 94:407–424

22. Natale A, Newby KH, Pisano E, Leonelli F, Fanelli R, Potenza D, Beheiry S, Tomassoni G (2000) Prospective randomized comparison of antiarrhythmic therapy versus first-line radiofrequency ablation in patients with atrial flutter. J Am Coll Cardiol 35:1898–1904

23. Ndrepepa G, Zrenner B, Deisenhofer I, Karch M, Schneider M, Schreieck J, Schmitt C (2000) Relationship between surface electrocardiogram characteristics and endocardial activation sequence in patients with typical atrial flutter. Z Kardiol 89:527–537

24. Olshansky B, Okumura K, Hess PG, Waldo AL (1990) Demonstration of an area of slow conduction in human atrial flutter. J Am Coll Cardiol 16:1639–1648

25. Ouali S, Anselme F, Savoure A, Cribier A (2002) Acute coronary occlusion during radiofrequency catheter ablation of typical atrial flutter. J Cardiovasc Electrophysiol 13:1047–1049

26. Puech P, Latour H, Grolleau R (1970) Les flutter et ses limites. Arch Mal Coeur 61:116–124

27. Roithinger FX, Karch MR, Steiner PR, Sippens-Groenewegen A, Lesh MD (1997) Relationship between atrial fibrillation and typical atrial flutter in humans: activation sequence changes during spontaneous conversion. Circulation 96:3484–3491

28. Saoudi N, Atallah G, Kirkorian G, Touboul P (1990) Catheter ablation of the atrial myocardium in human type I atrial flutter. Circulation 81:762–771

29. Saoudi N, Cosio F, Waldo A, Chen SA, Iesaka Y, Lesh M, Saksena S, Salerno J, Schoels W (2001) Classification of atrial flutter and regular atrial tachycardia according to electrophysiologic mechanism and anatomic bases: a statement from a joint expert group from the Working Group of Arrhythmias of the European Society of Cardiology and the North American Society of Pacing and Electrophysiology. J Cardiovasc Electrophysiol 12:852–866

30. Scavee C, Jais P, Hsu LF, Sanders P, Hocini M, Weerasooriya R, Macle L, Raybaud F, Clementy J, Haissaguerre M (2004) Prospective randomised comparison of irrigated-tip and large-tip catheter ablation of cavotricuspid isthmus-dependent atrial flutter. Eur Heart J 25:963–969

31. Scheinman MM, Yang Y, Cheng J (2004) Atrial flutter: Part II Nomenclature. Pacing Clin Electrophysiol 27:504–506

32. Scherf D, Reid EC, Chamsai DG (1957) Strophanthin therapy in atrial flutter. Am J Med Sci 234:180–184

33. Schmieder S, Ndrepepa G, Dong J, Zrenner B, Schreieck J, Schneider MA, Karch MR, Schmitt C (2003) Acute and long-term results of radiofrequency ablation of common atrial flutter and the influence of the right atrial isthmus ablation on the occurrence of atrial fibrillation. Eur Heart J 24:956–962

34. Schreieck J, Zrenner B, Kumpmann J, Ndrepepa G, Schneider MA, Deisenhofer I, Schmitt C (2002) Prospective randomized comparison of closed cooled-tip versus 8-mm-tip catheters for radiofrequency ablation of typical atrial flutter. J Cardiovasc Electrophysiol 13:980–985

35. Schwartzman D, Callans DJ, Gottlieb CD, Dillon SM, Movsowitz C, Marchlinski FE (1996) Conduction block in the inferior vena caval-tricuspid valve isthmus: association with outcome of radiofrequency ablation of type I atrial flutter. J Am Coll Cardiol 28:1519–1531

36. Shah D, Haissaguerre M, Takahashi A, Jais P, Hocini M, Clementy J (2000) Differential pacing for distinguishing block from persistent conduction through an ablation line. Circulation 102:1517–1522

37. Shah DC, Haissaguerre M, Jais P, Takahashi A, Clementy J (1999) Atrial flutter: contemporary electrophysiology and catheter ablation. Pacing Clin Electrophysiol 22:344–359

38. Steinberg JS, Prasher S, Zelenkofske S, Ehlert FA (1995) Radiofrequency catheter ablation of atrial flutter: procedural success and long-term outcome. Am Heart J 130:85–92

39. Timmermans C, Ayers GM, Crijns HJ, Rodriguez LM (2003) Randomized study comparing radiofrequency ablation with cryoablation for the treatment of atrial flutter with emphasis on pain perception. Circulation 107:1250–1252

40. Waldo AL, MacLean WA, Karp RB, Kouchoukos NT, James TN (1977) Entrainment and interruption of atrial flutter with atrial pacing: studies in man following open heart surgery. Circulation 56:737–745

41. Wells JL Jr, MacLean WA, James TN, Waldo AL (1979) Characterization of atrial flutter. Studies in man after open heart surgery using fixed atrial electrodes. Circulation 60:665–673

42. Zrenner B, Ndrepepa G, Schneider M, Karch M, Deisenhofer I, Schreieck J, Schomig A, Schmitt C (2000) Basket catheter-guided three-dimensional activation patterns construction and ablation of common type atrial flutter. Pacing Clin Electrophysiol 23:1350–1358

7 Atypical atrial flutter

Sonja Weyerbrock, Isabel Deisenhofer

7.1 Introduction

Atrial flutter with its characteristic sawtooth waves in the inferior ECG leads was first described by Jolie and Ritchie in 1911 [14], but despite its early clinical recognition it was not until recently that major advances have been made in terms of understanding the mechanisms, diagnosis, management and clinical significance of this macroreentrant atrial arrhythmia (see Chapter 6). Thus, the understanding of the typical atrial flutter circuit around the tricuspid valve paved the way for the understanding and subsequent treatment of other forms of macroreentrant atrial arrhythmias, or so-called atypical atrial flutters. As a result of recent advances, there is now a better understanding of the mechanisms of atypical atrial flutter forms and due to new mapping techniques and technologies, atypical atrial flutter has become even more amenable to catheter ablation with remarkable improvement in the acute and long-term success of the invasive therapy of this macroreentrant atrial arrhythmia.

7.2 Definitions

The easiest way to define atypical atrial flutter is its demarcation from typical atrial flutter: Any atrial reentry which does not circle around the tricuspid valve and does not use the cavotricuspid isthmus as a critical zone of slow conduction is called atypical atrial flutter. However, there are three isthmus-dependent atrial flutter forms (lower loop, double wave and intra-isthmus reentry) that are also subsummarized as atypical atrial flutter (see Chapter 7.5.1–7.5.3). Atypical atrial flutter may be divided into right and left atrial reentrant tachycardias, incisional

or macro- and microreentrant arrhythmias, depending on the anatomic location or the electrophysiological substrate of the respective reentrant circuit (Table 7.1).

Atypical atrial flutter typically presents with a variable flutter wave morphology and almost always faster atrial rates (160–220 ms cycle length) compared to typical atrial flutter [7, 25, 27]. Transitions from and to atrial fibrillation are frequent and atypical flutter may occur spontaneously or can be induced in the EP laboratory by atrial pacing maneuvers (burst pacing or programmed) with or without sympathomimetic drugs. Because atypcial atrial flutter does not necessarily depend upon a fixed anatomically defined reentrant pathway or critical isthmus, it is usually described by the anatomic and functional features of the underlying reentrant circuit. Thus, atypical atrial flutter circuits may occur due to macroreentry around larger central barriers such as right free-wall atriotomy incisions, the superior and inferior vena cava or crista terminalis in the right atrium, pulmonary veins or mitral annulus in the left atrium or (with variable locations in both atria)

Table 7.1. Classification of atypical atrial flutter

▮ Right atypical atrial flutter
– Lower loop reentry (LLR) ⎫
– Double wave reentry (DWR) ⎬ isthmus-dependent
– Intra-isthmus reentry (IIR) ⎭
– Upper loop reentry (ULR)
– Scar-related macroreentrant atrial tachycardia (MAT)
– Scar-related MAT without prior cardiac surgery
– Scar-related MAT with prior cardiac surgery
– Complex right atypical atrial flutter
▮ Left atypical atrial flutter
– Left septal atrial flutter
– Perimitral atrial flutter
– Scar- and pulmonary vein-related atrial flutter
– Coronary sinus atrial flutter

around the fossa ovalis or electrically silent areas (scars) of various etiology (e.g., mechanical, infectious or age-related fibrosis). In this perspective, the delineation of the circuit and possible slow conduction areas is indispensable in order to plan the ablation. Ablation lesions should be designed to cut the reentrant circuit by connecting two nonconductive structures with an ideally short line, thus, allowing a relatively easy creation of a complete conduction block in the reentry circuit [35].

7.3 Diagnostic criteria

7.3.1 ECG criteria

Differentiation between typical and atypical flutter solely based on the surface ECG pattern may be difficult and sometimes even misleading. Due to the variability of the flutter wave morphology in different atypical atrial flutter forms, there are no established ECG features distinguishing between right and left atypical atrial flutter. However, a 12-lead surface ECG with clearly visible and synchronously recorded flutter waves is often helpful for further diagnosis. In fact, recent studies by Bochoeyer et al. [1] and Jais et al. [12] demonstrated that in left atypical atrial flutter the flutter (or P) wave in V1 is predominantly positive, often prominent with a large amplitude, and often associated with relatively flat flutter waves in the other leads, especially low-amplitude signals (frequently upright due to predominantly craniocaudal activation) in the inferior leads (II,III, aVF). In addition, in right atrial flutter Bochoeyer et al. [1] also found atypical ECG surface patterns that were cavotricuspid isthmus-dependent and vice versa. However, it has to be kept in mind that in patients with atrial fibrillation and a distinct biatrial activation pattern (e.g., left atrial fibrillation with regular right atrial activation), the surface ECG may present with patterns of coarse atrial fibrillation mimicking other supraventricular tachycardias, especially atrial flutter [17, 22].

7.3.2 Mapping strategies

∎ Entrainment pacing

Successful ablation of atypical atrial flutter depends on exact identification of the responsible reentrant circuit and its critical isthmus. The aim of mapping is to determine the complete reentrant circuit with tracing of the activation throughout the complete cycle length of the tachycardia, in order to define its narrowest, technically accessible areas that could be optimal ablation targets. Kalman et al. [16] described the use of entrainment maneuvers as an essential step in establishing the mechanism and defining the critical zone of conduction for ablation of atypical atrial flutter. They defined atypical atrial flutter as a macroreentrant atrial arrhythmia with a flutter-like surface ECG pattern and an endocardial activation sequence and response to attempted entrainment inconsistent with counterclockwise or clockwise typical atrial flutter [16]. In addition, double and multiple reentry circuits were defined by the presence of more than one activation front that fulfills the above conditions and by demonstration of entrainment of the tachycardia from more than one region in the atria requiring multiple radiofrequency applications.

For clinical practice, entrainment mapping should be performed in all patients at a cycle length of 10 to 30 ms less than the flutter cycle length and concealed entrainment is diagnosed when the difference between the tachycardia cycle length (TCL) and the postpacing interval (PPI) is less than 30 ms with identical intracardiac and surface flutter wave morphology. However, it has to be kept in mind that pacing at very short cycle lengths can induce significant conduction delay within the entrained circuit with prolongation of the postpacing interval within the circuit. Thus, the measurements should always be performed at the longest cycle length capable of entraining the tachycardia. In addition, pacing and entrainment maneuvers should be used sparingly just for the identification of precise areas in the circuit, because it can result in disruption or interruption of the tachycardia with possible noninducibility of the tachycardia or transformation to another flutter circuit, change in cycle length or morphology or may even lead to degeneration of flutter to atrial fibrillation.

Pacing and entrainment maneuvers may be useful not only to distinguish atypical from typical atrial flutter but also in differentiating right from left atypical atrial flutter [2]. Thus, coronary sinus activation often but not always (e.g., septal circuits) proceeds from distal to proximal in left atrial flutter circuits. Even more important, a right atrial atypical flutter circuit can be excluded on the basis of the following right atrial mapping criteria [12, 13]:

▌ Postpacing interval in the right atrium is longer than the tachycardia cycle length by ≥40 ms at ≥3 different sites in the right atrium, including the cavotricuspid isthmus and the right atrial free-wall, but with exception of the septal area due to possible capture of the left atrium

▌ Spontaneous variations of >100 ms in the right atrium with concomitant variations of <20 ms in the left atrium as determined by coronary sinus recording

▌ Right atrial activation time as determined by sequential conventional mapping at ≥8 different sites accounting for <50% of the arrhythmia cycle length according to a reference placed in the coronary sinus

Another possibility is direct mapping of the left atrium via a transseptal approach to demonstrate the reentrant circuit during left atrial atypical flutter using entrainment mapping combined with 3D electroanatomical mapping. However, taking all the observations above into account, it has to be noted that perfect concordance between ECG criteria, the mechanism of the reentrant atrial arrhythmia and its critical isthmus dependence – as assessed by entrainment mapping techniques – does not exist [16].

▌ **New mapping systems**

New mapping approaches such as 3D mapping systems using electroanatomical mapping with the CARTO system (Carto Biosense Webster), EnSite system (Endocardial Solutions), Basket catheters or ultrasound system (Cardiac Pathways) have certainly revolutionized our understanding of macroreentrant circuits in atypical atrial flutter. Due to large experience with 3D mapping systems in atypcial atrial flutter forms, these mapping systems are recommended to be used not only in the absence of understandable flutter circuits but also – due to the complexity of the circuit(s) – in all left atrial flutters as the

first line mapping strategy. In these cases, pacing and entrainment maneuvers should be used only if they are required to improve further understanding of the macroreentrant atrial arrhythmia circuit(s) in order to avoid interruption, noninducibility or transformation to another flutter circuit. A nice example for the successful use of 3D mapping systems is the characterization of scar-related atypical atrial flutter after surgical repair of congenital heart disease. The use of electroanatomical mapping with the Carto system combined with entrainment mapping allowed the identification of conductive "channels" in or between scars [8, 21]. Scars in this context are defined as electrically silent areas with no recordable atrial activity/potential distinguishable from noise (generally voltage amplitude ≤0.03 mV). The density of points has to be high enough – in general ≥80 recorded points per LA or RA map are recommended – in order to allow the understanding of the atrial flutter circuit(s) and to define the precise isthmus(es) as target(s) for successful ablation. Using the atrial electroanatomic maps constructed during the mapping procedures, the macroreentrant atrial circuits could be ablated successfully with a "focal" ablation directed to the conductive channel. Similarly, the use of noncontact mapping simplified the characterization of the reentry circuits in patients with single loop or double loop figure-of-eight right macroreentrant atrial tachycardias and led to precise localization of the free-wall channels and/or crista terminalis gaps with subsequently successful elimination of these arrhythmias by RF ablation scars [33]. However, the use of new 3D mapping systems, especially the electroanatomical Carto mapping, is limited by its reliance on stable rhythms. Thus, in case of nonsustained atrial flutter or the occurrence of variable circuits, new maps have to be performed to identify new and possibly different reentrant circuits.

7.4 Ablation procedure

7.4.1 Ablation strategy

If the mapping procedure leads to a conclusive demonstration of an underlying reentrant circuit, radiofrequency (RF) ablation should be performed by either targeting the critical isthmus and/or the most accessible part of the macroreentrant circuit allowing the best electrode-tissue contact along the desired line. Besides these technical considerations, the possibility of damaging structures such as the phrenic nerve (lateral high RA) or conducting tissue (e.g., sinus and AV node) with an ablation line across a critical isthmus has to be kept in mind, otherwise an alternative ablation site has to be considered. Target sites for successful ablation are identified by early, fragmented or double potentials and by concealed entrainment [9] using conventional mapping techniques. To define the critical isthmus(es) to target, additional guidance by 3D mapping systems can be particularly helpful. The ablation line should either connect two nonconductive structures (e.g., the mitral annulus and a pulmonary vein) and interrupt by this the circuit conduction or it should transect an area critical for the circuit and connect to an anatomic area of block. Lesion continuity can be achieved by progressively pulling back the catheter across the critical isthmus (dragging lesions) to produce stable lesions from one part to the other. The creation of stable RF lesions is best assessed by reduction of the target electrogram amplitude by 80% or splitting into wide double potentials indicating local conduction block.

For RF ablation of atypical atrial flutters, usually conventional large tip RF catheters (8 mm tip; target temperature of 50–55 °C; power limit 50/70 W) are used. More recently, irrigated tip catheters (4 mm tip; target temperature of 45–50 °C; power limit 30–50 W; infusion rate of 30 ml/min) have been used for difficult cases with resistant gaps in the ablation line and/or especially for left atrial atypical flutters [12, 13, 24]. Due to its high efficacy and safety profile, the use of irrigated tip catheters is also helpful in patients with structural heart disease and an enlarged left atrium.

7.4.2 Definition of success

Procedural success is defined as: **1.** termination of atypical atrial flutter, **2.** complete and stable conduction block across the critical tachycardia isthmus, and **3.** non-inducibility of atypical atrial flutter.

Conduction block across the target isthmus is verified by pacing close on either side of the ablation line and demonstration of marked delay and reversal in the direction of activation on the opposite side of the ablation line. In addition, differential pacing (Chapter 6) is a further useful parameter for demonstrating a complete line of block. The absence of any atrial activation and/or demonstration of widely split double potentials on the ablation lesion are also an indicator of complete line of block. Although a residual very slow conduction over the ablation line can not be excluded in all cases, combined fulfillment of the above mentioned criteria will provide good evidence for complete conduction block. The exact site of pacing and recording during pacing maneuvers for confirmation of conduction block is crucial for the reliability of the obtained results. As mentioned above, pacing as well as recording sites should be as close to the ablation line as possible and at least two recording sites – one closer, one more distant to the assumed line of block – should be chosen, to evaluate a complete reversal of activation sequence (activation front from more distant to the line to more close to the line).

Long-term success is assumed, if the targeted atrial flutter morphology and/or intracardiac reentrant activation does not occur anymore without or with previously ineffective antiarrhythmic drugs if they were required for persistent atrial flutter or in case of concomitant occurrence of atrial fibrillation.

7.4.3 Success rate

As a result of new mapping techniques and technologies, atypical atrial flutter has become amenable to catheter ablation with significant improvement in acute and long-term therapy of this macroreentrant atrial arrhythmia. The success rates of RF ablation of right and left atypical atrial flutter in different studies are listed in Table 7.2.

7.4.4 Pre- and postablation management

Since patients with atrial flutter carry the same embolic risk as patients with atrial fibrillation [10], oral anticoagulation is recommended for at least one month prior to the ablation and for 3 to 6 months after the ablation procedure in patients without an additional indication for anticoagulation. Afterwards, ambulatory ECG re-

Table 7.2. Summary of atypical atrial flutter studies

Study	Patients (n)	Structural HD (n/n)	Arrhythmia substrate	Mapping	Acute Success (n/n,%)	Recurrences (n/n,%)	Follow-up (months)
Jais et al. (2000) [13]	22	17/22	LA flutter	Carto	20/22 (91%)	6/22 (27%)	15±7
Delacretaz et al. (2001) [8]	20	20/20	Lesion right MAT	Carto	18/20 (90%)	4/20 (20%)	19±14
Nakagawa et al. (2001) [21]	16	16/16	Lesion right MAT	Carto	16/16 (100%)	3/16 (19%)	13.5
Ouyang et al. (2002) [24]	28	25/28	Left MAT	Carto	25/28 (89%)	4/28 (14%)	14
Della et al. (2002) [9]	19	17/19	Right and left MAT	Conventional	15/19 (79%)	4/19 (21%)	15±10
Tai et al. (2004) [33]	15	5	RA flutter	Noncontact	13/15 (87%)	3/15 (20%)	19±14
Stevenson et al. (2005) [31]	8	0/0	Scar-related right MAT	Carto	7/8 (88%)	2/8 (25%)	20±13

HD heart disease, *LA* left atrium, *MAT* macroreentrant atrial tachycardia, *RA* right atrium, *Carto/Noncontact* 3D mapping systems

cordings should be obtained on a regular basis during follow-up visits either in the outpatient clinic or by the referring physician. Only if these recordings show no relapse of arrhythmia or any other arrhythmia requiring oral anticoagulation, the anticoagulation can be stopped 3 to 6 months after the ablation procedure.

In order to rule out existing left atrial thrombi, it is recommended to perform systematically transesophageal echocardiography prior to the procedure in all patients. Besides this, patients should be monitored by telemetry and ambulatory ECG recordings until discharge.

7.5 Right atypical atrial flutter

7.5.1 Lower loop reentry (Figure 7.1)

▌ **Definition.** Lower loop reentry is defined as an isthmus-dependent atypical atrial flutter with a counterclockwise or less commonly clockwise wave front short-circuiting through the low posterior right atrium around the inferior vena cava with early breakthrough(s) over the crista terminalis [4, 39]. Lower loop reentry can alternate with typical atrial flutter and occurs either spontaneously or after pacing. Due to its activation path with short-circuiting the crista terminalis with simultaneous conduction up the septum and the lateral wall – with subsequently wave front collision over the high lateral right

atrium or the septum – as well as conduction over the cavotricuspid isthmus, the cycle length of lower loop reentry tends to be shorter because of the smaller size of the reentry circuit.

▌ **ECG criteria.** The ECG pattern of lower loop reentry resembles mostly that of typical counterclockwise atrial flutter with flutter (P) waves positive in V1 and negative in the inferior leads, which can be explained by the identical caudocranial wave front direction of both flutter circuits. However, depending on the site of wave front breakthrough(s) over the crista terminalis or in case of multiple cristal breakthroughs, the surface ECG morphology can be different or even unusual [1]. Thus, high cristal breakthroughs can be associated with a clockwise surface ECG pattern (flutter wave positive in inferior leads and negative in V1) due to its craniocaudal activation of the septum and left atrium over Bachmann's bundle. In contrast, the surface ECG morphology in lower loop circuits with multiple cristal breakthroughs is neither consistent with the counterclockwise nor clockwise ECG pattern. Independent of the surface ECG pattern, the cavotricuspid isthmus is defined as central part of all lower loop reentry tachycardias [4, 36, 39] .

▌ **Mapping and ablation strategies.** The isthmus-dependence of the lower loop reentry mechanism can be demonstrated by the presence of concealed entrainment at the isthmus, termination of the tachycardia by cavotricuspid isthmus

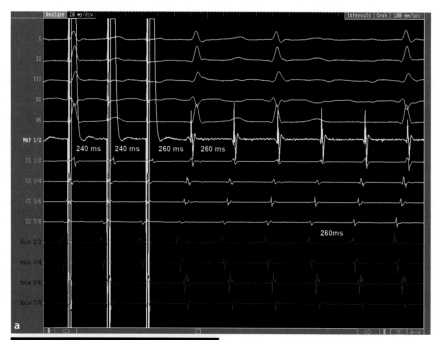

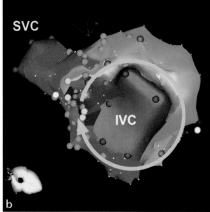

Fig. 7.1. Lower loop reentry (LLR). Patient presenting in our EP lab with sustained atypical atrial flutter several years after mitral valve replacement due to severe mitral regurgitation following chordal rupture. **a** shows simultaneous recordings of 5 surface ECG recordings (I, II, III, V1 and V6) and intracardiac electrograms (MAP, CS and Halo catheter) during atypical atrial flutter with 2:1 to 3:1 conduction (CL 260 ms) while performing an entrainment maneuver from the cavotricuspid isthmus over the MAP catheter. Despite concealed entrainment in the cavotricuspid isthmus the surface ECG morphology does not resemble typical atrial flutter; the flutter wave morphology rather looks unusual (P wave positive in I, biphasic in II/III and almost flat in V1/V6). The intracardiac activation sequence proceeds from distal to proximal on the Halo catheter and from proximal to distal on the CS catheter.

The exact site(s) of cristal breakthrough(s) can not be obtained by conventional mapping because only an 8-pole electrode catheter (Halo) is positioned along the TA (higher cristal break(s) most likely). The corresponding 3D electroanatomical (Carto) map of the right atrium under a modified inferior view (**b**) shows a clockwise direction of activation around the IVC with no participation of activation wave front rotation around the TA. Because the cavotricuspid isthmus is still a necessary part of the reentry circuit, the LLR could be successfully ablated by cavotricuspid isthmus ablation (red tags). *Red tags* ablation sites, *blue tags* double potentials (zones of slow conduction), *brown tags* negative entrainment, *yellow tags* phrenic nerve, *pink tags* tricuspid annulus, *SVC* superior vena cava, annotated as scar (grey surface), *IVC* inferior vena cava, *TA* tricuspid annulus

ablation and lack of inducibility after achievement of bidirectional block.

7.5.2 Double wave reentry

∎ **Definition.** Double wave reentry is characterized by two wave fronts circulating in the same direction in the flutter circuit with both using the cavotricuspid isthmus as its arrhythmia substrate [3]. Double wave reentry is usually nonsustained and may be induced in patients with typical atrial flutter by critically timed atrial premature complexes (APCs) induced in the EP lab resulting in generation of a second wave front during tachycardia. The cycle length of each wave front is approximately 70% of the original flutter cycle length and almost always spontaneously reverts back into single wave typical atrial flutter by block of one wave front in the isthmus.

∎ **ECG criteria.** The ECG pattern of double wave reentry is identical to that of the underlying typical atrial flutter pattern, because the intracardiac activation sequences are identical during acceleration and spontaneous typical atrial flutter. Of note, double wave reentry presents as a more rapid and irregular arrhythmia in comparison to typical atrial flutter.

∎ **Mapping and ablation strategies.** Double wave reentry, if generated by critically timed APCs, usually spontaneously converts into typical atrial flutter or triggers atrial fibrillation. Successful ablation of the cavotricuspid isthmus prevents further occurrence of double wave reentry.

7.5.3 Intra isthmus reentry (IIR)

∎ **Definition.** Intra isthmus reentry is defined as a reentrant circuit within the cavotricuspid isthmus itself, which is bounded by the septal cavotricuspid isthmus and the coronary sinus ostium but without any involvement of the lateral cavotricuspid isthmus [38].

∎ **ECG criteria.** The predominant surface ECG pattern is similar to that of typical counterclockwise atrial flutter, but also clockwise surface ECG patterns or unusual ECG patterns may be seen in patients with IIR. In addition, IIR may present with slower rates in comparison to typical atrial flutter [38].

∎ **Mapping and ablation strategies.** Different intracardiac activation patterns (e.g., simultaneous or near simultaneous activation at the CS and low lateral right atrium) may occur in patients with IIR, but all have several features in common [38], which will further distinguish this reentrant circuit from typical atrial flutter: 1) concealed entrainment from the medial (septal) cavotricuspid isthmus and CS ostium but not from the lateral cavotricuspid isthmus or other right atrial sites along the tricuspid annulus, 2) recording of fractionated and/or double potentials at the cavotricuspid isthmus just outside the CS ostium, which can be entrained. Thus, a linear RF lesion across the septal – not the lateral – cavotricuspid isthmus, where double potentials or fractionated potentials and concealed entrainment can be demonstrated, leads to a cure of IIR.

7.5.4 Upper loop reentry (Figure 7.2)

∎ **Definition.** Upper loop reentry is defined as noncavotricuspid isthmus-dependent atrial flutter with rotation of activation between the tricuspid annulus and superior vena cava (SVC) in the upper portion of the right atrium [36]. Using noncontact 3D mapping, Tai et al. [32, 33] could further delineate the circuit in showing clockwise or less commonly counterclockwise activation around a functional and anatomic central obstacle consisting of the crista terminalis and the SVC. Due to early breakthrough(s) over the lateral annulus during upper loop reentry, wave front collision can be documented over the isthmus or low lateral right atrial wall. Upper loop reentry may occur either spontaneously, by pacing or emerge spontaneously from typical atrial flutter and/or lower loop reentry.

∎ **ECG criteria.** The surface ECG pattern of upper loop reentry resembles either clockwise (flutter (P) wave morphology positive in inferior leads and negative in V1) or less commonly counterclockwise (flutter (P) wave morphology negative in inferior leads and positive in V1) atrial flutter depending on the rotation of the activation front around the SVC.

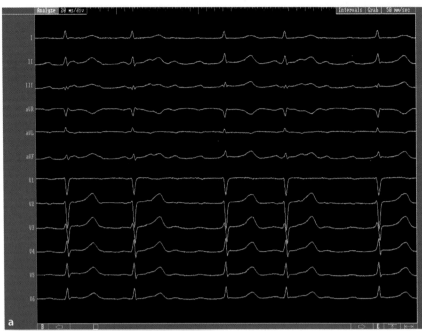

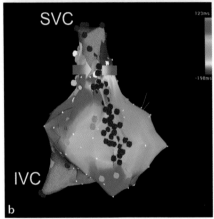

Fig. 7.2. Upper loop reentry (ULR). Upper panel shows a surface ECG in a patient with sustained clockwise ULR several years after cardiac surgery with mitral and aortic valve replacement. Note the positive flutter waves in the inferior leads and slightly negative flutter wave in V1. The lower panel presents the corresponding 3D electroanatomical (Carto) map of the right atrium under a modified posterior-anterior (PA) to lateral projection of the same patient. The activation map shows an 'early-meets-late' zone (colliding of dark red and violet color) with clockwise rotation of the activation front around the SVC. Zones of slow conduction represented by double potentials (blue tags) are located inferolateral (former atriotomy incision). A linear ablation line connecting the SVC to the former atriotomy incision terminated ULR. *Red tags* ablation sites, *blue tags* double potentials, *SVC* superior vena cava, *IVC* inferior vena cava, both annotated as scar (grey surface)

∎ **Mapping and ablation strategies.** Mapping and entrainment maneuvers during reentry should be performed for exact identification of the circuit and critical isthmus. Depending on the cristal breakthrough(s), concealed entrainment can be demonstrated anywhere between the fossa ovalis area and the SVC and/or the inferior vena cava (IVC) [36]. Thus, RF applications connecting the fossa ovalis to the SVC and/or the IVC may result in successful termination of this arrhythmia. However, if a conduction gap along the crista terminalis is found critical for maintenance of this reentrant circuit, linear ablation of the conduction gap in the crista terminalis is effective in eliminating upper loop reentry tachycardia [32].

7.5.5 Scar-related right macroreentrant atrial tachycardia (MAT)

▪ Scar-related (nonincisional) MAT without prior cardiac surgery

▪ **Definition.** Scar-related macroreentrant atrial tachycardia in the absence of a surgical atriotomy represents an unusual cause of multiple macroreentrant atrial tachycardias of different locations, most commonly right atrial free-wall circuits or cavotricuspid isthmus-dependent atrial flutter, which occur due to extensive spontaneous scarring of the right atrium. In most cases, the macroreentry rotates around a free-wall "scar", which is defined as a central obstacle with areas of electrical silence or low-voltage (≤0.03 mV). Accordingly, "channels" of conduction with consistently recorded low amplitude signals between the scars could be identified as the underlying source of this arrhythmia [31]. Interestingly, most patients with scar-related (nonincisional) macroreentrant tachycardia present with more than one tachycardia mechanism and the spontaneous "scarring" occurs independent of the underlying heart disease [26, 29, 31].

▪ **ECG criteria.** Surface ECG morphology in patients with scar-related (nonincisional) macroreentrant atrial tachycardia without prior cardiac surgery varies depending on the presence of preexisting cavotricuspid isthmus block [31]. Thus, in the absence of preexisting cavotricuspid isthmus block, the most common ECG pattern is characterized by inverted (negative) flutter waves in leads V1–V6 with inverted flutter waves in the inferior leads and isoelectric or upright (positive) flutter waves in leads I and aVL. On the other hand, if cavotricuspid isthmus block can be already documented at baseline or occurs following successful isthmus ablation, the most common ECG pattern presents with upright flutter waves in the inferior leads and an inverted or biphasic flutter wave in V1 with transition to upright flutter waves in leads V4–V6.

▪ **Mapping and ablation strategies.** Entrainment and especially 3D electroanatomical mapping are helpful tools not only in identifying the mechanisms of these arrhythmias but also in guiding the successful ablation procedure. However, in case of entrainment maneuvers, it has to be kept in mind that it should be used only cautiously as it carries a risk of termination or change to a different macroreentrant atrial tachycardia, especially due to the fact that difficulties to capture might occur at sites of "scarred" regions in the right atrium. Target sites for linear ablation should be the narrowest identifiable portion of the circuit such as between the posterolateral or lateral "scar areas" and the IVC or the SVC or tricuspid annulus depending on the underlying mechanisms of these arrhythmias. Less commonly a successful "focal" ablation can be achieved between two electrically silent or scarred areas within identified conducting channel(s). Because patients with scar-related (nonincisional) macroreentrant atrial tachycardia without prior cardiac surgery frequently have more than one underlying tachycardia mechanism including possible involvement of the cavotricuspid isthmus, RF ablation of the cavotricuspid isthmus is recommended in all patients without preexisting bidirectional isthmus block, independent of the clinical or presenting tachycardia. Interestingly, these patients also present with a high incidence of sinus node dysfunction with indication to pacemaker implantation most likely due to involvement of the sinoatrial node by extensive spontaneous scaring of the right atrium [31].

▪ Scar-related (incisional) MAT with prior cardiac surgery
(Figures 7.3 and 7.4)

▪ **Definition.** Scar-related incisional macroreentrant atrial tachycardia is a result of previous cardiac surgery in patients with congenital heart disease [15, 21] but may as well occur in patients after valvular surgery [18]. In addition, in some cases the creation of a block secondary to linear catheter ablation may serve as a central obstacle and conduction gaps in the ablation line are often the underlying arrhythmia substrate in these macroreentrant atrial tachycardias [11]. The precise reentry course is determined by the location of the scars and the associated anatomic barriers. The most common reentry loop in patients with arrhythmogenic atriotomy scars after surgical closure of an atrial septal defect (ASD) is cavotricuspid isthmus-dependent atrial flutter, followed by periatriotomy reentrant tachycardia and by far less commonly

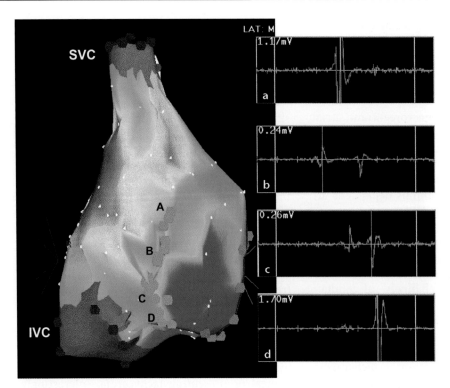

Fig. 7.3. Electroanatomical map of a 'scar' in sinus rhythm. In a modified PA view of a patient with prior cardiac surgery a line of widely split double potentials (blue tags) identifies the scar of the former atriotomy incision. The inserted elec-trogram windows on the right show representative locations (**a–d**) within the scared area. *Blue tags* double potentials, *pink tags* tricuspid annulus, *SVC* superior vena cava, *IVC* inferior vena cava, both annotated as scar (grey surface)

reentry using the prosthetic patch as the central obstacle for its reentrant circuit [34, 41]. Of note, factors predisposing to either cavotricuspid or periatriotomy reentrant circuits are determined by the atriotomy properties [30]. Thus, a posterior atriotomy, a transverse or short atriotomy and a low atriotomy extending to the inferior vena cava predispose to cavotricuspid reentry. On the other hand, periatriotomy reentry is frequently observed if the scar is a relatively long vertical line, however incomplete at the inferior vena cava and anteriorly placed. Patients with complex atrial surgery due to Mustard, Senning or Fontan procedures present with even a wider spectrum of macroreentrant atrial tachycardias depending not only on the extent of surgery within both atria but also on electrical and structural remodeling processes, which will be described in further detail in Chapter 12.

■ ECG criteria. There is no typical surface ECG pattern existing for scar-related or incisional macroreentrant atrial tachycardia. However, be-

cause typical atrial flutter is often associated with periatriotomy reentrant tachycardia – in fact, it is even the most common underlying reentrant circuit in these patients – the ECG pattern often resembles that of typical atrial flutter.

■ Mapping and ablation strategies. Using conventional mapping, the scar can be identified by an area of electrical silence, low voltage electrograms or most commonly a line of widely split double potentials (Figure 7.4). The activation front usually moves in opposite directions on either side of the central obstacle. Entrainment mapping techniques are essential for further identification of the reentrant circuits and for defining the critical isthmus, where wide and often fragmented potentials can be recorded. Thus, isthmuses in the circuit can be found between the IVC and the inferior end of the scar, the SVC and the superior end of the scar, the atriotomy lesion and the tricuspid annulus or even within the scars [21]. The additional use of 3D mapping systems is often helpful for identification and localization of the reentrant circuits

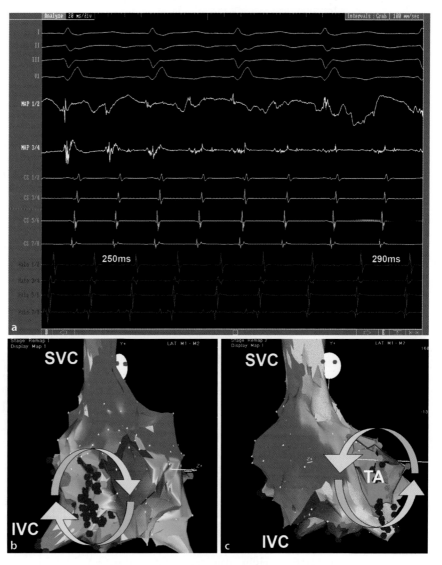

Fig. 7.4. Scar-related (incisional) macroreentrant atrial tachycardia (MAT) with prior cardiac surgery. Patient after surgical closure of an ostium secundum atrial septal defect with a patch, who presented in our EP lab with flutter transformation from atypical atrial flutter around the atriotomy to typical isthmus-dependent atrial flutter during RF ablation. **a** shows simultaneous recordings of four surface ECG recordings (I, II, III and V1) and intracardiac electrograms (MAP, CS and Halo catheter) with sudden prolongation of the flutter cycle length from 250 ms to 290 ms during creation of a linear lesion between the inferior end of the scar (atriotomy) and the IVC. Of note, the flutter waves of the surface ECG did not change in morphology (negative P waves in the inferior leads, positive P wave in V1) during transformation from atypical to typical atrial flutter. **b, c** present the corresponding 3D electroanatomical maps, with clockwise rotation of atypical atrial flutter around the atriotomy (**b** modified right lateral view) and counterclockwise typical atrial flutter (**c** modified AP view). Both flutter types could be successfully ablated by linear ablation from the inferior end of the atriotomy to the IVC and by cavotricuspid isthmus ablation, respectively. *Red tags* ablation sites, *blue tags* double potentials, *SVC* superior vena cava, *IVC* inferior vena cava, both annotated as scar (grey surface), *TA* tricuspid annulus

around scars, especially in the absence of an underlying arrhythmia. Different approaches are proposed for ablation depending on the mechanisms of the macroreentrant circuits:

▮ Reentry circuit around the atriotomy scar: creation of linear lesion(s) between the scar and an anatomic barrier (e.g., inferior vena cava, tricuspid annulus or superior vena cava, the latter with some caveat since the sinus node and/or phrenic nerve are in close proximity)

∎ Reentry circuit(s) within the scar itself: "focal" ablation of isolated, conducting channels.

In order to avoid potential damage of either the right phrenic nerve while performing ablation on the right atrial free wall or of the sinus node during RF applications to the high right atrium, special precautions in terms of ablation site and RF settings have to be taken. Namely maximal output pacing in planned ablation sites to check for phrenic nerve capture and a sinus rhythm electroanatomical map to define the area of sinus node depolarization are helpful to avoid complications. In addition, ablation of the cavotricuspid isthmus should be performed in all patients because typical atrial flutter may occur after initial ablation due to creation of new obstacles.

7.5.6 Complex right atypical atrial flutter

Complex right atrial flutter rhythms usually present with one or more flutter circuits (e.g., single loop or double loop, figure-of-eight reentry) due to multiple transverse breakthroughs at the level of the crista terminalis [40]. Depending on the mode of septal and left atrial activation as well as on the degree of stability of these complex rhythms, the surface ECG pattern usually shows variable flutter wave morphologies. It is also interesting to note that a significantly increased incidence of atrial fibrillation has been demonstrated in right atypical atrial flutter, especially complex right atrial flutter circuits, compared to typical atrial flutter [37]. In case of double or multiple reentry circuits, the presence of more than one activation front can be documented using combined entrainment and 3D mapping, which allows further identification of the reentry mechanisms and permits the precise localization of possible ablation targets or ablation lines [33].

7.6 Left atypical atrial flutter

The presence of underlying heart disease (e.g., cardiomyopathy; mitral valve disease including mitral valve replacement) can be frequently seen in patients with left atypical atrial flutter [12]. If left atrial flutter is suspected by ECG criteria, a distal to proximal coronary sinus activation and/or right atrial mapping criteria (see above), 3D mapping systems should be used as the first line mapping strategy for further identification of underlying flutter circuit(s) and localization of critical isthmus(es) as potential target sites for successful ablation. Due to the risk of transformation of the clinical arrhythmia to another morphology or into atrial fibrillation, additional entrainment maneuvers should be performed only sparingly, if necessary at all. Single, double or even multiple loop circuits could be demonstrated in patients with left macroreentrant atrial tachycardia [12, 24, 28] with rotation around anatomic or functional barriers such as the mitral annulus, pulmonary veins or electrically silent areas or lines of block (characterized by widely separated double potentials), respectively. The presence of electrically silent area(s) – acting either as the central obstacle or lateral barrier depending on the location and underlying reentrant mechanism – is observed relatively often in patients with left atypical atrial flutter [12, 13]. Atrial fibrosis, severe myocardial damage but also scars due to cardiac surgery or secondary to catheter ablation might be responsible for the occurrence of variably located electrically silent areas within the left atrium. Preferred target ablation sites should be the isthmuses shared by more than one circuit, if double or multiple circuits are identified as underlying macroreentrant mechanism(s). Single or linear RF applications across the critical isthmus(es) should be placed between two anatomic barriers or an anatomic barrier and electrically silent area(s) or zone(s) of block, respectively. It has to be kept in mind that interruption of one circuit may lead to another macroreentrant circuit with a different target isthmus. Complete block of the target isthmus(es) can be confirmed by mapping and pacing on either side of the ablation line after successful ablation. The demonstration of widely split double potentials or the absence of electrograms all along the ablation line is a further indicator of a complete line of block. An additional ablation of the cavotricuspid isthmus is further recommended in almost all left atypical atrial flutter circuits in order to avoid confusion with 'pseudo atypical atrial flutter forms' (typical atrial flutter with atypical flutter wave morphology) after successful left atrial flutter ablation [13].

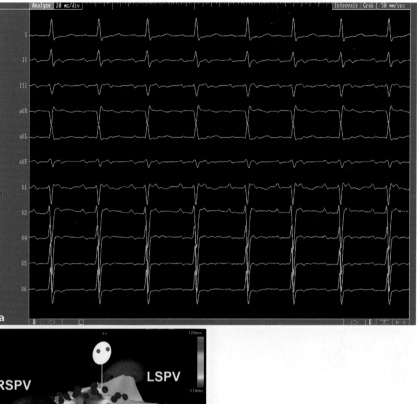

Fig. 7.5. Left septal atrial flutter. Patient with a history of paroxysmal atrial fibrillation in whom left septal atrial flutter occurred after successful isolation of the pulmonary veins. The surface ECG pattern in the upper panel (**a**) shows a large, dominant positive flutter (P) wave in V1 with almost flat or isoelectric flutter waves in the other leads. A septal reentry could be demonstrated by 3D electroanatomical mapping (**b** modified AP view) and the flutter circuit terminated by creation of a linear ablation from the right superior pulmonary vein to the mitral annulus. *Red tags* ablation sites, *blue tags* double potentials, *pink tags* mitral annulus, *PV* pulmonary vein, *LSPV* left superior PV, *RSPV* right superior PV, *RIPV* right inferior PV, *MA* mitral annulus

7.6.1 **Left septal atrial flutter** (Figure 7.5)

▌ **Definition.** Left septal atrial flutter is characterized by counterclockwise or clockwise rotation around the fossa ovalis which serves as central barrier. The circuit involves the left atrial septum with the right superior and/or inferior pulmonary veins as posterior and the mitral annulus as anterior functional barrier(s) [1, 19].

▌ **ECG criteria.** The surface ECG pattern shows typically a large, dominant positive flutter (P) wave in V1 with almost flat or isoelectric flutter waves in the other leads.

▌ **Mapping and ablation strategies.** Coronary sinus activation from distal to proximal is not always present in septal circuits. However, using entrainment combined with 3D mapping allows for identification of the target isthmus(es) in

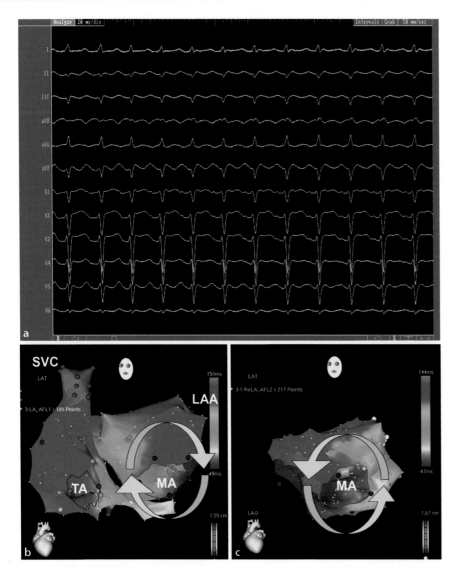

Fig. 7.6. Peri-mitral atrial flutter. Patient presenting with peri-mitral atrial flutter several months after PV isolation for paroxysmal atrial fibrillation. The 12-lead surface ECG (**a**) shows atypical atrial flutter (positive P waves in V1/V2 accompanied by diminished flutter (P) waves in the inferior leads) with 2:1 conduction. The electroanatomical map of both atria and the coronary sinus (**b**) and the left atrium alone (**c**) in a modified LAO view shows a reentry around the mitral valve (MA) with either clockwise (left lower panel) or counterclockwise (right lower panel) rotation around the annulus (round arrows). The right atrium is activated passively via the coronary sinus, in which activation spreads from distally to proximally. The reentrant tachycardia stopped after cycle length prolongation by drawing a "left isthmus line" from the ostium of the left inferior PV to the lateral mitral annulus. *MA* mitral annulus, *TA* tricuspid annulus, *LAA* left atrial appendage, *SVC* superior vena cava, annotated as scar (grey surface)

left septal circuits. Thus, linear ablation should be performed in the critical isthmus between the fossa ovalis and right pulmonary vein(s) or mitral annulus, respectively, where concealed entrainment is demonstrable.

7.6.2 Perimitral atrial flutter
(Figures 7.6 and 7.7)

▐ **Definition.** Perimitral atrial flutter presents with either clockwise or counterclockwise rotation around the mitral annulus and may occur either as a single loop reentry or as part of a double or multiple loop reentry circuit.

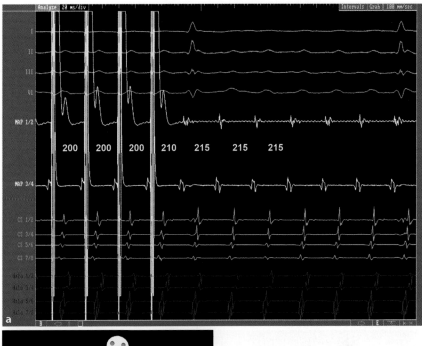

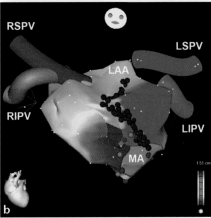

Fig. 7.7. Perimitral atrial flutter. Patient with perimitral atrial flutter 8 months after successful cavotricuspid isthmus ablation for typical atrial flutter. **a** shows simultaneous recordings of four surface ECG recordings (I, II, III and V1) and intracardiac electrograms (MAP, CS and Halo catheter) during atypical atrial flutter with 3:1 to 6:1 conduction (CL 215 ms) while performing an entrainment maneuver from the anterior mitral annulus over the MAP catheter. A prominent, positive P wave is seen in V1 accompanied by flat positive P waves in leads I–III. Of note is also, that the coronary sinus activation proceeds from proximal to distal and that the earliest atrial activation is seen almost simultaneously on CS 7/8 and Halo 7/8. Concealed entrainment from the anterior mitral annulus (but also from lateral and inferior MA (not shown) verifies the diagnosis of perimitral atrial flutter. The electroanatomical map of the left atrium (**b**) in a modified LAO view shows a counterclockwise reentry around the mitral valve (MA), which could be successfully ablated by creating an anterior lesion from the anterior MA to the base of the left atrial appendage (LAA). **b** *Red tags* ablation sites, **b** *green tags* positive entrainment points, *light red tags* mitral annulus, *MA* mitral annulus, *LAA* left atrial appendage, *PV* pulmonary vein, *LSPV* left superior PV, *LIPV* left inferior PV, *RSPV* right superior PV, *RIPV* right inferior PV

∎ **ECG criteria.** The surface ECG pattern shows prominent, positive P waves in V1/V2 accompanied by diminished or multiphasic flutter (P) waves in the inferior leads [1].

∎ **Mapping and ablation strategies.** In perimitral atrial flutter, concealed entrainment can be often documented from both the mitral annulus and the coronary sinus. Depending on the critical isthmus(es), successful ablation can be

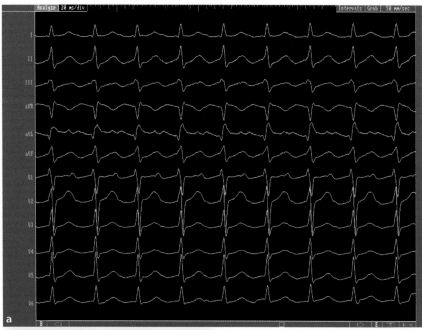

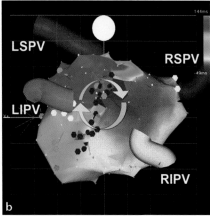

Fig. 7.8. Posterior wall 'scar' circuit. Left atypical atrial flutter with a posterior wall 'scar' circuit occurred secondary to circumferential left atrial catheter ablation for paroxysmal atrial fibrillation. The surface ECG pattern (**a**) shows atypical atrial flutter (positive P wave in V1) with 2:1 conduction. The PA view (**b**) of the 3D electroanatomical map shows a spreading of activation in a clockwise direction on the posterior wall of the left atrium (arrows). This reentrant circuit is most probably related to gaps in the posterior wall part of the for-merly applied ablation line encircling the left-sided PVs. Entrainment mapping confirmed the diagnosis (brown tags) and successful ablation could be achieved by linear ablation connecting the inferior and superior gap on the posterior wall of the LA. *Red tags* ablation sites, *blue tags* double potentials, *brown tags* positive entrainment points, *pink tags* mitral annulus, *LA* left atrium, *PV* pulmonary vein, *LSPV* left superior PV, *LIPV* left inferior PV, *RSPV* right superior PV, *RIPV* right inferior PV

achieved by dragging a line connecting the mitral annulus to an anatomic barrier such as a pulmonary vein (e.g., the left isthmus between the mitral annulus and the left inferior pulmonary vein) or to electrically silent areas variably located within the left atrium.

7.6.3 Scar- and pulmonary vein-related atrial flutter

∎ **Posterior wall 'scar' circuits** (Figure 7.8)

∎ **Definition.** Posterior wall 'scar' circuits are characterized by macroreentry propagating around low voltage or scarred areas located over the left atrial posterior wall. Atrial fibrosis or atrial myopathy but also scars due to cardiac surgery or secondary to left atrial catheter ablation might be responsible for the occurrence of these electrically silent areas/zones of block within the posterior wall of the left atrium. Interestingly, comparing locations of silent areas within the left atrium, most of them are posteriorly located [13].

■ **ECG criteria.** The surface ECG pattern is variable and might be even sometimes mimicking typical counterclockwise atrial flutter. However, the occurrence of low-amplitude signals in the inferior leads and a prominent, positive voltage in lead 1 is suggestive of posterior wall 'scar' circuits [1].

■ **Mapping and ablation strategies.** Using conventional mapping, the 'scar' can be identified by an area of electrical silence, low voltage electrograms or a line of double potentials. After verifying posterior wall 'scar' circuits by entrainment combined with 3D mapping, the circuits can be interrupted by connecting the 'scars' to either the right or left pulmonary veins or to the posterior mitral annulus.

■ **Peripulmonary vein (PV) circuits** (Figures 7.9)

■ **Definition.** Peri-PV circuits may present as single and/or double loop reentrant circuits rotating around one or more ipsilateral PV. Atrial tissue between the PV(s) but also gaps in ablation line(s) following left atrial ablation for atrial fibrillation [6, 20] may serve as underlying arrhythmia substrate for potential peri-PV circuits.

■ **ECG criteria.** Peri-PV circuits demonstrate with variable surface ECG patterns depending on the location (e.g., left versus right PVs) of these arrhythmias and the activation spreading pattern in a LA potentially transected by linear lesions.

■ **Mapping and ablation strategies.** For identification of peri-PV circuits and their critical isthmus(es), 3D mapping should be used. Depending on the location of the peri-PV circuits successful ablation can be achieved by joining the PV to the mitral annulus and/or to the contralateral superior PV across the roof of the left atrium.

7.6.4 Coronary sinus atrial flutter

■ **Definition.** Atypical atrial flutter within the coronary sinus (CS) is defined by a macroreentrant atrial tachycardia involving the myocardium of CS as a critical component of its circuit [23]. This special form of atypical atrial flutter might occur in up to 25% of patients after left atrial circumferential ablation for atrial fibrillation [5].

■ **ECG criteria.** The most common surface ECG pattern seen in patients with atypical atrial flutter involving the coronary sinus shows positive flutter (P) wave morphology in V1 and the inferior leads concomitant with an isoelectric flutter wave in lead 1 and negative flutter wave in aVL [5].

■ **Mapping and ablation strategies.** Using entrainment mapping techniques, the CS should be considered as part of the reentrant circuit if the postpacing interval in the CS is within 25 ms of the tachycardia cycle length. Based on entrainment and/or activation mapping using an electroanatomical mapping system, the target site for successful ablation should be either the proximal, mid or distal CS. RF delivery within the CS or its branches is highly effective but should be used with caution. In our experience, use of an irrigated tip catheter, which should be limited to 25 W/43 °C maximum power and temperature, respectively, lowers the potential risks of any complications, such as damage to the coronary arteries (mainly RCA and/or LCx) as well as esophagus and/or CS perforation or stenosis, to an acceptable level.

7.7 Conclusion

Atypical atrial flutter represents a large variety of macroreentrant atrial tachycardias utilizing flutter circuits in both the right and the left atrium. The combined use of 3D mapping and entrainment pacing provides insight into the course of the reentrant circuit(s) and facilitates the identification of the critical isthmus(es) as potential ablation targets. Thus, atypical atrial flutter has become amenable to catheter ablation with remarkable improvement in the acute and long-term efficacy of this therapy for this macroreentrant atrial arrhythmia.

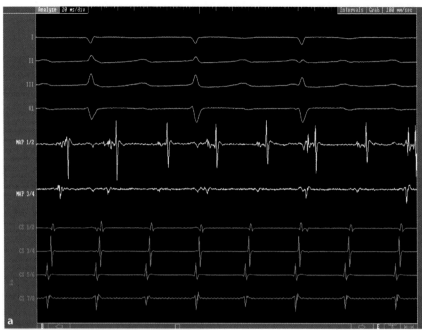

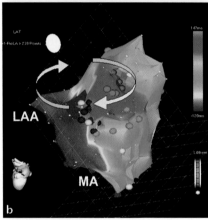

Fig. 7.9. Peripulmonary vein (PV) circuit. Patient with peri-PV circuit around the left PVs after circumferential PV ablation for paroxysmal atrial fibrillation. **a** shows simultaneous recordings of four surface ECG recordings (I, II, III and V1) and intracardiac electrograms (MAP, CS catheter) during 2:1 atypical atrial flutter. Note the fractionated potentials on the mapping catheter while mapping an area between the left PV and the LAA. **b** presents the corresponding 3D electro-anatomical map in a modified left lateral view of the left atrium, where the ostia of the LSPV and LIPV are marked with green and purple tags, respectively. A reentry with a clockwise activation front around the LSPV could be demonstrated and the ablation was orientated to the critical isthmus of this reentry. *Red tags* ablation sites, *blue tags* double potentials, *brown tags on ablation line* positive entrainment, *bright red tags* mitral annulus (MA), *LAA* left atrial appendage, *green tags* LSPV (left superior PV), *purple tags* LIPV (left inferior PV)

■ References

1. Bochoeyer A, Yang Y, Cheng J, Lee RJ, Keung EC, Marrouche NF, Natale A, Scheinman MM (2003) Surface electrocardiographic characteristics of right and left atrial flutter. Circulation 108:60–66
2. Chang KC, Lin YC, Chou HT, Hung JS (2000) Electrophysiologic characteristics and ablation of an atypical atrial flutter in the right atrium. J Cardiovasc Electrophysiol 11:334–338
3. Cheng J, Scheinman MM (1998) Acceleration of typical atrial flutter due to double-wave reentry induced by programmed electrical stimulation. Circulation 97:1589–1596
4. Cheng J, Cabeen WR, Jr., Scheinman MM (1999) Right atrial flutter due to lower loop reentry: mechanism and anatomic substrates. Circulation 99:1700–1705
5. Chugh A, Oral H, Good E, Han J, Tamirisa K, Lemola K, Elmouchi D, Tschopp D, Reich S, Igic P, Bogun F, Pelosi F, Jr., Morady F (2005) Catheter ablation of atypical atrial flutter and atrial tachycardia within the coronary sinus after left atrial ablation for atrial fibrillation. J Am Coll Cardiol 46:83–91
6. Chugh A, Oral H, Lemola K, Hall B, Cheung P, Good E, Tamirisa K, Han J, Bogun F, Pelosi F, Jr., Morady F (2005) Prevalence, mechanisms, and clinical significance of macroreentrant atrial tachycardia during and following left atrial ablation for atrial fibrillation. Heart Rhythm 2:464–471
7. Cosio FG, Martin-Penato A, Pastor A, Nunez A, Goicolea A (2003) Atypical flutter: a review. Pacing Clin Electrophysiol 26:2157–2169
8. Delacretaz E, Ganz LI, Soejima K, Friedman PL, Walsh EP, Triedman JK, Sloss LJ, Landzberg MJ, Stevenson WG (2001) Multi atrial macro-reentry circuits in adults with repaired congenital heart disease: entrainment mapping combined with three-dimensional electroanatomic mapping. J Am Coll Cardiol 37:1665–1676
9. Della BP, Fraticelli A, Tondo C, Riva S, Fassini G, Carbucicchio C (2002) Atypical atrial flutter: clinical features, electrophysiological characteristics and response to radiofrequency catheter ablation. Europace 4:241–253
10. Gallagher MM, Hennessy BJ, Edvardsson N, Hart CM, Shannon MS, Obel OA, Al-Saady NM, Camm AJ (2002) Embolic complications of direct current cardioversion of atrial arrhythmias: association with low intensity of anticoagulation at the time of cardioversion. J Am Coll Cardiol 40:926–933
11. Haissaguerre M, Jais P, Shah DC, Gencel L, Pradeau V, Garrigues S, Chouairi S, Hocini M, Le Metayer P, Roudaut R, Clementy J (1996) Right and left atrial radiofrequency catheter therapy of paroxysmal atrial fibrillation. J Cardiovasc Electrophysiol 7:1132–1144
12. Jais P, Shah DC, Haissaguerre M, Hocini M, Peng JT, Takahashi A, Garrigue S, Le Metayer P, Clementy J (2000) Mapping and ablation of left atrial flutters. Circulation 101:2928–2934
13. Jais P, Hocini M, Weerasoryia R, Macle L, Scavee C, Raybaud F, Shah DC, Clementy J, Haissaguerre M (2002) Atypical left atrial flutters. Card Electrophysiol Rev 6:371–377
14. Jolly WA, Ritchie WT (2003) Auricular flutter and fibrillation. 1911. Ann Noninvasive Electrocardiol 8:92–96
15. Kalman JM, VanHare GF, Olgin JE, Saxon LA, Stark SI, Lesh MD (1996) Ablation of 'incisional' reentrant atrial tachycardia complicating surgery for congenital heart disease. Use of entrainment to define a critical isthmus of conduction. Circulation 93:502–512
16. Kalman JM, Olgin JE, Saxon LA, Lee RJ, Scheinman MM, Lesh MD (1997) Electrocardiographic and electrophysiologic characterization of atypical atrial flutter in man: use of activation and entrainment mapping and implications for catheter ablation. J Cardiovasc Electrophysiol 8:121–144
17. Karch MR, Ndrepepa G, Schneider MA, Weber S, Schreieck J, Schmitt C (2003) Single chamber atrial fibrillation involving only the left atrium: implications for maintenance and radiofrequency ablation therapy. Pacing Clin Electrophysiol 26:883–891
18. Markowitz SM, Brodman RF, Stein KM, Mittal S, Slotwiner DJ, Iwai S, Das MK, Lerman BB (2002) Lesional tachycardias related to mitral valve surgery. J Am Coll Cardiol 39:1973–1983
19. Marrouche NF, Natale A, Wazni OM, Cheng J, Yang Y, Pollack H, Verma A, Ursell P, Scheinman MM (2004) Left septal atrial flutter: electrophysiology, anatomy, and results of ablation. Circulation 109:2440–2447
20. Mesas CE, Pappone C, Lang CC, Gugliotta F, Tomita T, Vicedomini G, Sala S, Paglino G, Gulletta S, Ferro A, Santinelli V (2004) Left atrial tachycardia after circumferential pulmonary vein ablation for atrial fibrillation: electroanatomic characterization and treatment. J Am Coll Cardiol 44:1071–1079
21. Nakagawa H, Shah N, Matsudaira K, Overholt E, Chandrasekaran K, Beckman KJ, Spector P, Calame JD, Rao A, Hasdemir C, Otomo K, Wang Z, Lazzara R, Jackman WM (2001) Characterization of reentrant circuit in macroreentrant right atrial tachycardia after surgical repair of congenital heart disease: isolated channels between scars allow "focal" ablation. Circulation 103:699–709
22. Ndrepepa G, Zrenner B, Schreieck J, Karch MR, Schneider MA, Schomig A, Schmitt C (2000)

Left atrial fibrillation with regular right atrial activation and a single left-to-right electrical interatrial connection: multisite mapping of dissimilar atrial rhythms. J Cardiovasc Electrophysiol 11:587–592

23. Olgin JE, Jayachandran JV, Engesstein E, Groh W, Zipes DP (1998) Atrial macroreentry involving the myocardium of the coronary sinus: a unique mechanism for atypical flutter. J Cardiovasc Electrophysiol 9:1094–1099

24. Ouyang F, Ernst S, Vogtmann T, Goya M, Volkmer M, Schaumann A, Bansch D, Antz M, Kuck KH (2002) Characterization of reentrant circuits in left atrial macroreentrant tachycardia: critical isthmus block can prevent atrial tachycardia recurrence. Circulation 105:1934–1942

25. Ricard P, Imianitoff M, Yaici K, Coutelour JM, Bergonzi M, Rinaldi JP, Saoudi N (2002) Atypical atrial flutters. Europace 4:229–239

26. Sanders P, Morton JB, Davidson NC, Spence SJ, Vohra JK, Sparks PB, Kalman JM (2003) Electrical remodeling of the atria in congestive heart failure: electrophysiological and electroanatomic mapping in humans. Circulation 108:1461–1468

27. Scheinman MM, Cheng J, Yang Y (1999) Mechanisms and clinical implications of atypical atrial flutter. J Cardiovasc Electrophysiol 10:1153–1157

28. Schmitt C, Ndrepepa G, Zrenner B (2001) Reentry circuit location and left atrial three-dimensional activation patterns in left atrial flutter. Z Kardiol 90:292–296

29. Schreieck J, Zrenner B, Dong J, Ndrepepa G, Schmitt C (2002) Dissimilar atrial rhythms: coexistence of reentrant atrial tachycardia, atrioventricular nodal reentrant tachycardia and interatrial conduction block. Z Kardiol 91:68–73

30. Shah DC JP, Hocini M (2002) Catheter ablation of atypical right atrial flutter. Catheter ablation of Arrhythmias, 2nd Edition. Futura Inc., Armonk, NY

31. Stevenson IH, Kistler PM, Spence SJ, Vohra JK, Sparks PB, Morton JB, Kalman JM (2005) Scar-related right atrial macroreentrant tachycardia in patients without prior atrial surgery: electroanatomic characterization and ablation outcome. Heart Rhythm 2:594–601

32. Tai CT, Huang JL, Lin YK, Hsieh MH, Lee PC, Ding YA, Chang MA, Chen SA (2002) Noncontact three-dimensional mapping and ablation of upper loop reentry originating in the right atrium. J Am Coll Cardiol 40:746–753

33. Tai CT, Liu TY, Lee PC, Lin YJ, Chang MS, Chen SA (2004) Non-contact mapping to guide radiofrequency ablation of atypical right atrial flutter. J Am Coll Cardiol 44:1080–1086

34. Weyerbrock S, Zrenner B, Dong J, Deisenhofer I, Schreieck J, Schmitt C (2005) Mapping und Ablation atrialer Tachyarrhythmien nach operativem Verschluss eines Vorhofseptumdefektes. Z Kardiol 94 (Suppl 1):V971

35. Wu RC, Berger R, Calkins H (2002) Catheter ablation of atrial flutter and macroreentrant atrial tachycardia. Curr Opin Cardiol 17:58–64

36. Yang Y, Cheng J, Bochoeyer A, Hamdan MH, Kowal RC, Page R, Lee RJ, Steiner PR, Saxon LA, Lesh MD, Modin GW, Scheinman MM (2001) Atypical right atrial flutter patterns. Circulation 103:3092–3098

37. Yang Y, Mangat I, Glatter KA, Cheng J, Scheinman MM (2003) Mechanism of conversion of atypical right atrial flutter to atrial fibrillation. Am J Cardiol 91:46–52

38. Yang Y, Varma N, Keung EC, Scheinman MM (2005) Reentry within the cavotricuspid isthmus: an isthmus dependent circuit. Pacing Clin Electrophysiol 28:808–818

39. Zhang S YG, Hariharan R, Ho J, Yang Y, Ip J, Thakur RK, Seger J, Scheinman MM, Cheng (2004) Lower loop reentry as a mechanism of clockwise right atrial flutter. Circulation 109: 1630–1635

40. Zrenner B, Ndrepepa G, Schneider M, Karch M, Hofmann F, Schomig A, Schmitt C (1999) Computer-assisted animation of atrial tachyarrhythmias recorded with a 64-electrode basket catheter. J Am Coll Cardiol 34:2051–2060

41. Zrenner B, Ndrepepa G, Schneider MA, Karch MR, Brodherr-Heberlein S, Kaemmerer H, Hess J, Schomig A, Schmitt C (2001) Mapping and ablation of atrial arrhythmias after surgical correction of congenital heart disease guided by a 64-electrode basket catheter. Am J Cardiol 88: 573–578

8 Focal atrial tachycardia

CLAUS SCHMITT, ALEXANDER PUSTOWOIT, MICHAEL SCHNEIDER

Focal atrial tachycardias are a relative rare rhythm disorder, seen in less than 10% of electrophysiological studies. In general, two types of atrial tachycardias can be defined based on their electrophysiological mechanisms [33]:

- Focal atrial tachycardia (due to an automatic, triggered, or microreentrant mechanism)
- Macroreentrant atrial tachycardia (including typical isthmus-dependent atrial flutter) and other macroreentrant tachycardia (in the right and left atrium).

This chapter concentrates on focal mechanisms although in some instances a clear distinction between a circumscribed reentrant circuit and a focal pattern of atrial activation cannot be made.

8.1 Definition

Focal atrial tachycardia is due to an automatic, triggered or microreentrant mechanism [3].

- Enhanced (or abnormal) automaticity cannot be initiated or terminated by programmed electrical stimulation. It cannot be entrained but it may be transiently suppressed with atrial overdrive stimulation but will resume with a gradual increase in rate. It usually can be elicited by administration of intravenous isoproterenol. A classical phenomenon is "warming up" and "cooling down" of the arrhythmia.
- Triggered activity is clinically less well characterized. It can be initiated and terminated by pacing but no entrainment is found. Tachycardia initiation is cycle length dependent. Verapamil and adenosine may suppress triggered activity.
- Atrial tachycardias based on microreentrant mechanisms are inducible by techniques of

programmed electrical stimulation and are circumscribed to small areas of scar or fibrosis. In these regions, entrainment stimulation may be possible. It may respond to adenosine.

On clinical grounds these distinctions are not very helpful. The electrophysiological characteristics of focal atrial tachycardia are based on accepted criteria [26]:

- Radial spreading in all directions from a single site of earliest activation
- Range of activation less than the tachycardia cycle length (in macroreentrant tachycardia it would span over the whole tachycardia cycle length)
- Elimination of atrial tachycardia by focal ablation at the site of earliest activation.

Focal atrial tachycardias may be unifocal or multifocal (10%) and may have confusing electrocardiographic features. Posteroseptal atrial tachycardia may mimic fast-slow AV nodal reentrant tachycardia or AV reentrant tachycardia involving an accessory bypass tract, e.g., permanent junctional reentry tachycardia. The atrial rate is less than 250 beats per minute with an isoelectric baseline between P waves (in contrast to atrial flutter). They occur with and without structural heart disease and can be incessant or paroxysmal. The following electrophysiological criteria are used to make a diagnosis of focal atrial tachycardia:

- P wave configuration different from that of sinus rhythm (for clarification of P wave morphology brief ventricular pacing (Figure 8.1) or intravenous adenosine may be helpful)
- Occurrence of tachycardia independent of critical atrial-His interval
- Spontaneous termination in the absence of AV block

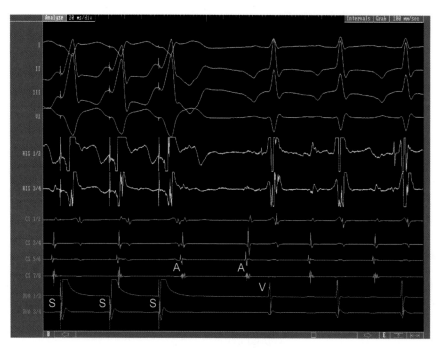

Fig. 8.1. Brief right ventricular stimulation (S) to clarify P wave morphology. After cessation of pacing, the onset of the P wave in lead I can clearly be delineated

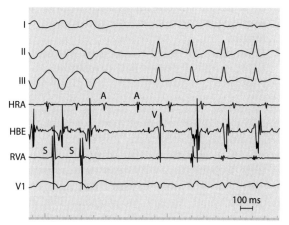

Fig. 8.2. The response to ventricular pacing with 1:1 ventriculoatrial conduction during tachycardia in a patient with atrial tachycardia. Shown are the leads I, II, III and V1 and the intracardiac electrograms recorded at the high right atrium (HRA), His bundle electrogram (HBE) and the right ventricular apex (RVA). The tachycardia cycle length is 260 ms. Ventricular pacing at a cycle length of 230 ms results in 1:1 ventriculoatrial conduction. The electrogram response upon cessation of ventricular pacing is atrial-atrial-ventricle (A-A-V). From Knight et al. [4] with permission

▮ Upon cessation of ventricular pacing with a cycle length shorter than the tachycardia cycle length and retrograde capture of the atria an "A-A-V" response [21] occurs (Figure 8.2).

This is highly sensitive and specific and virtually diagnostic of atrial tachycardia [31]. The atrioventricular node is refractory for anterograde conduction for the last retrograde atrial complex (resulting from ventricular pacing) leading to an "A-A-V" response.

▮ In case of VA conduction, the atrial activation sequence is different from that of the tachycardia

▮ A variable VA relationship during tachycardia. In AVNRT or AVRT, the VA interval is fixed as this retrograde limb is an integral part of the reentry circuit.

▮ VA dissociation (Figure 8.3) during ventricular pacing. The inability to capture the atria retrogradely during ongoing tachycardia had a positive predictive value of 80% for atrial tachycardia [31].

▮ Exclusion of accessory pathways, AV nodal reentrant tachycardia. Positive P waves in inferior leads (inferior P wave axis) excludes AVNRT and AVRT because this suggests a superior origin of an atrial tachycardia. A potential exception is the retrograde limb of an anteroseptal bypass tract which may result in an inferior P wave axis. Negative P waves in the inferior leads (superior P wave axis) and a long R-P interval occur in atypical AVNRT and a concealed bypass tract with a slow ret-

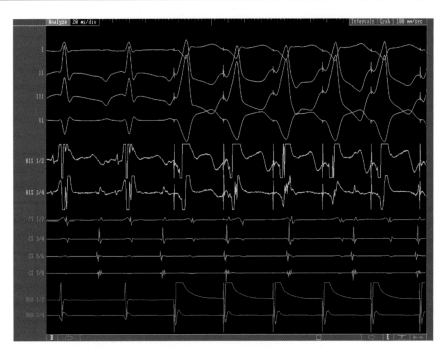

Fig. 8.3. VA dissociation during ventricular pacing. Independent atrial activation sequence despite ventricular pacing

rograde conduction. In the latter condition advancement of the atrial complex during His bundle refractoriness proves the presence of an accessory pathway. The diagnosis of atypical AVNRT is favored by dual retrograde conduction properties and inducibility of the arrhythmia with ventricular pacing (see Chapter 5).

Termination of tachycardia after intravenous adenosine administration unfortunately does not allow differentiation between AV nodal reentrant tachycardias and tachycardias with a focal mechanism [11, 15]. The majority of focal tachycardias, especially those with a septal origin, will terminate after a bolus of intravenous adenosine; however, block between the atrium and His makes a diagnosis of tachycardias dependent on AV conduction more likely.

To what extent focal tachycardia is a precursor of focal atrial fibrillation or a distinct clinical problem is discussed controversially. Currently there is more evidence for the concept that focal atrial tachycardia is a different entity as ablation of focal atrial tachycardia may not prevent atrial fibrillation in patients with a prior history of both arrhythmias [19, 30].

8.2 Electrocardiographic features

Focal atrial tachycardia occurs from the right and left atrium. Preferential sites of origin in the right atrium are the crista terminalis, the tricuspid annulus, the coronary sinus ostium and less common the right atrial appendage, the parahisian region and the junction with the superior vena cava. In the left atrium, the region of the pulmonary veins, the mitral annulus and less common the left atrial septum, the left atrial roof and left atrial appendage are preferential sites of origin. Before planing catheter ablation, the analysis of P wave morphology is very helpful to guide the electrophysiological procedure (Figure 8.4). The most helpful ECG leads are aVL and V1 in distinguishing right from left atrial foci [18, 38, 39, 42]:

▪ A *positive or biphasic P wave in aVL* is most likely associated with a RA focus (sensitivity of 88%, specificity of 79%) [18]
▪ A *positive P wave in V1* is closely associated with a LA focus (sensitivity 93%, specificity 88%) [18].

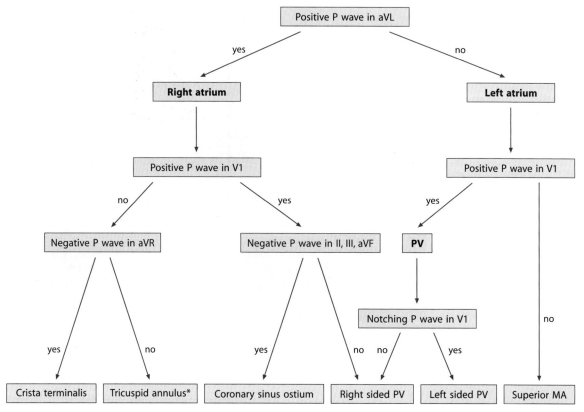

Fig. 8.4. Simplified algorithm for determination of origin of focal atrial tachycardia by P wave morphology. (*) Deep negative P waves in II, III, aVF and V1 are typically seen in atrial tachycardias arising from the inferoanterior tricuspid ring. *MA* mitral annulus

8.3 Catheter ablation

Catheter ablation of focal atrial tachycardias is challenging because there is a wide variety of possible sites of origin [1, 4]. The reliability of the proposed ECG algorithms has limitations; thus, one should always be prepared for a transseptal left-sided approach especially in situations where a high crista terminalis or a septal origin is presumed. P wave onset can be masked by the superimposed QRS and T waves. Even after intracardiac mapping, there is sometimes uncertainty about a left or right atrial origin. As a general rule one has to consider a left-sided origin if the earliest right atrial signal precedes the P wave by less than 20 ms. If this is the case in the region of typical interatrial connections along the interatrial septum, a left-sided origin of the focus is highly likely. Typical interatrial connections are the Bachmann's bundle (high anteroseptal), the fossa ovalis (mid posterior) and the coronary sinus ostium (low

posterior). The situation is further complicated by the fact that there are distinct muscle bridges between the posterior left atrium and the intercaval area of the right atrium as described by Ho et al. [12]. Recent work from our group [6] confirmed that posterior interatrial connections to the intercaval area play a major role in interatrial electrical propagation during pulmonary vein tachycardias, sometimes mimicking a right atrial tachycardia (Figure 8.5).

Various approaches have been tried to improve the efficacy of radiofrequency catheter ablation. A standard approach uses a multipolar Halo catheter along the tricuspid ring, a catheter to record the His bundle electrogram, a multipolar coronary sinus catheter and a roving catheter. A distal to proximal activation along the CS catheter clearly implies a left-sided origin. However, a proximal to distal activity in the CS catheter (Figure 8.8) does not exclude a left-sided origin (e.g., a focus in the right pulmonary veins or a focus at the anterior mitral ring).

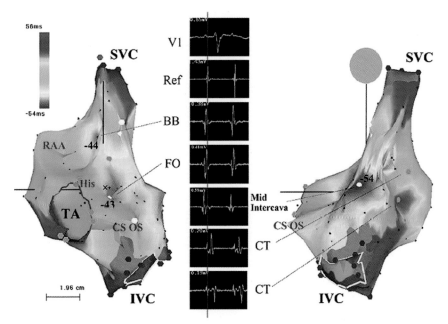

Fig. 8.5. Multiple right atrium (RA) breakthrough sites in a patient with a focal tachycardia originating from deep inside the right superior pulmonary vein. Carto activation map of the RA in left lateral view (left) and posteroanterior view (right) shows a posterior breakthrough at the midintercaval area preceding two other breakthrough sites at the high RA: the presumed insertion site of the Bachmann bundle (BB) and the fossa ovalis (FO), respectively. Bipolar potentials recorded from the breakthrough site at the mid intercaval area are discrete and sharp, indicating local potential rather than far field potentials from the left atrium. Double potentials (blue tags) recorded from posterolateral RA indicates the crista terminalis (CT). Red indicates earliest activation; purple indicates latest activation. Numbers indicate the local activation time (in milliseconds) relative to the reference catheter (Ref) placed in the coronary sinus. *CS OS* coronary sinus ostium, *His* His bundle position, *IVC* inferior vena cava, *RAA* right atrial appendage, *SVC* superior vena cava, *TA* tricuspid annulus. From Dong et al. [17] with permission

Another approach uses a crista terminalis catheter. This looks like a "C" along the posterolateral right atrium and picks up electrical activity between the border of smooth and the trabeculated right atrium, a preferential site of RA foci. Further approaches are the deployment of multipolar basket catheters (Figure 8.6) [32, 34, 37] or the use of the noncontact mapping technique (Figure 8.7) [10, 35, 36].

Basket catheter mapping and noncontact mapping are simultaneous mapping techniques. They have special advantages for short-lived or unstable arrhythmias. For stable, sustained atrial tachycardias we currently prefer the electroanatomic mapping technique [6] because only one catheter is needed for mapping and ablation; furthermore, the Carto system enables more detailed reconstructions of the right and left atrial anatomy [22, 24, 27, 41]. Modern three-dimensional mapping tools are extremely helpful in localizing and ablation of right and left atrial foci (see Chapter 3).

The characteristics of the local potential at the target site are not uniform. Lesh et al. [23] observed fractionated potentials in 7 of 11 successful ablation sites (64%) of focal atrial tachycardia. In our experience double potentials, fractionated potentials and small prepotentials (Figure 8.8) were found in 24 of 35 left atrial focal atrial tachycardias (69%) at the earliest site of atrial activation [6]. The activation times found are generally in the range of 30–100 ms before the onset of the P wave.

8.4 Localizations

8.4.1 Right atrium

▮ Crista terminalis

▮ **ECG criteria.** The so-called "cristal tachycardias" [16] arise from the junction of the smooth septal with the trabeculated right atrium. This

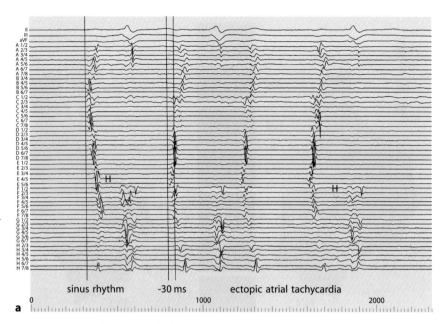

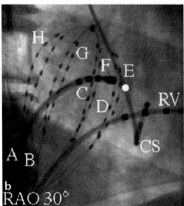

Fig. 8.6. Fluoroscopic appearance (RAO 30°) of a multipolar basket catheter (MBC) and other standard catheters in RA. Letters A to H identify basket splines. CS and RVA indicate standard catheters placed in the coronary sinus and right ventricular apex. Initiation of a short episode of right atrial tachycardia. Standard lead II, III, and aVF and MBC bipolar electrograms are displayed. First beat is sinus; the three consecutive beats are ectopic originating from midseptal region. The P wave in inferior leads is predominantly negative with terminal positive forces. Activation sequence of RA is reversed. The earliest activity recorded from basket electrodes is 30 ms in advance of the beginning of the P wave. From Schmitt et al. [18] with permission

is an area of marked anisotropy favoring the development of focal atrial tachycardias. The crista terminalis originates in the interatrial groove and traverses the right atrium posterolaterally into the eustachian ridge. Cristal tachycardias arising from the superior crista terminalis may mimic persistent sinus tachycardia. Whether or not the syndrome of inappropriate sinus tachycardia represents an independent disease entity has been challenged recently [31]. Probably, it can be included within the category of atrial tachycardias arising from the superior crista terminalis. Accordingly, a focus high in the crista has upright P waves, foci at the inferior crista terminalis have inverted P waves in leads II, III and aVF. V1 is inverted or biphasic. A hallmark of cristal tachycardias is a negative P wave in aVR [38] (Figure 8.9). A differentiation of a focus at the high crista terminalis from the right upper pulmonary vein can be very difficult because of the close anatomic proximity. An upright (and not a biphasic) P wave in V1

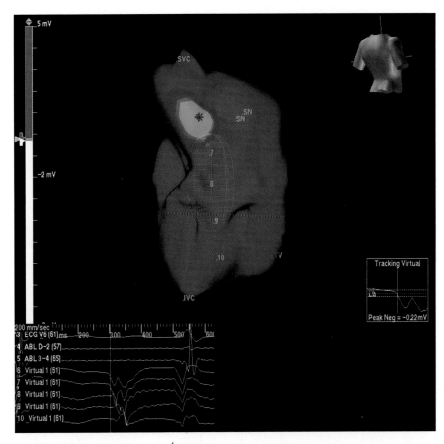

Fig. 8.7. Noncontact mapping of right atrial tachycardia. Documentation of the ectopic focus close to the sinus node in the right atrium. A 3D map of the right atrium is shown. In the virtual map of the right atrium, the earliest spot of activation was located close to the sinus node. Insert: Conventional and virtual electrograms. *IVC* inferior vena cava, *SVC* superior vena cava, *SN* sinus node

indicates an focus adjacent to the right upper pulmonary vein.

▮ **Mapping and ablation strategies.** The crista terminalis can be visualized nicely by intracardiac ultrasound (ICE) (Figure 8.10) which has been used for delineation and ablation of these tachycardias. However, the use of ICE is costly and time consuming. A multipolar crista terminalis catheter has been used in various studies [16]. It is estimated that approximately two-thirds of focal right atrial tachycardias arise along the terminal crest. A high success rate (>95%) has been reported with radiofrequency catheter ablation (Figure 8.11). Ablation of critical tachycardias arising from the superior crista terminalis can damage the right phrenic nerve leading to right diaphragmatic paralysis. Therefore, it is mandatory to perform atrial pacing at a high output from the planned ablation site. In case of phrenic nerve stimulation, ablation should not be performed at that site.

▮ **Tricuspid annulus**

▮ **ECG criteria.** Preferential site of origin along the tricuspid ring is the inferoanterior region [25]. Characteristic electrocardiographic features are deep negative P waves in the inferior leads and V1 (Figure 8.13).

▮ **Mapping and ablation strategies.** In one series [25] of 64 patients with right focal atrial tachycardias, 9 (13%) arose from the tricuspid annulus. In 7 cases the annular focus was localized to the inferoanterior region of the tricuspid ring (Figure 8.12). Mean activation time was −43 ±11 ms prior to P wave onset. A high success rate (100%) and only one recurrence within nine months were reported.

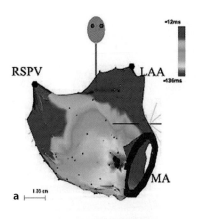

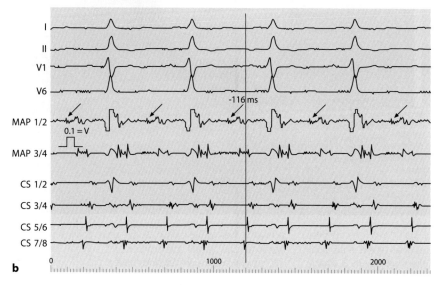

Fig. 8.8. Prepotentials recorded from the earliest activation site during left atrial focal tachycardia. **a** Electroanatomic activation map of the left atrium during tachycardia in right anterior oblique 30° view. The arrhythmogenic focus (red) was located at the midseptal mitral annulus (MA). **b** Surface leads I, II, V1, and V6 and intracardiac electrograms from the mapping and ablation catheter (MAP1/2, MAP3/4) and coronary sinus catheter (CS 1/2–7/8) recorded during tachycardia.

The CS was activated from proximal to distal. From the distal bipole of the mapping and ablation catheter (MAP1/2), prepotentials (red arrows) with an amplitude of 0.04 mV were recorded 116 ms before P wave onset at the site of earliest atrial activation. The prepotential was followed by a rounded potential with relatively high amplitude. *LAA* left atrial appendage, *RSPV* right superior pulmonary vein. From Dong et al. [17] with permission

▮ Coronary sinus ostium

▮ ECG criteria. Atrial tachycardias arising near the coronary sinus ostium have P wave characteristics similar to counterclockwise flutter with negative P waves in the inferior leads and a positive P wave in V1 (Figure 8.13). Electrocardiographic differentiation from right and left septal origin is difficult and sometimes impossible. The best discriminator is a positive P wave in V1 [7] for left septal sites (which in general is an uncommon localization).

▮ Mapping and ablation strategies. In the largest reported series of patients referred for ablation of focal atrial tachycardia, 13 of 193 patients (6.7%) had the site of origin at the ostium of the coronary sinus [17]. Mean activation time at the successful ablation site was −36 ± 8 ms. Catheter ablation was acutely successful in 11 cases with no recurrences over a median follow-up of 25 months. There are some case reports with elimination of foci far inside the coronary sinus (after failed left atrial attempts) [28, 29, 40].

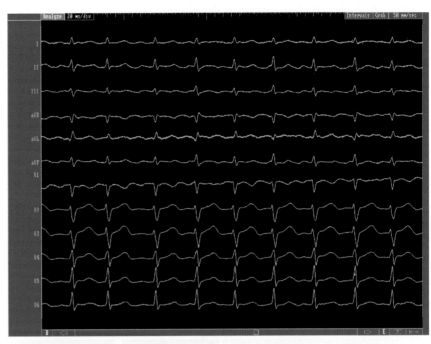

Fig. 8.9. ECG from a patient with a focal atrial tachycardia from the crista terminalis (CT). Please note negative P waves in aVR and V1

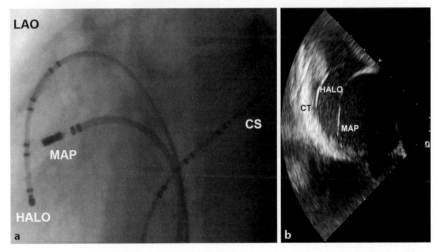

Fig. 8.10. Left (LAO) anterior oblique fluoroscopic projection and intracardiac echocardiography in a patient with a focal atrial tachycardia originating from the crista terminalis (CT).

MAP mapping (ablation) catheter, *CS* coronary sinus catheter, *Halo* multipolar catheter along the tricuspid annulus

▌ Uncommon sites

▌ **ECG criteria.** In 1997, Iesaka et al. [14] reported about a new entity of adenosine sensitive atrial tachycardia probably due to focal reentry within the atrioventricular nodal transitional area. They observed 11 patients with atrial tachycardias mimicking electrocardiographically atypical AV nodal tachycardias. The ECG showed long RP intervals and the P waves were characteristically inverted in the inferior limb leads.

▌ **Mapping and ablation strategies.** The induction was not related to a jump in the AH interval nor was its perpetuation dependent on conduc-

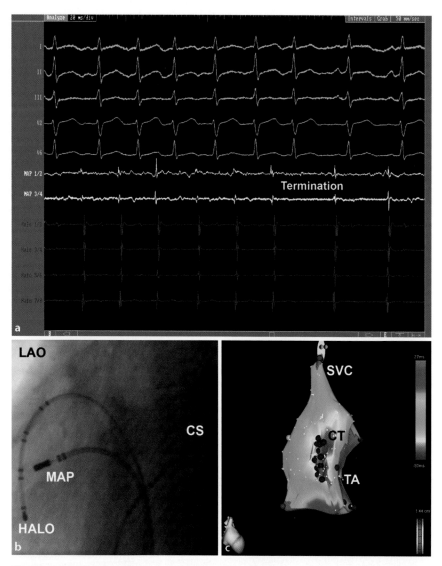

Fig. 8.11. Cristal tachycardia. Intracardiac recordings from a patient with termination under ablation of the crista terminalis (CT). **b** (LAO) fluoroscopic view of ablation catheter (MAP), a multipolar Halo catheter along the tricuspid ring and a multipolar catheter in coronary sinus (CS). Lower right electroanatomic mapping of the right atrium with earliest atrial activation in the CT (red). Same patient as in Figures 8.9 and 8.10. *LAO* left anterior oblique, *SVC* superior vena cava, *TA* tricuspid annulus

tion in the AV node. The tachycardia can be terminated with very small amounts of adenosine [2]. The earliest atrial activation was in the low anterior right atrial septum. Ventricular pacing during tachycardia resulted in AV dissociation or in an "A-A-V" response (Figures 8.2 and 8.3). Successful ablation sites often show low amplitude His signals and have typically fractionated potentials (Figure 8.14). The presumed (micro)-reentrant circuit appears limited close to the AV node and is not linked to dual AV nodal conduction.

Other uncommon sites of focal atrial conduction are those originating from the superior vena cava [5] (Figure 8.15). This is also a potential source for focal atrial fibrillation.

8.4.2 Left atrium

The most common site of origin of left focal atrial tachycardias are the pulmonary veins and the mitral annulus [6, 9]. Left atrial appendage, the roof of the left atrium, a focus deep inside

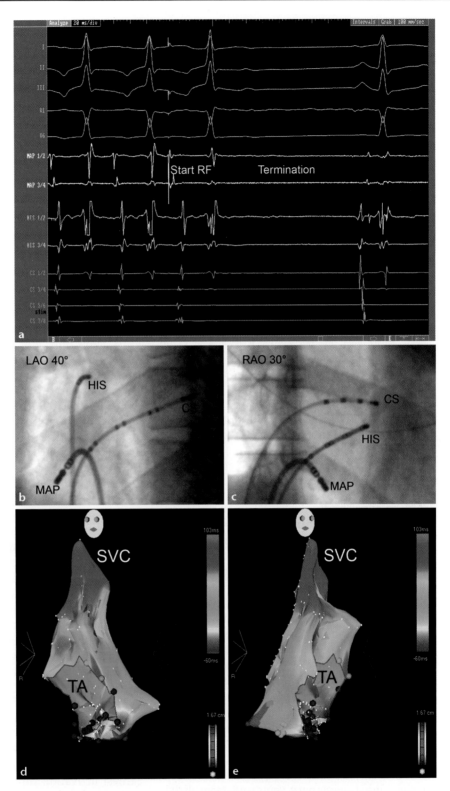

Fig. 8.12. Intracardiac ECG, fluoroscopy and Carto image from a patient with a focal atrial tachycardia from the tricuspid annulus. *LAO* left anterior oblique, *RAO* right anterior oblique, *RF* radiofrequency ablation, *HIS* His catheter, *CS* coronary sinus catheter, *MAP* mapping (ablation) catheter, *SVC* superior vena cava, *TA* tricuspid annulus

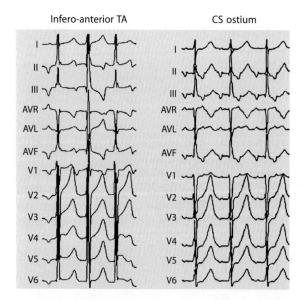

Fig. 8.13. ECG from patients with a focal atrial tachycardia originating from the coronary sinus ostium and the tricuspid annulus. Please note that the P wave is positive in V1 in tachycardias arising from the coronary sinus ostium. From Kistler et al. [10] with permission

the coronary sinus and left septal sites are less common origins of left focal atrial tachycardias.

▌ Pulmonary veins

▌ ECG criteria.
The P wave in V1 is always positive. In left-sided pulmonary vein tachycardias a negative P wave is observed in aVL; a positive P wave in aVL may be a specific marker of right pulmonary vein origin [42]. In addition, broad notched P waves in V1 favor left-sided veins. The inferior leads are markedly positive in all superior veins with a characteristic notching in the left-sided pulmonary veins.

▌ Mapping and ablation strategies.
In the majority of cases, the source of focal left atrial tachycardia is the pulmonary veins, most of them at ostial sites. The largest series comprise 27 patients, 33 patients and 51 patients with an incidence of 78%, 54% and 46%, respectively, of all focal left atrial tachycardias mapped [6, 9, 19]. CS activation occurred from proximal to distal for right-sided pulmonary veins and from distal to proximal for left-sided pulmonary veins. There was a propensity for upper veins, in one series FAT originated in 62.5% in the right upper pulmonary vein [9]. A minority of pul-

monary vein foci arises from deep inside the veins. Catheter ablation can be achieved with a high rate of success (>95%) (Figure 8.17). There is controversy in as far a focal ablation or complete pulmonary vein isolation is necessary. The occurrence of concomitant atrial fibrillation is surprisingly low which suggests that focal atrial tachycardia originating from the pulmonary veins is a distinct clinical problem from atrial fibrillation. Interestingly, pulmonary vein tachycardias seem to have a preferential interatrial connection to the intercaval area (Figure 8.5) of the right atrium through small muscle bridges (see above) [6].

▌ Mitral annulus

▌ ECG criteria.
The superior aspect of the mitral annulus is the region most often responsible for the origin of focal tachycardias. Whereas the limb leads show low amplitudes, the electrocardiographic sign most often described is a characteristic P wave in V1 with an initial negative component followed by an upright component (Figure 8.18). The initial negative component is probably due to the relatively anterior position of the superior mitral ring with electrical activation spreading initially away from V1, followed by activation of the remainder of the left atrium with an activation front directed towards V1 [20].

▌ Mapping and ablation strategies.
Focal atrial tachycardia arising from the mitral annulus [8, 19] is the second most frequent location inside the left atrium. When mapping the right atrium, the earliest atrial endocardial activity occurs at the His bundle region (up to −20 ms!); the CS activation is most often proximal to distal (Figure 8.8) as there is a propensity for FAT origin at the superior aspect of the mitral annulus. The typical P wave characteristics (Figure 8.18) with a negative initial deflection and a larger positive deflection in the precordial leads (V1) should prevent futile ablation attempts in the His bundle region. In the series of patients by Hachiya et al. [9], the mean cycle length of pulmonary vein tachycardias was shorter compared to those of mitral annulus origin. The earliest activation time compared to P wave onset was around 40 ms.

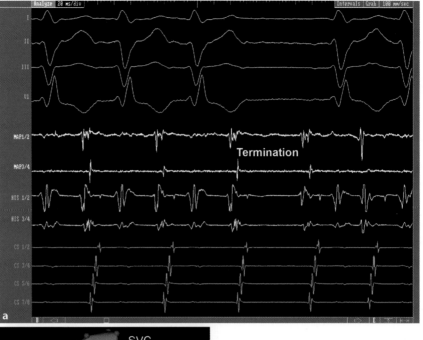

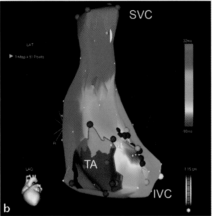

Fig. 8.14. Intracardiac ECG, fluoroscopy and Carto image from a patient with a focal atrial tachycardia originating close to the AV node. Please note the close proximity of the ablation spots (red dots) to the location of the His bundle (yellow dots). The border of the tricuspid annulus is also marked with red dots. *SVC* superior vena cava, *IVC* inferior vena cava, *TA* tricuspid annulus

8.4.3 Efficacy and safety of catheter ablation

In an analysis of pooled data of 514 patients [13], the success rate of catheter ablation of focal atrial tachycardias was 86%, the recurrence rate was 8% and the complication rate 2%. Severe complications specific for ablation of focal atrial tachycardias comprised cardiac perforation (during transseptal puncture, perforation of the left atrial appendage), damage to the right or left phrenic nerve and AV block (septal tachycardias).

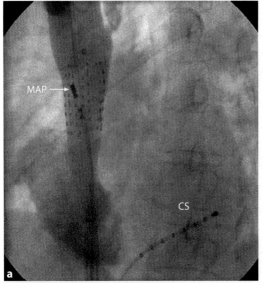

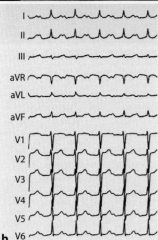

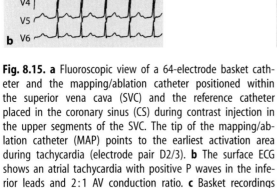

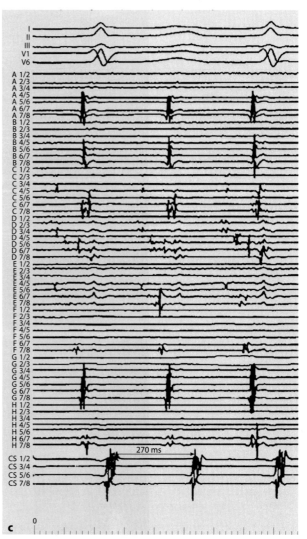

Fig. 8.15. a Fluoroscopic view of a 64-electrode basket catheter and the mapping/ablation catheter positioned within the superior vena cava (SVC) and the reference catheter placed in the coronary sinus (CS) during contrast injection in the upper segments of the SVC. The tip of the mapping/ablation catheter (MAP) points to the earliest activation area during tachycardia (electrode pair D2/3). **b** The surface ECG shows an atrial tachycardia with positive P waves in the inferior leads and 2:1 AV conduction ratio. **c** Basket recordings from the superior vena cava (SVC) during ongoing tachycardia from the coronary sinus. During ongoing tachycardia, the earliest activation is observed in electrode pair D2/3. Low amplitude, fragmented potentials are seen over the entire spline D located in the anterior aspect of the SVC. Double potentials are seen in spline E. The posterior (spline G) and septal (spline A) walls of the SVC show high amplitude, sharp potentials, which indicate rapid conduction and healthy muscle in those regions. From Dong et al. [38] with permission

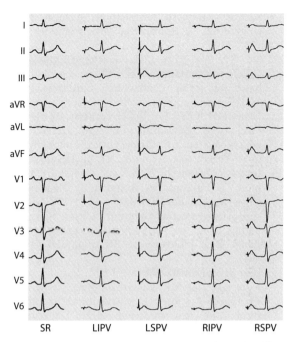

Fig. 8.16. P wave morphology during pacing from the different pulmonary veins. Please note marked notching of P waves in V1 in the left-sided pulmonary veins. *SR* sinus rhythm, *LIPV* left inferior pulmonary vein, *LSPV* left superior pulmonary vein, *RIPV* right inferior pulmonary vein, *RSPV* right superior pulmonary vein

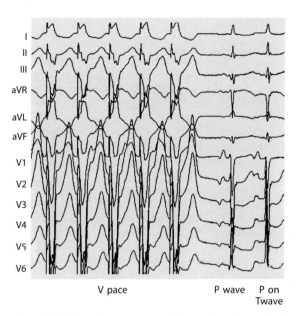

Fig. 8.18. Ventricular pacing for isolating the tachycardia P wave in a patient with a focal atrial tachycardia from the superior mitral annulus at the aortomitral continuity. From Kistler et al. [10] with permission

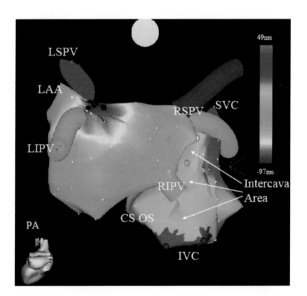

Fig. 8.17. Carto image from a patient with a focal atrial tachycardia from the left superior pulmonary vein. *LSPV* left superior pulmonary vein, *LAA* left atrial appendage, *LIPV* left inferior pulmonary vein, *PA* posterior-anterior, *RSPV* right superior pulmonary vein, *SVC* superior vena cava, *RIPV* right inferior pulmonary vein, *CS OS* coronary sinus ostium, *IVC* inferior vena cava

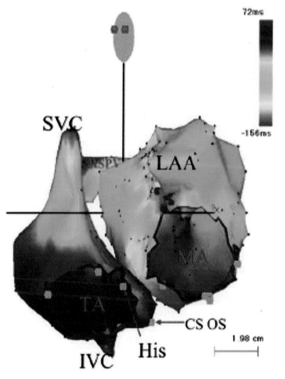

Fig. 8.19. Carto image from a patient with a focal atrial tachycardia from the superior mitral annulus. *SVC* superior vena cava, *LAA* left atrial appendage, *MA* mitral annulus, *TA* tricuspid annulus, *IVC* inferior vena cava, *HIS* His bundle, *CS OS* coronary sinus ostium. From Dong et al. [17] with permission

∎ References

1. Anguera I, Brugada J, Roba M, Mont L, Aguinaga L, Geelen P, Brugada P (2001) Outcomes after radiofrequency catheter ablation of atrial tachycardia. Am J Cardiol 87:886–890
2. Chen CC, Tai CT, Chiang CE, Yu WC, Lee SH, Chen YJ, Hsieh MH, Tsai CF, Lee KW, Ding YA, Chang MS, Chen SA (2000) Atrial tachycardias originating from the atrial septum: electrophysiologic characteristics and radiofrequency ablation. J Cardiovasc Electrophysiol 11:744–749
3. Chen SA, Chiang CE, Yang CJ, Cheng CC, Wu TJ, Wang SP, Chiang BN, Chang MS (1994) Sustained atrial tachycardia in adult patients. Electrophysiological characteristics, pharmacological response, possible mechanisms, and effects of radiofrequency ablation. Circulation 90:1262–1278
4. Chen SA, Tai CT, Chiang CE, Ding YA, Chang MS (1998) Focal atrial tachycardia: reanalysis of the clinical and electrophysiologic characteristics and prediction of successful radiofrequency ablation. J Cardiovasc Electrophysiol 9:355–365
5. Dong J, Schreieck J, Ndrepepa G, Schmitt C (2002) Ectopic tachycardia originating from the superior vena cava. J Cardiovasc Electrophysiol 13:620–624
6. Dong J, Zrenner B, Schreieck J, Deisenhofer I, Karch M, Schneider M, Von Bary C, Weyerbrock S, Yin Y, Schmitt C (2005) Catheter ablation of left atrial focal tachycardia guided by electroanatomic mapping and new insights into interatrial electrical conduction. Heart Rhythm 2:578–591
7. Frey B, Kreiner G, Gwechenberger M, Gossinger HD (2001) Ablation of atrial tachycardia originating from the vicinity of the atrioventricular node: significance of mapping both sides of the interatrial septum. J Am Coll Cardiol 38:394–400
8. Gonzalez MD, Contreras LJ, Jongbloed MR, Rivera J, Donahue TP, Curtis AB, Bailey MS, Conti JB, Fishman GI, Schalij MJ, Gittenberger-de Groot AC (2004) Left atrial tachycardia originating from the mitral annulus-aorta junction. Circulation 110:3187–3192
9. Hachiya H, Ernst S, Ouyang F, Mavrakis H, Chun J, Bansch D, Antz M, Kuck KH (2005) Topographic distribution of focal left atrial tachycardias defined by electrocardiographic and electrophysiological data. Circ J 69:205–210
10. Higa S, Tai CT, Lin YJ, Liu TY, Lee PC, Huang JL, Hsieh MH, Yuniadi Y, Huang BH, Lee SH, Ueng KC, Ding YA, Chen SA (2004) Focal atrial tachycardia: new insight from noncontact mapping and catheter ablation. Circulation 109:84–91
11. Higa S, Tai CT, Lin YJ, Liu TY, Lee PC, Huang JL, Yuniadi Y, Huang BH, Hsieh MH, Lee SH, Kuo JY, Lee KT, Chen SA (2004) Mechanism of adenosine-induced termination of focal atrial tachycardia. J Cardiovasc Electrophysiol 15:1387–1393
12. Ho SY, Anderson RH, Sanchez-Quintana D (2002) Atrial structure and fibres: morphologic bases of atrial conduction. Cardiovasc Res 54:325–336
13. Hsieh MH, Chen SA (2002) Catheter ablation of focal atrial tachycardia. In: Zipes DP, Haissaguerre M (eds) Catheter ablation of arrhythmias. Futura Inc., Armonk, NY, pp 185–201
14. Iesaka Y, Takahashi A, Goya M, Soejima Y, Okamoto Y, Fujiwara H, Aonuma K, Nogami A, Hiroe M, Marumo F, Hiraoka M (1997) Adenosine-sensitive atrial reentrant tachycardia originating from the atrioventricular nodal transitional area. J Cardiovasc Electrophysiol 8:854–864
15. Iwai S, Markowitz SM, Stein KM, Mittal S, Slotwiner DJ, Das MK, Cohen JD, Hao SC, Lerman BB (2002) Response to adenosine differentiates focal from macroreentrant atrial tachycardia: validation using three-dimensional electroanatomic mapping. Circulation 106:2793–2799
16. Kalman JM, Olgin JE, Karch MR, Hamdan M, Lee RJ, Lesh MD (1998) "Cristal tachycardias": origin of right atrial tachycardias from the crista terminalis identified by intracardiac echocardiography. J Am Coll Cardiol 31:451–459
17. Kistler PM, Fynn SP, Haqqani H, Stevenson IH, Vohra JK, Morton JB, Sparks PB, Kalman JM (2005) Focal atrial tachycardia from the ostium of the coronary sinus: electrocardiographic and electrophysiological characterization and radiofrequency ablation. J Am Coll Cardiol 45:1488–1493
18. Kistler PM, Kalman JM (2005) Locating focal atrial tachycardias from P-wave morphology. Heart Rhythm 2:561–564
19. Kistler PM, Sanders P, Fynn SP, Stevenson IH, Hussin A, Vohra JK, Sparks PB, Kalman JM (2003) Electrophysiological and electrocardiographic characteristics of focal atrial tachycardia originating from the pulmonary veins: acute and long-term outcomes of radiofrequency ablation. Circulation 108:1968–1975
20. Kistler PM, Sanders P, Hussin A, Morton JB, Vohra JK, Sparks PB, Kalman JM (2003) Focal atrial tachycardia arising from the mitral annulus: electrocardiographic and electrophysiologic characterization. J Am Coll Cardiol 41:2212–2219
21. Knight BP, Zivin A, Souza J, Flemming M, Pelosi F, Goyal R, Man C, Strickberger SA, Morady F (1999) A technique for the rapid diagnosis of atrial tachycardia in the electrophysiology laboratory. J Am Coll Cardiol 33:775–781
22. Kottkamp H, Hindricks G, Breithardt G, Borggrefe M (1997) Three-dimensional electromag-

netic catheter technology: electroanatomical mapping of the right atrium and ablation of ectopic atrial tachycardia. J Cardiovasc Electrophysiol 8:1332–1337

23. Lesh MD, Van Hare GF, Epstein LM, Fitzpatrick AP, Scheinman MM, Lee RJ, Kwasman MA, Grogin HR, Griffin JC (1994) Radiofrequency catheter ablation of atrial arrhythmias. Results and mechanisms. Circulation 89:1074–1089

24. Marchlinski F, Callans D, Gottlieb C, Rodriguez E, Coyne R, Kleinman D (1998) Magnetic electroanatomical mapping for ablation of focal atrial tachycardias. Pacing Clin Electrophysiol 21:1621–1635

25. Morton JB, Sanders P, Das A, Vohra JK, Sparks PB, Kalman JM (2001) Focal atrial tachycardia arising from the tricuspid annulus: electrophysiologic and electrocardiographic characteristics. J Cardiovasc Electrophysiol 12:653–659

26. Naccarelli GV, Shih HT, Jalal S (1995) Clinical arrhythmias: mechanisms, clinical features, and management of supraventricular tachycardia. In: Zipes DP, Jalife J (eds) Cardiac Electrophysiology. From Cell to Bedside. WB Saunders, Philadelphia, pp 607–619

27. Natale A, Breeding L, Tomassoni G, Rajkovich K, Richey M, Beheiry S, Martinez K, Cromwell L, Wides B, Leonelli F (1998) Ablation of right and left ectopic atrial tachycardias using a three-dimensional nonfluoroscopic mapping system. Am J Cardiol 82:989–992

28. Navarrete AJ, Arora R, Hubbard JE, Miller JM (2003) Magnetic electroanatomic mapping of an atrial tachycardia requiring ablation within the coronary sinus. J Cardiovasc Electrophysiol 14:1361–1364

29. Pavin D, Boulmier D, Daubert JC, Mabo P (2002) Permanent left atrial tachycardia: radiofrequency catheter ablation through the coronary sinus. J Cardiovasc Electrophysiol 13:395–398

30. Reithmann C, Dorwarth U, Fiek M, Matis T, Remp T, Steinbeck G, Hoffmann E (2005) Outcome of ablation for sustained focal atrial tachycardia in patients with and without a history of atrial fibrillation. J Interv Card Electrophysiol 12:35–43

31. Roberts-Thomson KC, Kistler PM, Kalman JM (2005) Atrial tachycardia: mechanisms, diagnosis, and management. Curr Probl Cardiol 30:529–573

32. Rodriguez E, Callans D, Kantharia B, Gottlieb C, Marchlinski FE (2000) Basket catheter localization of the origin of atrial tachycardia with atypical morphology after atrial flutter ablation. Pacing Clin Electrophysiol 23:269–272

33. Saoudi N, Cosio F, Waldo A, Chen SA, Iesaka Y, Lesh M, Saksena S, Salerno J, Schoels W (2001) Classification of atrial flutter and regular atrial tachycardia according to electrophysiologic mechanism and anatomic bases: a statement from a joint expert group from the Working Group of Arrhythmias of the European Society of Cardiology and the North American Society of Pacing and Electrophysiology. J Cardiovasc Electrophysiol 12:852–866

34. Schmitt C, Zrenner B, Schneider M, Karch M, Ndrepepa G, Deisenhofer I, Weyerbrock S, Schreieck J, Schomig A (1999) Clinical experience with a novel multielectrode basket catheter in right atrial tachycardias. Circulation 99:2414–2422

35. Schmitt H, Weber S, Schwab JO, Voss RM, Kneller R, Tillmanns H, Waldecker B (2001) Diagnosis and ablation of focal right atrial tachycardia using a new high-resolution, non-contact mapping system. Am J Cardiol 87:1017–1021, A1015

36. Schneider MA, Ndrepepa G, Weber S, Deisenhofer I, Schomig A, Schmitt C (2004) Influence of high-pass filtering on noncontact mapping and ablation of atrial tachycardias. Pacing Clin Electrophysiol 27:38–46

37. Simon RD, Rinaldi CA, Baszko A, Gill JS (2004) Electroanatomic mapping of the right atrium with a right atrial basket catheter and three-dimensional intracardiac echocardiography. Pacing Clin Electrophysiol 27:318–326

38. Tada H, Nogami A, Naito S, Suguta M, Nakatsugawa M, Horie Y, Tomita T, Hoshizaki H, Oshima S, Taniguchi K (1998) Simple electrocardiographic criteria for identifying the site of origin of focal right atrial tachycardia. Pacing Clin Electrophysiol 21:2431–2439

39. Tang CW, Scheinman MM, Van Hare GF, Epstein LM, Fitzpatrick AP, Lee RJ, Lesh MD (1995) Use of P wave configuration during atrial tachycardia to predict site of origin. J Am Coll Cardiol 26:1315–1324

40. Volkmer M, Antz M, Hebe J, Kuck KH (2002) Focal atrial tachycardia originating from the musculature of the coronary sinus. J Cardiovasc Electrophysiol 13:68–71

41. Wetzel U, Hindricks G, Schirdewahn P, Dorszewski A, Fleck A, Heinke F, Kottkamp H (2002) A stepwise mapping approach for localization and ablation of ectopic right, left, and septal atrial foci using electroanatomic mapping. Eur Heart J 23:1387–1393

42. Yamane T, Shah DC, Peng JT, Jais P, Hocini M, Deisenhofer I, Choi KJ, Macle L, Clementy J, Haissaguerre M (2001) Morphological characteristics of P waves during selective pulmonary vein pacing. J Am Coll Cardiol 38:1505–1510

9 Ventricular tachycardia

Jürgen Schreieck, Gabriele Hessling, Alexander Pustowoit, Claus Schmitt

▌ Introduction

During the last two decades, catheter ablation of ventricular tachycardia (VT) has shifted from an option only for selected patients with focal VT in the absence of structural heart disease to a treatment strategy for a large number of patients with ischemic and nonischemic ventricular tachyarrhythmias.

With the development of implantable cardioverter defibrillators (ICD), the impact of VT ablation had come to question in the large population of VT patients with ischemic heart disease. In fact, during long-term survival, many of those patients (with an ICD) develop complex substrates for ventricular arrhythmias that are amenable to catheter ablation. VT ablation has proven to be a valuable tool in this patient population with the goal of reducing ICD shock deliveries due to the arrhythmia. Catheter ablation has also shown its value in the management of patients with polymorphic ventricular tachycardia, ventricular fibrillation or in an electrical storm.

Major steps concerning technical aspects of VT ablation were the development of new 3D mapping systems for exact electroanatomical mapping of the individual underlying substrate, irrigated tip radiofrequency ablation and the epicardial ablation approach. The better understanding of trigger and substrate in ventricular tachyarrhythmias led to new ablation strategies and an expanding indication for VT ablation. Today, most ventricular arrhythmogenic substrates are approachable by catheter ablation.

9.1 Classification of VT: according to mechanism or substrate?

Although coronary artery disease is the most common condition associated with VT, there are other entities that are important when approaching VT ablation. The following classification regarding the VT mechanism has widely been used:

- ▌ "Idiopathic VT" in the structurally normal heart (right or left nonreentrant outflow tract tachycardia, left ventricular "verapamil-sensitive" reentrant tachycardia)
- ▌ Bundle branch reentrant tachycardia
- ▌ VT related to ischemic heart disease (coronary artery disease/myocardial infarction)
- ▌ VT in nonischemic heart disease (idiopathic dilated CMP, arrhythmogenic right ventricular cardiomyopathy, tetralogy of Fallot after cardiac surgery, muscular dystrophies and neuromuscular disease)
- ▌ VT in channelopathies (long QT syndrome, Brugada syndrome, catecholaminergic VT).

When thinking in terms of catheter ablation, defining the substrate ("approaching the target") is at least as important as defining the underlying mechanism. There are three substrate types that can be distinguished:

- ▌ *Single fibers* near or above the ventricular valves (from which idiopathic nonreentrant ventricular arrhythmias predominantly originate)
- ▌ *Fascicular arrhythmias* involving specific parts of the conduction system. These arrhythmias appear mostly monomorphic (verapamil-sensitive idiopathic left ventricular tachycardia and bundle branch reentrant tachycardia)
- ▌ *Scar-related* ventricular tachycardia originating from low voltage areas with signs of anisotropic and delayed conduction (usually related to structural heart disease).

In the following, the "substrate" approach to VT ablation will be shown in detail taking into consideration underlying pathology and arrhythmia mechanism. A short outlook on ablation of ventricular fibrillation will round off this chapter.

9.2 General considerations in VT mapping and catheter ablation

The key question in VT ablation is whether the underlying substrate is fixed or dynamically changing. Functional myocardium that only exhibits transient ectopy due to reversible causes such as inflammation or electrolyte imbalance should not be targeted by catheter ablation. The paradigm for the concept of single fiber ("focal") VT ablation is the group of idiopathic monomorphic VT from the outflow tracts of both ventricles or the tricuspid and mitral annulus. Patients with dilated cardiomyopathy might also suffer from focal VT from the valves [25, 48]. Ablation of a focal VT in the absence of scars is targeted close to the valves where pump function is less compromised. This is also applicable for some focal VT with ischemic heart disease. Ablation of a focus in the ventricular free wall or at the papillary muscles in the absence of scars should be performed very cautiously.

Scar-related reentrant VT typically depends on delayed conduction in scarred myocardial areas and ablation should primarily target scarred tissue (usually in the border zone of low voltage areas) before an ablation of healthy tissue is attempted. Although voltage mapping is an accepted approach for mapping those scars, it is important to remember that electrical viability is not identical with myocardial cell viability. In case of ischemia and inflammation a reduced voltage may be reversible. The presentation of multiple types of right ventricular VT, low voltage areas in the right ventricle or proven reentrant VT should raise suspicion of arrhythmogenic right ventricular cardiomyopathy (Figures 9.17 and 9.18).

∎ **Right ventricular mapping** is delicate due to large trabecular muscles and a sickle-shaped narrow volume of the ventricle. A large curve catheter might pass the tricuspid valve directly via a transfemoral venous access. However, a more reliable way for right ventricular apex mapping is often the use of a catheter with a small curve placed over a long vascular guiding sheath with a 90–150° angle. To map the right

ventricular outflow tract (RVOT), the catheter is moved into the pulmonary artery and then drawn back through the pulmonary valve. Mapping of the tricuspid annulus from the ventricular side remains a challenge. Drawing back a small C-curved catheter guided by a preshaped long vascular sheath (angle 60–90°) for the superior parts of the tricuspid annulus or by a more curved sheath (angle 120–150°) for the inferior tricuspid annulus offers a reliable solution. Mapping of the tricuspid annulus should be performed in the LAO view to follow the catheter movement around the complete tricuspid ring.

∎ **Left ventricular mapping** is challenging as it is the most forcefully contracting chamber of the heart. It can be approached by retrograde access via the aortic valve (preferred in our lab) or by a transseptal approach. The transseptal access is primarily performed if significant aortic valve stenosis or a prosthetic aortic valve is present.

The mapping catheter in the left ventricle is straightened and centered contact-free in the middle of the left ventricular cavity. It is then moved forward orthogonal to the corresponding ventricular wall or curved, rotated and drawn back to touch the base of the ventricle and the mitral annulus. Placement of a diagnostic right-sided His bundle catheter gives a good orientation for the level of the aortic valve. Catheter movement is limited by the mitral apparatus when mapping the base and the mitral annulus. A curved catheter should never turn more than 180° in that position to avoid rolling up and rupture of the chordae and mitral leaflets. Mapping with a small curve (C-curve) catheter has the advantage of easier access over the aortic valve but it is often difficult to map the entire anterior wall with this technique.

There are three reasons for an epicardial approach to VT ablation: 1) failed endocardial ablation, 2) contraindications to endocardial mapping such as a prosthetic valve in the aortic or mitral position and 3) the ECG suggesting an epicardial VT origin. There are conditions such as Chagas disease and cardiac sarcoidosis with a preferential epicardial VT manifestation.

Figure 9.1 shows the different approaches for left ventricular mapping.

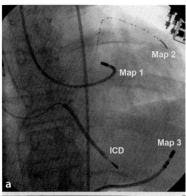

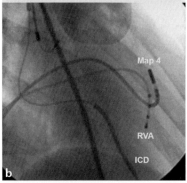

Fig. 9.1. Fluoroscopic views of different approaches to LV mapping. **a** (AP) shows a Map catheter (Map 1) positioned in the left ventricle retrograde via the aortic valve. Map 2 is a 2F 16-polar epicardial mapping electrode introduced via the coronary sinus. Map 3 is an ablation catheter positioned epicardially after pericardial puncture. **b** (RAO) shows a map catheter (Map 4) positioned in the left ventricle via a transseptal approach. *ICD* electrode of an internal cardioverter defibrillator, *RVA* right ventricular apex

9.3 Specific VT entities: idiopathic nonreentrant ventricular tachycardia ("single fibers")

The predominant origin of this VT type is the right ventricular outflow tract (RVOT) but it is also found at the left ventricular outflow tract (LVOT) or at the mitral and tricuspid annulus. Patients are mostly young or middle-aged with the symptom of palpitations during exercise or a condition of stress. Tachycardia presents clinically as repetitive monomorphic nonsustained or as paroxysmal monomorphic sustained. Both forms are currently thought to reflect different clinical manifestations of an identical cellular mechanism. Idiopathic monomorphic nonreentrant VT is probably due to a cyclic-AMP mediated, triggered, catecholamine-related arrhythmia mechanism. Empirical data from catheter mapping and ablation suggest that single myocardial fibers from muscle extensions near or above heart valves are responsible for focal activity [40, 55]. Prognosis is usually good although rare cases of sudden death have been reported [53].

▮ Differentiating idiopathic RVOT and LVOT tachycardia from the surface ECG

Generally, the surface ECG of idiopathic non-reentrant tachycardia is characterized by an inferior axis and a left bundle branch block pattern (Figure 9.2).

Several criteria for differentiation of a left-sided from a right-sided origin of idiopathic outflow tract tachycardia have been suggested [13, 19, 20, 27, 28, 30, 40]. ECG differentiation is mainly based on the R/S transition in the precordial leads. A *left-sided* origin typically has an R/S transition in leads V1 or V2. A *right-sided* origin is associated with an R/S transition in V4 or beyond. An R/S transition in V3 can indicate an *interventricular wall origin* as well as an endocardial right- or left-sided origin. An algorithm for defining the ablation site by VT morphology on the surface ECG is shown in Figure 9.3.

A posteroseptal origin near the pulmonary valve or from the left aortic cusp is quite frequent. VT can also arise from a supravalvular origin in the aortic root or the pulmonary artery [19, 20, 28, 40]. The conjunction between the right and left ventricular septal wall is continuously turned to a close proximity between the posterior wall of the pulmonary artery and the anterior wall of the aortic root. Therefore right-to left-sided differentiation on the infravalvular level is shifted to a posterior-anterior differentiation on the supravalvular level. Depending on the origin below or above the valve, ECG R/S transition criteria can vary considerably in lead V3. ECG criteria should therefore be applied with some limitations. Figure 9.4 shows some examples of idiopathic nonreentrant VT.

▮ ECG criteria for idiopathic VT from the atrioventricular valves

Idiopathic nonreentrant VT can also originate from tissue close to the mitral (MA) and tricuspid (TA) annulus [31, 54]. Idiopathic VT from

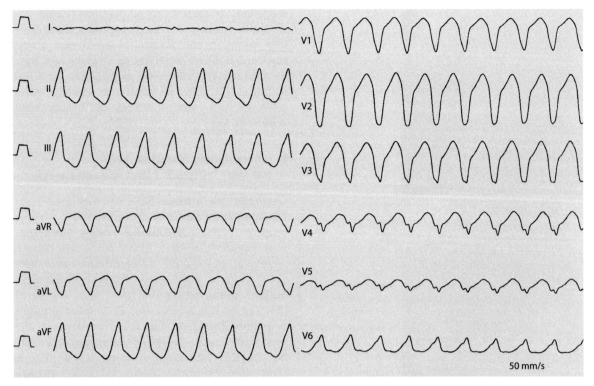

Fig. 9.2. *Right ventricular outflow tract (RVOT) tachycardia.* An inferior axis and a left bundle branch block pattern are present. Note the late R/S transition in V6 suggesting a right ventricular origin

the mitral annulus often shows a characteristic delta wave-like beginning of the QRS (177±19 ms) with a transitional zone of the R wave occurring exclusively between V1-V2 [31]. Delta wave-like QRS complexes can also be observed in VT of epicardial origin (see below).

VT from the anterior mitral annulus might display a similar ECG pattern as VT from the aortic cusp (inferior axis, early R/S transition in V1-V3). In the MA-VT group, the R wave amplitude in lead aVF tends to be smaller with a wider QRS complex compared to VT from the aortic cusp [31]. There is an overlap of ECG criteria due to a possible origin in the aortomitral continuity (left fibrous trigone).

TA-VT with an origin at the free wall tricuspid annulus has a R/S wave transition beyond V3 and shows a transition in V3 in case of a septal origin [54]. A delta wave-like pattern has not been described for VT arising from the tricuspid annulus. This is probably due to the thinner ventricular wall even in case of an epicardial origin. An inferoseptal or even interseptal origin at the annulus of an atrioventricular valve can show an R/S transition at lead V2. TA-VT from the free

wall with an anterior origin is reported to have a notched R wave in the inferior leads. In case of an inferior origin a notched Q wave in the inferior leads is observed [54].

It is important to remember that the R/S transition can not distinguish the origin of an idiopathic VT in the boundary regions between pulmonary artery and aorta, aortic and mitral valve and in the interseptal area between the atrioventricular valves.

For detailed localization of VT originating from the mitral or tricuspid annulus, the algorithms for ECG-based localization of accessory pathways are quite reliable [31].

∎ ECG criteria for the epicardial origin of left-sided idiopathic VT

The widening of the initial part of the QRS ("pseudo delta wave" ≥34 ms) due to the intramural conduction delay is quite specific for an epicardial VT origin. Various factors like muscle mass or nonuniform anisotropy can affect QRS width. A broad QRS (>200 ms) is typical for an epicardial origin of idiopathic VT in the ab-

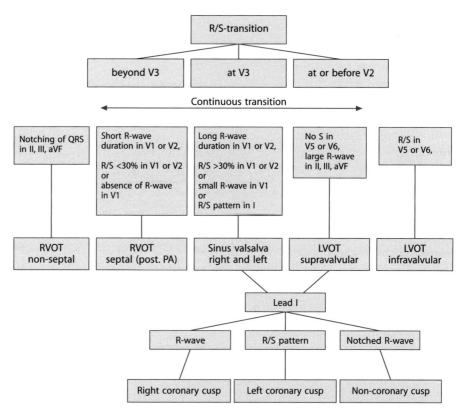

Fig. 9.3. Definition of the optimal ablation side by ECG morphology of idiopathic outflow tract VT. The R/S transition in the precordial leads is the key for differentiation of a right ventricular from a left ventricular origin. There is a continuous transition zone with an R/S transition at V3 from the posteroseptal RVOT to a VT origin from a sinus of Valsalva. Lead I has the greatest importance for differentiation between the coronary cusps. (Criteria for this algorithm were derived from [20, 27, 30, 40])

sence of other causes of conduction delay. ECG criteria for an epicardial origin have been suggested including a broad pseudo delta wave, broad RS complex and long QRS duration [6]. ECG examples of two forms of epicardial VT are shown in Figure 9.5.

In some cases of LVOT tachycardia, percutaneous pericardial instrumentation has proven that the earliest sites were epicardial [28, 39, 46]. It is assumed that the arrhythmogenic substrate of LVOT tachycardia with supravalvular origin is epicardially linked to the left ventricle. However, VT could be successfully ablated from the endoluminal side of the left coronary cusp [46]. An epicardial origin of idiopathic VT from left ventricular areas other than the outflow tract has also been observed [6]. RVOT or septal tachycardias are mostly not suitable for epicardial ablation.

It is important to remember that criteria for an epicardial origin overlap with those for VT from the mitral annulus (broad QRS, delta

wave-like beginning, delayed intrinsic deflection time) [31]. VT from the mitral annulus may be linked to a primarily epicardial activation; however, most forms can be ablated from the endocardial side [31]. The mitral annulus should be mapped in detail before switching to an epicardial ablation approach. Successful ablation has been reported at the mitral annulus even with an endocardial activation time of 0 ms before the onset of the QRS complex leading to the conclusion that epicardial fibers at this location are successfully ablated by endocardial RF application.

▪ Mapping and ablation of idiopathic nonreentrant ventricular tachycardia

▪ **RVOT tachycardia.** Success rates for RF catheter ablation of RVOT tachycardia range from 80 to 100% with a low procedural complication rate [10]. The origin of RVOT tachycardia is pre-

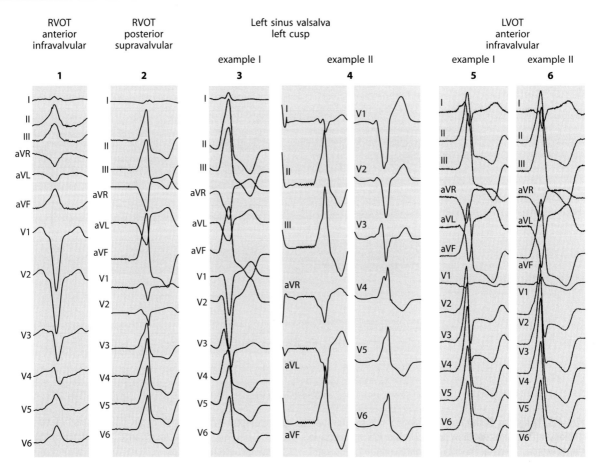

Fig. 9.4. ECG examples of idiopathic nonreentrant RVOT and LVOT tachycardia with a supra- or infravalvular tachycardia origin. Suggested ECG criteria for differentiating left and right origin can sometimes be misleading. VT in example 2 shows criteria for a LVOT origin although arising from the pulmonary artery. The ECG of VT in example 3 points to an RVOT origin although VT originates from the left sinus of Valsalva

dominately the septal aspect in a narrow area just below the pulmonary valve [10, 26, 36]. Successful ablation sites are usually determined with the help of pace and activation mapping.

Pace mapping is performed by identifying a pacing site that gives a QRS configuration identical to that of the VT. An example is shown in Figure 9.6.

Algorithms for an ECG-guided approach have tried to identify the portion of the RVOT septum where detailed pace mapping should be directed [18, 26, 36]. We use a simple pace mapping algorithm after positioning the ablation catheter just below the pulmonary valve annulus (see also Figure 9.7).

∎ If the R wave in leads V3-V4 is too small, the catheter is moved posteriorly. If it is too large, the catheter is moved anteriorly.

∎ If the QRS complex in lead I is too large or too positive, the catheter is moved to the more lateral aspect of the pulmonary valve.

∎ If the amplitude of the R wave in the inferior limb leads has to be reduced for pace map matching, the catheter tip is drawn downwards (proximal outflow tract). If an enlargement of the amplitude has to be achieved, the catheter is moved upwards (distal outflow tract), in some cases above the level of the pulmonary valve.

After the area of interest has been defined by pace mapping, *activation mapping* is performed. Usually an electroanatomical mapping system is used (see Chapter 3). Successful ablation sites are associated with demonstration of a discrete potential before the onset of the earliest surface

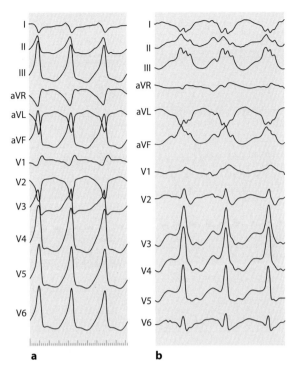

Fig. 9.5. a *Epicardial VT near the trigonum fibrosum.* Earliest endocardial activation was found near the trigonum fibrosum between the aortic and mitral valve with an activation time of −4 ms. **b** *Epicardial VT from the anterolateral left ventricle* in a patient with cardiac sarcoidosis. Earliest endocardial activation time was determined with −18 ms

QRS complex. A mean activation time of only −15 ms ± 18 ms to QRS onset has been reported for successful ablation sites. If the earliest activation time to QRS onset is less than −20 ms, the pulmonary artery should be checked carefully for earlier activated fibers. In our experience, a catheter position with an earliest activation time to QRS onset of more than −20 ms justifies an ablation attempt. If the earliest activation is posteroseptal at the conjunction to the aortic root, a detailed LVOT mapping should be performed before starting RF ablation in the RVOT. A primary ablation attempt in the posteroseptal region seems justified without left-sided mapping if endocardial activation times ≥ −30 ms are observed. If ectopy does not terminate quickly (or is not temporarily heated up) after achieving a sufficient ablation temperature (>50 °C in the power controlled mode), the position of the earliest activation should be revised. If there is not enough ectopy for further mapping, a pace map matching of ≥11 leads [41] can justify further ablation attempts [18].

If VT originates supravalvular from the root of the pulmonary artery, ablation is often painful and bears a considerable risk of artery dissection. A small ablation line below the pulmonary valve just below the focus isolates the arrhythmogenic fiber. Careful energy titration during RF application is mandatory to avoid overheating and the "popping" phenomenon by trapping the catheter tip in a pulmonary cusp.

The endpoint for ablation is the complete suppression of ectopy also during provocative maneuvers like isoprenaline or burst pacing. Even a single typical VPB might indicate recurrence. It is our policy to apply a security RF application guided by electroanatomical mapping as this might reduce the recurrence rate.

It is important to note that electroanatomical mapping systems bear a location error in strongly contracting areas such as the RVOT. An anatomically defined point recorded during a VPB or tachycardia compared to sinus rhythm can differ in the 3-dimensional localization (see Figure 9.7). Therefore, the anatomical position of the earliest activation and of the primary successful ablation points should be recorded during the arrhythmia and during sinus rhythm.

▮ **LVOT tachycardia.** Endocardial activation times to QRS onset at successful ablation sites in the LVOT have been reported to be greater than in RVOT-VT (mean −30 ± 14 ms, range −5 to −58 ms)[41]. Especially VT originating from the sinus of Valsalva is reported to have earlier local activation times in the range of −35 to −60 ms [28] or −23 to −97 ms [40]. Similar to RVOT mapping, pace map matching of ≥11 ECG leads is predictive for ablation success [41]. Ectopy below the aortic valve is approached very similar to RVOT ectopy. The arrhythmogenic fiber in coronary cusp VT might be detected during sinus rhythm as delayed local potentials which can guide a successful ablation [40].

Several "security" features for ablating inside the sinus of Valsalva have been suggested. We recommend aortic and coronary angiography to localize the aortic valve and the coronary ostia and to exclude anatomic abnormalities. During ablation inside the left or right aortic cusp the corresponding coronary artery should be visualized by angiography. If there is only a small distance between ablation site and coronary ostium, the coronary artery should be cannulated. Ablation is performed under continuous fluoro-

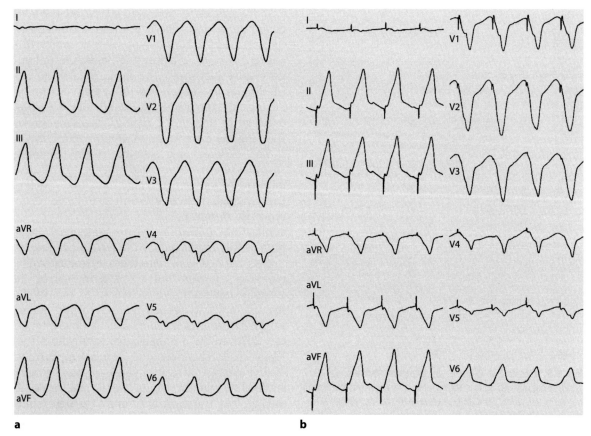

a

b

Fig. 9.6. *Pace mapping in RVOT tachycardia.* **a** RVOT tachycardia with an inferior axis and a left bundle branch block pattern (see also Figure 9.2). **b** shows the pace map from a location in the RVOT just below the pulmonary valve that matches the QRS complexes of the clinical tachycardia in all 12 ECG leads

scopic visualization to avoid a dislocation of the ablation catheter into the coronary ostium during RF application (Figure 9.8). As RF application has been reported to terminate VT from the coronary cusp in less than 8 seconds [40], RF application is usually titrated from 15 to 30 Watts and stopped after 10 seconds. Studies have shown that RF ablation at the aortic cusps can be performed safely and effectively with only a small risk of aortic valve, aortic root or coronary artery damage [28, 40, 42, 47].

∎ **VT from the atrioventricular valves.** VT originating from the tricuspid or mitral annulus can be ablated endocardially with a high success rate [31, 54]. Pace mapping and mapping of presystolic small potentials at the valve annulus are prerequisites for successful ablation [31, 54]. In our experience pace mapping is an important guide

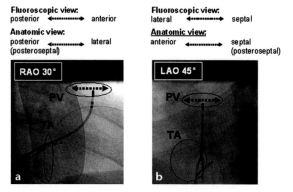

Fig. 9.7 a–g. *Mapping and ablation of idiopathic monomorphic VT from the RVOT.* **a** The mapping catheter in the RAO 30° view is fluoroscopically guided to an anatomically lateral or posterior-posteroseptal position (*TA* tricuspid annulus, *PV* pulmonary valve). **b** The mapping catheter in the LAO 45° view is fluoroscopically guided to an anatomically septal/posteroseptal or anterior position in the RVOT

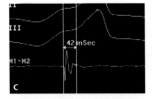
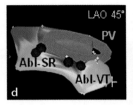
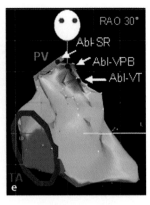
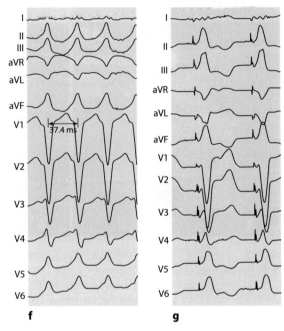

Fig. 9.7. c Earliest bipolar mapping showing a presystolic potential (42 ms before onset of QRS complex) beginning with a typically negative deflection as the target for ablation in the RVOT. **d** Electroanatomical activation mapping of focal activity at the level of the pulmonary valve (PV). There is a shift of catheter position during VT (Abl-VT) and sinus rhythm (Abl-SR) due to movement of the strong contracting ventricular area. Two primarily successful ablation points were applied anteriorly (red ablation dots Abl-VT). After ablation a few spontaneous VPBs occurred from the same localization, which were successfully ablated by two more RF applications during sinus rhythm (Abl-SR). On the map, the ablation position during SR was more than one centimeter apart from the position during VT although the catheter was positioned at the same anatomical site. **e** Complete electroanatomical activation map of RVOT tachycardia originating anterolaterally below the pulmonary valve. Earliest endocardial activation is shown in red and preceded the onset of QRS by 28 ms. Again please note the virtual shift of ablation points acquired during VT (Abl-VT), during a typical VPB (Abl-VPB) and during sinus rhythm (Abl-SR), although all RF applications were directed to the same anatomical site. **f** 12-lead surface ECG during VT. **g** Corresponding pace map close to the ablation site

for successful ablation. In contrast to outflow tract tachycardia, there is a significant change of the paced surface ECG within small distances along the annulus. The endocardial local activation time of small distinct prepotentials of ectopic activity from the mitral annulus have been reported in the range of –20 to –90 ms [31]. Two examples of MA-VT are shown in Figures 9.9 and 9.10.

The ablation technique is very similar to the ablation of accessory pathways from the ventricular side at the atrioventricular valves. Stable

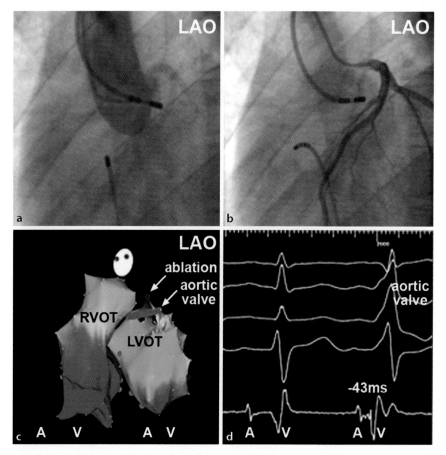

Fig. 9.8. *Mapping and ablation of idiopathic monomorphic VT from the left sinus Valsalva.* **a** Aortography in the LAO view with the ablation catheter at the successful ablation position at the left aortic cusp. **b** Angiography of the left coronary artery in the LAO view with the ablation catheter at the successful ablation site. **c** Color-coded electroanatomical activation map of the right and left ventricular outflow tract during VT in a LAO 45°/caudally angulated view. Red color illustrates earliest activation from above the aortic valve. Three red points below the valve are unsuccessful ablation sites with an endocardial activation time of 18–22 ms before QRS.

The brown dot above the aortic valve marks the successful ablation site with an activation time of –43 ms. RF application of 20 W with a maximal temperature of 55 °C for 20 s with a standard 4 mm electrode abolished the ectopy. **d** Mapping catheter recording of a sinus beat followed by a typical VPB at the successful ablation site. A low amplitude fractionated presystolic potential preceded the onset of QRS by 43 ms. Note that atrial electrograms (A) from the left atrial appendage were recorded at the aortic cusp and may overlap with the ventricular activation (V)

contact pressure under the valve leaflet of the catheter tip is crucial for ablation success. We recommend a security burn around the primary successful ablation site as ectopic activity may recur with a little shift of origin. An origin at the septal aspect of the atrioventricular valves can be challenging and in many cases an electroanatomical mapping system helps in differentiating a right or left origin.

9.4 Specific VT entities: "fascicular" VT

9.4.1 Idiopathic verapamil-sensitive VT

This type of reentrant left VT is usually terminated by verapamil administration and is therefore called "verapamil-sensitive". The ECG during tachycardia shows right bundle branch block with left (common) or right (uncommon) axis deviation (Figure 9.11). Clinically, VT is of-

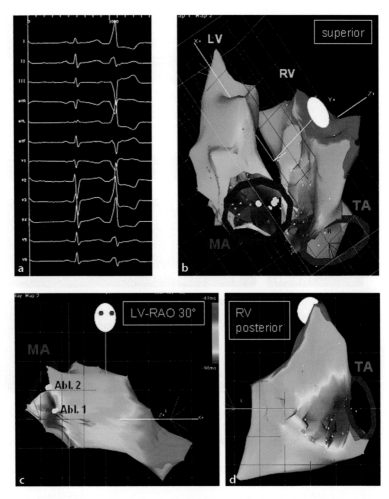

Fig. 9.9. *Mapping and ablation of idiopathic monomorphic VT from the inferoseptal mitral annulus (MA) using right and left ventricular electroanatomical activation mapping.* **a** Ventricular premature beat (VPB) originating from the inferoseptal mitral annulus. **b** Electroanatomical activation map (superior view) of the left (LV) and right (RV) ventricle during VPB/VT. Note the simultaneous right and left ventricular endocardial activation (early activation in red). **c** Activation map of the left ventricle from a right anterior oblique (RAO) view. Earliest activation is shown in red. First RF application (Abl-1, white points) at the inferoseptal mitral annulus was performed during nonsustained VT and abolished VT. The second RF application, a "security burn" was performed during sinus rhythm and abolished the remaining single VPBs. As the geometry of the map was constructed during sinus rhythm, the two ablation points at the mitral annulus differed by a distance of one centimeter due to the shift in diastolic dimension of the left ventricle between sinus rhythm and VPB/VT. **d** Right ventricular activation map during VPB/VT viewed from posterior-lateral. The earliest endocardial activation time was only 8 ms less than at the left ventricular septum. However, the front of early activation was much broader in the right than in the left ventricle making a left ventricular origin more likely. The comparison of a detailed 3D right and left electroanatomical map is the most powerful tool for the differentiation of a left and right ventricular origin

ten sustained for a long period (often for days). Idiopathic fascicular VT occurs predominantly in males and onset is usually before the age of 30 years. It is almost always well tolerated with an excellent long-term prognosis. Therapy is more a relief of symptoms than a life-saving approach. The mechanism is currently believed to be reentry in the inferoseptal region of the left ventricle. Purkinje potentials and diastolic potentials (perhaps originating from a false tendon) observed during VT are believed to be involved in the reentrant circuit [1, 38]. In this concept, idiopathic reentrant VT with RBBB and left axis deviation (Figure 9.11) corresponds to an origin within the Purkinje network of the posterior division of the left bundle branch,

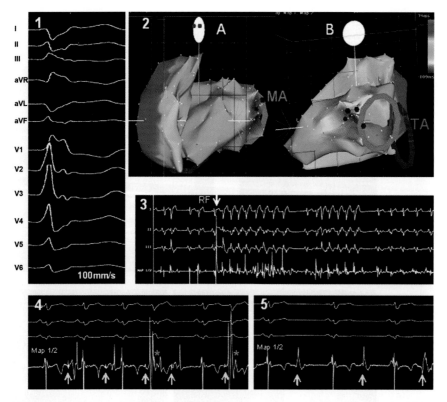

Fig. 9.10. *Mapping and ablation of idiopathic monomorphic VT from the lateral mitral annulus.* **1** QRS morphology of clinical VT. **2** Electroanatomical activation map of left and right ventricle, A) view from LAO 60°, B) posterior view (*MA* mitral annulus, *TA* tricuspid annulus). **3** Ablation at the mitral annulus with an endocardial activation time of –35 ms. The RF application induces an accelerated repetitive VT with the typical QRS morphology of the clinical VT (*RF* start of radiofrequency application). **4** At the ablation point sharp electrograms (yellow arrow) followed by larger, slightly smoother electrograms are recorded after the T wave corresponding to delayed afterdepolarizations as the probable mechanism of triggered activity. In two cases, the sharp potential seems to induce a VPB with the QRS morphology of the clinical VT (orange asterisk). **5** After successful ablation, electrograms suggesting delayed afterdepolarization are still present (yellow arrow) but these do not induce a VPB

while VT with RBBB and right axis deviation originates from the anterior division.

∎ Mapping and ablation of idiopathic verapamil-sensitive ("fascicular") VT

The assumption that this type of VT is based on a reentrant mechanism is supported by the fact that tachycardia can be induced and terminated by pacing, entrainment mapping can be performed and diastolic potentials are recorded. Catheter ablation has a high success and a low complication rate. It is guided by pace mapping or (more often) by activation mapping of a Purkinje potential and a diastolic potential (Figure 9.12). The Purkinje potential precedes the QRS during VT by 15–42 ms at successful ablation sites. It also precedes ventricular activation during sinus rhythm [37].

It has been reported that VT was also successfully ablated at sites far away from the Purkinje potential. A distinct diastolic potential preceding the Purkinje potential during VT had been found at those sites [58]. This potential is of small amplitude with a low frequency component. It is often recorded together with a Purkinje potential and precedes the QRS complex by 52 ± 22 ms [1]. The diastolic potential is often found in the basal and middle septal regions during VT.

The optimal ablation site for this type of tachycardia had been defined as a site where an isolated Purkinje potential preceding the QRS complex by 30–40 ms was found [37]. Often a

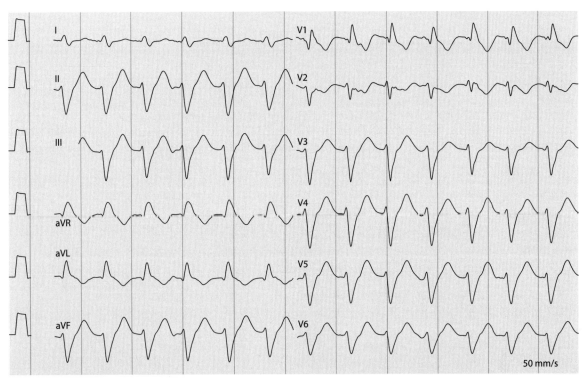

Fig. 9.11. Idiopathic verapamil-sensitive fascicular VT. Tachycardia shows a right bundle branch pattern with a left superior axis

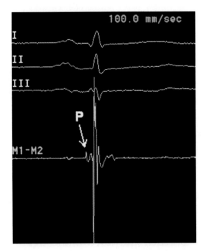

Fig. 9.12. *Mapping of idiopathic verapamil-sensitive VT* originating from the inferoseptal left ventricle. Left ventricular endocardial activation at the posterior and inferior septum was preceded by a distinct potential during sinus rhythm, consistent with a Purkinje potential (P) of a segment of the left posterior fascicle. Radiofrequency energy (30 W, 60 s) was applied in this region and ventricular ectopy declined. Further RF applications were then applied at this level of the ventricular septum along a line of 1.5 cm until no typical ventricular activity was provoked

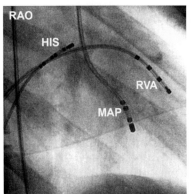

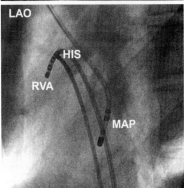

Fig. 9.13. Fluoroscopic image (RAO and LAO views) of the successful ablation site (MAP catheter). The MAP catheter is positioned in the left ventricle at the postero-inferior aspect of the ventricular septum

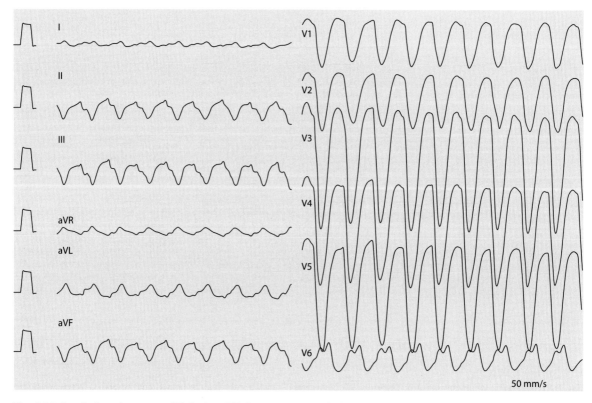

Fig. 9.14. Bundle branch reentrant VT. Surface ECG from a patient with dilated cardiomyopathy. VT shows a left bundle branch block pattern with a heart rate of 220/min

single RF application at this site is successful. Recently, the diastolic potential preceding the Purkinje potential has been reported to be a marker for ablation success with only one or two RF lesions. Successful ablations were often associated with a disappearance of the diastolic but not the Purkinje potential [56, 58].

A left-sided linear ablation approach has been proposed recently, if tachycardia is not inducible or nonsustained during the EP study using an ablation line along the mid to inferior septum that seems to be effective to control tachycardia [33].

9.4.2 Bundle branch reentrant VT

Bundle branch reentrant tachycardia (BBR-VT) is rare, accounting for 5–6% of all sustained monomorphic VT during an EP study [7]. It involves a macroreentrant circuit including the bundle branches and the interventricular septum. It almost exclusively occurs in patients

with structural heart disease (coronary artery disease, nonischemic dilated cardiomyopathy, aortic regurgitation) and is rarely found in patients with structurally normal hearts. All patients with BBR-VT seem to suffer from His-Purkinje disease [7]. Tachycardia rate is usually fast (>200/min) and patients present with presyncope or syncope. In the most common type, excitation travels up the left and down the right bundle branch and then through the interventricular septum to reach the left bundle again. Therefore, tachycardia is monomorphic with a "typical" LBBB pattern. An ECG example of the typical form of BBR-VT is shown in Figure 9.14. Besides the typical form of BBR-VT, two other forms have been described. The second type involves the same reentrant circuit in the opposite direction leading to a right bundle branch block pattern. The third type of BBR-VT reflects a circuit with the excitation wave front conducting retrograde via one left-sided fascicle and antegrade over the other fascicle (interfascicular) [5].

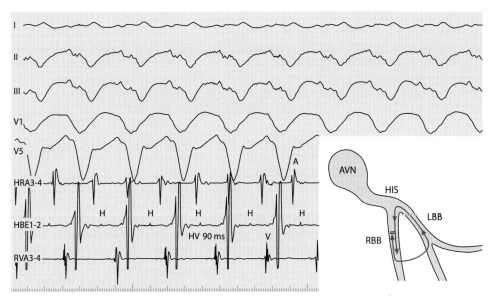

Fig. 9.15. Bundle branch reentrant VT (surface and intracardiac recordings). Note the long HV interval (90 ms) during tachycardia. Concomitant atrial flutter is recorded from the high right atrium (HRA 3–4) (*AVN* atrioventricular node, *HBE* His bundle, *RVA* right ventricular apex). Schematic drawing of the presumed mechanism of BBR-VT: conduction is blocked retrograde in the right bundle branch (RBB) and conducted transseptally up the left bundle branch (LBB). The excitation wavefront then reenters the RBB in the antegrade direction

▪ Mapping and ablation of bundle branch reentrant VT

The concept of BBR-VT is that an impulse (that usually dies out after activation of both ventricles) persists in the His-Purkinje system. The reentrant circuit is induced by a premature ventricular complex that produces a unidirectional block in a branch of the His-Purkinje system (most commonly a retrograde block in the right bundle branch). The excitation wave can then ascend using the left bundle to activate the His bundle retrogradely. If there is a critical delay through the septal ventricle and retrograde left bundle branch, antegrade activation occurs via the right bundle branch to complete the reentrant circuit (Figure 9.15). In patients without structural heart disease, BBR-VT is usually nonsustained because conduction time through the bundle branches is too fast and the prerequisites of reentry (slow conduction of the circuit and unidirectional block) are not fulfilled. Dilated hearts with long conduction times or hearts with His-Purkinje disease are prone to this VT type. BBR-VT is often inducible with programmed ventricular stimulation. During tachycardia, a His bundle and branch potential (with a prolonged HV interval) precede ventricular activity.

Ablation of BBR-VT has been performed by ablating the right bundle branch (Figure 9.16) [7]. The success of the procedure corresponds to the development of right bundle branch block. The ablation site is defined by first identifying the site of maximal His deflection and then moving the catheter superiorly until a right bundle potential is recorded. The interval

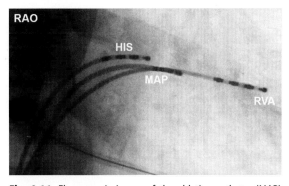

Fig. 9.16. Fluoroscopic image of the ablation catheter (MAP) placed at the recording site of a RBB potential in a patient with BBR-VT. *HIS* catheter placed in His position, *RVA* right ventricular apex

between His recording and BB potential should be at least 15 ms. RF application is started with low energy (15–20 W) which is gradually increased. Success rates are high with a low incidence of complete AV block [7, 14, 32]. There is limited experience with left bundle ablation in this setting which is technically more demanding.

Although BBR-VT is curable by catheter ablation, it should be kept in mind that in this patient population other VT forms might coexist due to the underlying structural heart disease. It was suggested that patients with BBR-VT are still at risk for other ventricular arrhythmias after RF ablation [7]. The indication for an ICD must therefore be reviewed in the individual patient.

9.5 Specific VT entities: scar-related VT

Scar-related VT is associated with underlying structural heart disease that should be characterized before starting an ablation. The potential for ischemia in patients with coronary ar-

tery disease or the severity of ventricular dysfunction has to be assessed by echocardiography, cardiac MRI or angiography. A mobile left ventricular thrombus is a contraindication for mapping and ablation that must be ruled out before the procedure.

The arrhythmia mechanism is a reentrant circuit linked to circumscript arrhythmogenic myocardium. Most forms of sustained monomorphic VT in the setting of coronary artery disease involve a reentry around a scar. Scar-related VT can also occur in arrhythmogenic right ventricular cardiomyopathy, nonischemic cardiomyopathies, after ventricular surgery as in tetralogy of Fallot or in cardiac sarcoidosis. An example of a scar-related VT in arrhythmogenic right ventricular cardiomyopathy (ARVC) is shown in Figures 9.17 and 9.18.

Due to the complexity of the underlying substrate, different VT types are often induced during the EP study. Dynamic substrate changes can lead to acceleration and degeneration of VT and therefore stable and unstable VT forms are commonly found in this setting as well.

Areas of myocardial scar usually contain regions of dense, inexcitable fibrosis that act as conduction barriers and regions of surviving

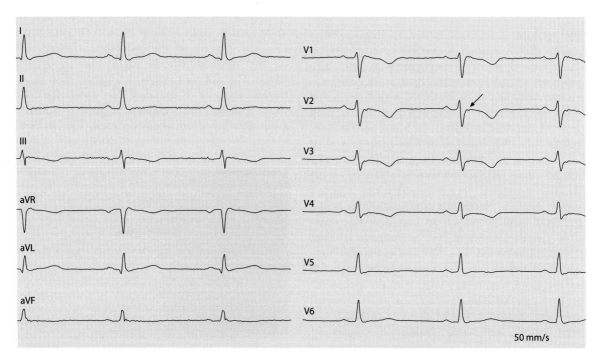

Fig. 9.17. Surface ECG during sinus rhythm of a patient with arrhythmogenic right ventricular cardiomyopathy. Note the epsilon potential (corresponding to delayed conduction) at the end of the QRS complex in lead V2 (arrow) and the negative T waves in leads V1 to V4

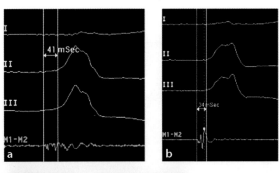

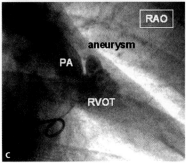

Fig. 9.18. Repetitive nonsustained VT originating from a small aneurysm in the anterior right ventricular outflow tract in a patient with arrhythmogenic right ventricular cardiomyopathy (ARVC). **a** Mapping catheter recordings (green electrograms) of the earliest endocardial activation during VT in the ARVC patient compared to recordings of a patient with idiopathic outflow tract tachycardia (**b**). The presystolic potentials in ARVC VT are more fractionated, complex and delayed than in idiopathic VT. **c** Right ventricular angiogram of the ARVC patient revealing a small right ventricular aneurysm in the anterior outflow tract from where the VT originates. Cardiac MRI confirmed the diagnosis of ARVC

myocardium that create a corridor for reentry (Figure 9.19). Many circuits involve a relatively narrow central common pathway that is the target of ablation [33]. Depolarization within this channel generates low amplitude signals that do not contribute to the QRS complex on the surface ECG. The exit of activation from this channel to the surrounding myocardium will define the surface QRS morphology as all viable myocardium is activated from this point. The region proximal to the exit is the central or proximal region. After leaving the exit, the excitation wave front might return to the proximal region through a broad zone of myocardium along the border of the scar (outer loop). Inner loops are contained within the scar. Sites that are not in

Fig. 9.19. Scar-related VT with a rate of 170 bpm. The precordial leads (left panel) show a concordant (no R/S) pattern. Arrows point to P waves (VA dissociation). The right panel depicts schematically three theoretical reentrant circuits in a scar area. Shaded areas are nonexcitable scar regions. **a** A double loop reentry (two outer loops) with a common protected slow conduction isthmus is shown. Conduction through this corridor occurs during diastole and is not visible on the ECG. QRS onset starts when the wavefront emerges from the exit. Bystanders (Bys) are sites outside the reentrant circuit. *CP* central common pathway. **b** shows a circuit that is contained within the scar area (inner loop reentry). **c** shows a single outer loop reentrant circuit around the margins of the scar area. Modified from Stevenson et al. [51] with permission

▼

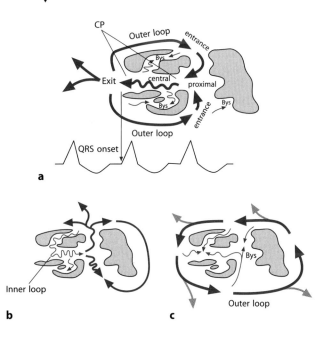

the reentry are called "bystanders". Figure 9.19 shows three theoretical reentrant circuits.

Assessment of the 12-lead ECG can help to localize the VT exit site of the reentrant circuit. VT with a RBBB pattern in V1 is likely to originate from the left ventricle. VT with a LBBB pattern in V1 is likely to originate from the LV septum or rarely from the right ventricle.

▮ Mapping of scar-related VT

Voltage, activation, entrainment and pace mapping techniques are commonly used in scar-related VT. While areas of scars with low amplitude electrograms can be identified by voltage mapping during sinus rhythm, the goal of activation and entrainment mapping is to identify critical portions of a reentrant circuit during VT that are protected by anatomic boundaries such as scars and valve structures ("isthmus of the ventricular tachycardia") [9].

The group of Marchlinski [34] suggested criteria for classifying a border zone of infarction and a dense scar area by *bipolar voltage mapping*. Scar-related tissue is classified by an abnormal low bipolar voltage of ≤1.5 mV measured by peak-to-peak amplitude of the electrogram (originally acquired by a 7F mapping catheter with a 4 mm tip electrode). Dense scar endocardium is described as areas mapped with a bipolar voltage of less than 0.5 mV. These criteria have been widely employed for voltage mapping of the left ventricle (Figure 9.20). Besides recording those potentials during sinus rhythm, anatomic landmarks are identified with the help of an electroanatomical mapping system. If an isthmus of slow conduction during the diastolic or presystolic period is identified in a low voltage area, linear ablation will often be successful. The identification of inexcitable scars surrounding a diastolic conduction isthmus make linear lesions most efficient. Inexcitable scars have been defined by the inability of capture with a pacing output of 10 mA and a pulse width of 2 ms [2, 3, 9, 49, 57]. They can be identified during tachycardia but also during sinus rhythm [2, 9, 49, 57]. In post infarction patients, VT that are well tolerated suggest a circuit size of more than 3–4 cm. Midisthmus and entrance sites are typically located within the region defined as densely infarcted myocardium (bipolar voltage <0.5 mV), whereas exit sites of the reentrant circuit are characteristically located in the border zone of low voltage areas [8].

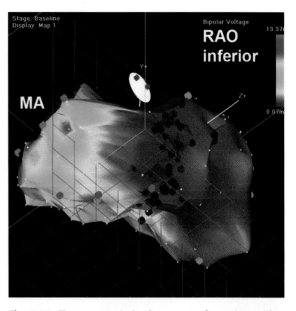

Fig. 9.20. Electroanatomical voltage map of a patient with a large anterior LV aneurysm (red = zone of low voltage – see scale in the right upper corner). A septal ablation line (marked with dark red dots) along the border zone of the low voltage area crossing the best pace map matching point of clinical VT (yellow dot) was created by rotation of a C-curved mapping catheter. *MA* mitral annulus

▮ Activation mapping

Activation mapping during VT should use the QRS complex with the sharpest deflection as reference for calculation of activation time of the local electrograms. An endocardial reference often dislocates during the EP study and is therefore less reliable. Of particular importance is the annotation of diastolic electrograms. In case of complex diastolic electrograms, the sharpest deflection should be tracked independent of the amplitude.

Standard entrainment criteria (Figure 9.21) can prove whether critical electrograms are inside the reentrant circuit (see Chapter 1). Entrainment pacing is performed during VT with a 10% shorter cycle length. Entrainment is positive if 1) the paced QRS is identical to the QRS of VT, 2) the stimulus to QRS interval approximates the interval from the onset of the recorded electrogram to VT QRS and 3) pacing at the site shows a return cycle length approximating VT cycle length (± 30 ms). The investigator should be aware that a negative entrainment does not exclude a reentrant mechanism due to several limitations of entrainment pacing (selected pacing cycle length too short, necessity of

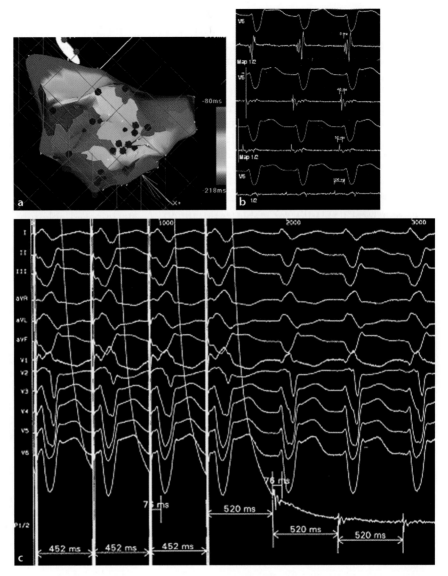

Fig. 9.21. *Linear VT ablation* of a protected slow conduction isthmus through an inferior myocardial scar. **a** Electroanatomical color-coded activation map of the left ventricle from a RAO/ inferior view during a slow and stable VT. Gray areas describe electrical scars (defined by bipolar voltage of less than 0.5 mV and inexcitability at maximum pacing output). **b** Typical electrograms with presystolic and diastolic potentials (arrow) inside the protected isthmus of slow conduction. **c** Positive entrainment with pacing at the exit point of the VT. The successful ablation line connects two scar areas (see **a**). Note that the paced QRS complex had an almost identical morphology as the QRS during tachycardia. The interval form the pacing stimulus to the upstroke of QRS is identical to the interval from the beginning of the local fractionated potential to the upstroke of QRS during tachycardia. Return cycle of the local electrogram is identical to tachycardia cycle length

high output pacing because of unstable catheter contact).

▮ **Pace mapping** can help to determine the region of interest or exit points of VT. In contrast to pace mapping for idiopathic VT ablation, it is important to note that pace mapping for scar-related reentrant VT provides only an approximation of the VT circuit [33]. Pacing with the VT cycle length can improve the congruence with spontaneous VT morphology. Several limitations remain for pace mapping-guided VT localization. False negative pace mapping can occur in the presence of functional unidirectional conduction block during spontaneous VT that may be absent during paced rhythm. Pacing in dead end pathways and outside the bounds of a protected isthmus but near the exit led to false positive pace map matching [33]. Pace mapping results should therefore be interpreted with caution and on the basis of a detailed substrate characterization.

■ Ablation of scar-related VT

■ Point ("focal") ablation for stable reentrant VT.
Stevenson et al. used arbitrary entrainment pacing sites (with concealed fusion according to stimulus-to-QRS interval) to subdivide the delayed protected conduction isthmus of a postinfarction reentrant tachycardia into an exit, central and proximal isthmus (Figure 9.19) [51].

Anatomy does not necessarily correspond to that description. The model is useful for conceptualizing findings during mapping and ablation of hemodynamically tolerated VT [51]. The most important finding is that a postpacing interval ±30 ms of VT cycle length with concealed fusion is associated with tachycardia termination by RF ablation (solid 4 mm tip catheters) and success is highest at the exit site of the isthmus [50, 51].

Exact concealed pace mapping of the exit site predicted the success of a single RF application if the following three criteria of concealed entrainment pacing were met: 1) an exact QRS match in the 12-lead ECG during entrainment, 2) a return cycle length of ≤10 ms of the VT cycle length, 3) presystolic potentials (<70% of the VT cycle length) with an activation time to the QRS within 10 ms of the stimulus-to-QRS interval [16].

The most important limitation for single point ablation is the low number (around 10%) of postinfarction patients with well-tolerated sustained VT which can be reproducibly induced by programmed stimulation [8]. In nonselected patients with a history of well-tolerated VT, ablation has been successful in 58% (when it was planned on an intention-to-treat basis by activation and entrainment mapping) [12].

A focal ablation approach targeting the earliest endocardial activation or just one point of positive entrainment without the understanding of the complete critical conduction isthmus is often useful for termination of incessant VT.

However, the long-term success of this approach is unclear even if the targeted VT is noninducible at the end of the procedure. Our recent data of postinfarction patients after focal ablation revealed a high recurrence rate of VT (70%) during long-term follow-up (ICD-controlled). This included clinical and nonclinical VT even in case of noninducibility at the end of the EP study [44]. The linear isthmus ablation approach with a significantly lower VT recurrence rate of 30% should therefore in our opinion be the preferred approach. If no diastolic conduction isthmus could be determined, a substrate-based ablation approach guided by potential or voltage criteria as outlined below should be performed in order to reduce the VT recurrence rate.

■ Substrate-based ablation of scar-related VT.
Substrate-based ablation of scar-related VT was developed for unstable VT forms [34]. It has also proven its value in the case of noninducible or polymorphic VT [33]. The understanding of the ventricular substrate enabling reentrant activation due to delayed conduction has been most extensively studied in postinfarction patients [33]. It can also be transferred to scar-related reentrant VT in patients with nonischemic cardiomyopathy [25, 34] or arrhythmogenic right ventricular cardiomyopathy [35]. Currently substrate-based ablation strategies are useful as part of the routine for almost all patients who undergo VT ablation [33, 59].

Substrate-based ablation relies on detailed electroanatomical mapping during sinus or paced rhythm and the determination of the region of interest or exit points of VT by pace mapping for documented VT. As outlined above, pace mapping results should be interpreted with caution and on the basis of a detailed substrate characterization. If no exact pace map matching site is found, a close approximation is useful to guide ablation.

Substrate-based ablation can be divided in two main strategies: 1) the linear ablation approach guided by voltage mapping and 2) a primary potential-guided ablation approach. Both strategies are frequently combined [33].

■ Linear substrate-based ablation guided by voltage mapping.
The basis for linear substrate-based ablation is endocardial bipolar voltage mapping during sinus rhythm or paced rhythm as outlined above to delineate a scar in a pa-

tient with coronary heart disease or an area of electrically abnormal myocardium in patients with cardiomyopathy. After completion of the bipolar voltage map, pace mapping is performed if VT is documented or inducible preferentially along the border zone of low voltage areas. The pace mapping matching point is thought to correspond to the area of the VT exit point in case of a short stimulation to QRS interval. In case of a longer stimulation-to-QRS interval time, an area of the diastolic conduction pathway is suspected [15, 34, 59].

After defining the area of interest by pace mapping, different linear ablation strategies have been suggested. Marchlinski et al. first described a perpendicular linear ablation crossing the border zone of a myocardial scar. The lesions extend from the areas demonstrating the lowest amplitude signals to areas demonstrating a distinctly normal signal (>1.5 mV) or to a valve continuity by crossing sites where pace mapping approximated the QRS morphology of the VT. A second approach is based on linear ablation parallel to the border zone of a low voltage area extending the best pace mapping site for a VT exit point for 1–2 cm (Figure 9.20) [15]. A third approach is a linear ablation line through the scar in case of delayed conduction or isolated potentials during sinus rhythm [17, 59] which can be present even in the dense scar area (bipolar voltage <0.5 mV). The common principle of all strategies is the extension of linear lesions to valve structures especially to the mitral annulus [15, 21, 33, 34, 59].

Endpoint for RF application is the inexcitability at the lesion site using a 2 ms pacing stimulus at 10 mA output and the noninducibility of VT by programmed stimulation [15, 34, 59]. If these criteria are not fulfilled, linear lesions are augmented, extended or more ablation lines are created guided by the remaining VT forms.

To avoid damage to viable tissue, substrate-based RF ablation has only been recommended at sites of voltage less than 1.5 mV [15] and more recently less than 1.8 mV [25, 33] to adjust factors such as hypertrophy. It has been well established that voltage mapping can accurately delineate a transmural myocardial infarction [11, 29]. However, the exact potential cut-off values for transmural infarction and more diffuse scarring have not been validated. Extensive ablation should be performed with caution and should be tailored to strategies which target the lowest voltage areas of local electrical activ-

ity. We currently perform a linear ablation approach even if a stable VT can be assessed by activation mapping as there seems to be evidence that substrate-based linear ablation also improves long-term success in stable, hemodynamically tolerated VT [44].

∎ **Potential-guided substrate ablation.** The potential-guided ablation approach has been reported to be successful in noninducible or unstable VT in patients with structural heart disease or even in an electrical storm of multiple unstable VT forms [43]. Arenal et al. ablated sites with isolated, delayed double or multiple components of the local electrograms separated by ≥50 ms during sinus rhythm or more frequently during right ventricular pacing in low voltage areas of less than 0.5 mV [3]. Isolated delayed electrograms were only targeted by ablation if pace mapping reproduced the clinical VT with stimulus-to-QRS interval of >50 ms or if isolated delayed electrograms became middiastolic during VT induction.

In a cohort of patients with ventricular infarction and frequent and partially unstable VT (mean of 2.7 ± 1.7 VT morphologies), ablation of sites with delayed and fractionated local potential in low voltage areas (<1.5 mV) led to a 69% VT-free long-term follow-up and to a significant reduction of VT episodes in 89% of patients [45]. The potential-guided RF applications were positioned 1.5 cm around best pace mapping match sites exclusively in areas of bipolar voltage <1.5 mV. The endpoint was the abolition of local fractionated electrograms and the noninducibility of clinically documented VT. This potential-guided substrate modification was also successful in VT patients in the situation of an electrical storm of multiple unstable VT forms [43] (Figure 9.22).

The analysis of isolated potentials during sinus rhythm in postinfarction patients is helpful to identify critical sites of the VT reentry circuit and can be incorporated into more conventional ablation strategies [8]. The presence of multipotential electrograms during atrial and ventricular paced rhythm [9] and the observation of slow conduction detected by pace mapping during sinus rhythm (>80 ms stimulus to QRS interval) proved to be a useful guide for identifying critical target areas for substrate-based ablation strategies [9].

In our experience, potential-guided substrate ablation can also be performed in patients with

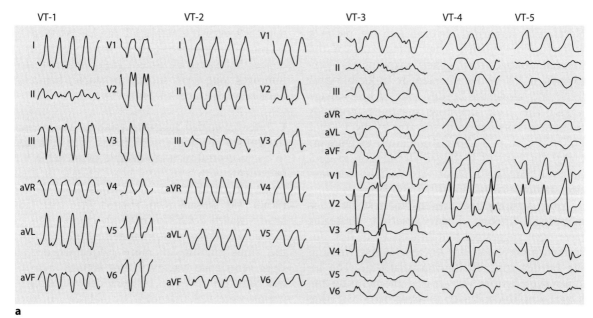

a

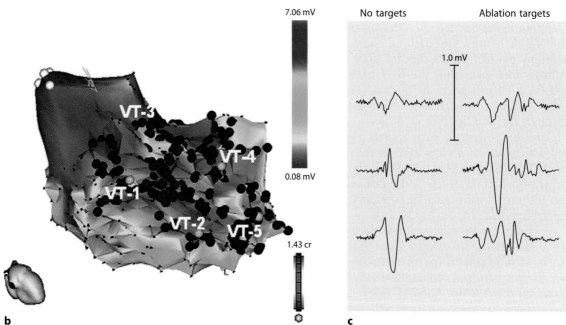

b

c

Fig. 9.22. Potential-guided substrate ablation of five forms of unstable VT in a severely compromised patient with a large inferior low voltage area. **a** ECG of five forms of unstable VT: Clinically documented VT-1 and VT-2 led to frequent ICD shock deliveries during an electrical storm, VT-3, VT-4 and VT-5 occurred during the EP study. From Schreieck et al. [43] with permission. **b** Voltage map of the left ventricle, inferior view. Yellow points mark best pace mapping match of the exit points of VT1–5. Around each VT exit point delayed fractionated electrograms were targeted by ablation in low voltage areas (bipolar voltage < 1.5 mV). **c** Low amplitude electrograms inside the inferior low voltage area. Targets for ablation were complex, delayed fractionated electrograms (RF application, irrigated tip 30–40 W). From Schreieck et al. [43] with permission

nonischemic cardiomyopathy (Figure 9.23), even in case of ventricular fibrillation (Figure 9.24). Especially in patients with dilated cardiomyopathy, the presence of delayed fractionated potentials seems to be more specific for delineation of the arrhythmogenic area than in postinfarction patients.

9.6 Ablation of ventricular fibrillation

A major challenge for catheter ablation of ventricular arrhythmias is the feasibility of eliminating episodes of ventricular fibrillation (VF). Studies in patients with idiopathic ventricular fibrillation [23, 24], ventricular fibrillation secondary to repolarization disorders (long QT and Brugada syndrome) [22] or ischemic heart disease [4, 35, 52] have provided insights into the role of focal triggers for VF that predominantly originate from the specialized intraventricular conduction system. In the majority of patients, isolated or repetitive premature ventricular

beats (VPB) occur that are identical to those triggering VF. This allows mapping and ablation of these VPBs.

In patients without structural heart disease, VF triggering VPBs originate mostly from peripheral Purkinje sources. These are located in the anterior right ventricle or in the left ventricle in a region of the lower septum from the ramifications of anterior and posterior fascicles and the intervening regions. At successful ablation sites of the Purkinje VPBs, the earliest Purkinje potential preceded local muscle activation by a conduction interval of 38 ± 28 ms [24]. Interestingly (although rare) an origin of these VPBs was also found in the RVOT and ablation strategy for these triggers was identical to that of VT from the RVOT [22, 24].

In patients after myocardial infarction, mapping and ablation of triggers for VF or polymorphic VT targets the most frequent VPB morphology originating exclusively from the left ventricular Purkinje network bordering the infarct zone [4, 35, 52]. Repetitive Purkinje activity with different conduction times to the earliest ventricular electrogram has been docu-

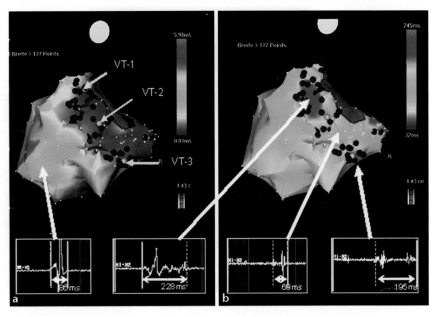

Fig. 9.23. Potential-guided, substrate-based VT ablation in a patient with dilated cardiomyopathy. **a** Voltage map of the left ventricle during right ventricular pacing, view from posterior and inferior. Yellow dots are the best pace map matching point for the exit of three forms of monomorphic VT (VT1–3). **b** Color-coded map of the electrogram duration during right ventricular pacing of the same patient. Electrogram duration was determined as the interval from the first to the last sharp deflection. Blue color encoded a delay of 180–230 ms. Note that the electrogram duration map more precisely delineated the arrhythmogenic areas than the voltage map in **a**. **c** Typical examples of electrograms with and without delayed local potentials

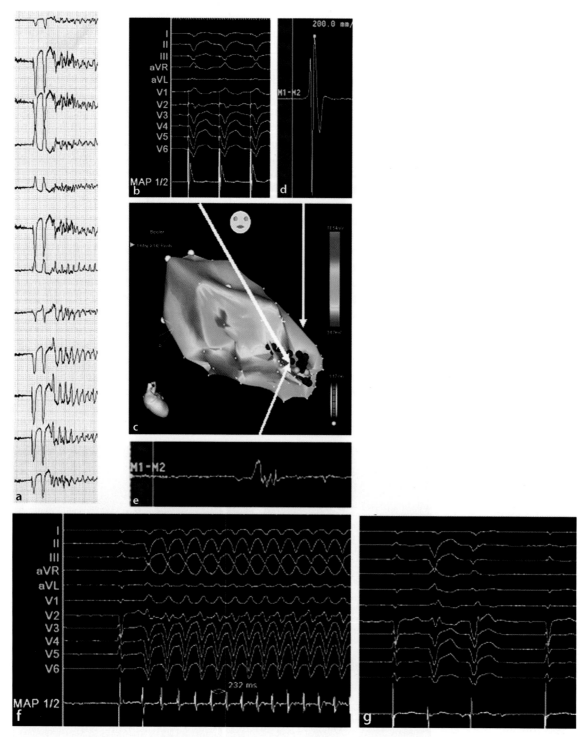

Fig. 9.24. Ablation of spontaneous ventricular fibrillation (VF) by a potential-guided, substrate-based ablation approach in a patient with dilated cardiomyopathy. **a** Spontaneous onset of VF documented on a 12-lead Holter ECG with a characteristic onset pattern. **b** Pace map matching of the VPBs triggering VF localized in the anteroapical left ventricle. **c** Voltage map of the left ventricle of the same patient. Yellow dots are best pace map matching points in a small low voltage area of less than 1.8 mV amplitude. Red dots: radiofrequency application sites (irrigated tip 40 W). **d** Electrogram far outside the critical area. **e** Electrogram within the critical area with multiple delayed fractionated potentials (amplitude <0.5 mV). **f** Accelerated ventricular rhythm with typical QRS morphology at the beginning of RF application at the successful ablation site. **g** Only single VPBs at the end of the RF application

mented during polymorphic VT [52]. In patients with ischemic heart disease, VPBs triggering VF not only have a QRS morphology mimicking fascicular VT (narrow RBBB complex, superior axis) but also the mapping and ablation strategy is similar to fascicular VT. Short, high frequency, low amplitude potentials precede the onset of VPBs and ventricular tachyarrhythmias by 20–160 ms [4, 35, 52]. During ablation, transient exacerbation of the arrhythmia (including VF) precedes the disappearance of VPBs. The endpoint of the ablation is the elimination of all local spontaneous VPBs by using multiple RF applications.

Besides approaching the triggers for VF, a combined approach for unstable VT/VF in ischemic heart disease targeting trigger and substrate seems reasonable [34]. Our group has shown recently that a potential-guided substrate-based approach can also establish VT/VF control in an unstable clinical situation (Figure 9.24) [43].

To summarize, catheter ablation of ventricular fibrillation represents one of the last challenges for interventional cardiac electrophysiology. So far the implantation of a cardioverter-defibrillator remains the cornerstone for primary and secondary prophylaxis of sudden cardiac death.

■ References

1. Aiba T, Suyama K, Aihara N, Taguchi A, Shimizu W, Kurita T, Kamakura S (2001) The role of Purkinje and pre-Purkinje potentials in the reentrant circuit of verapamil-sensitive idiopathic LV tachycardia. Pacing Clin Electrophysiol 24: 333–344

2. Arenal A, del Castillo S, Gonzalez-Torrecilla E, Atienza F, Ortiz M, Jimenez J, Puchol A, Garcia J, Almendral J (2004) Tachycardia-related channel in the scar tissue in patients with sustained monomorphic ventricular tachycardias. Circulation 110:2568–2574

3. Arenal A, Glez-Torrecilla E, Ortiz M, Villacastin J, Fdez-Portales J, Sousa E, del Castillo S, de Isla LP, Jimenez J, Almendral J (2003) Ablation of electrograms with an isolated, delayed component as treatment of unmappable monomorphic ventricular tachycardias in patients with structural heart disease. J Am Coll Cardiol 41:81–92

4. Bansch D, Oyang F, Antz M, Arentz T, Weber R, Val-Mejias JE, Ernst S, Kuck KH (2003) Successful catheter ablation of electrical storm after myocardial infarction. Circulation 108:3011–3016

5. Berger RD, Orias D, Kasper EK, Calkins H (1996) Catheter ablation of coexistent bundle branch and interfascicular reentrant ventricular tachycardias. J Cardiovasc Electrophysiol 7:341–347

6. Berruezo A, Mont L, Nava S, Chueca E, Bartholomay E, Brugada J (2004) Electrocardiographic recognition of the epicardial origin of ventricular tachycardias. Circulation 109:1842–1847

7. Blanck Z, Dhala A, Deshpande S, Sra J, Jazayeri M, Akhtar M (1993) Bundle branch reentrant ventricular tachycardia: cumulative experience in 48 patients. J Cardiovasc Electrophysiol 4: 253–262

8. Bogun F, Li Y-G, Groenefeld G, Hohnloser SH, Schuger C, Oral H, Pelosi F, Knight B, Strickberger SA, Morady F (2002) Prevalence of a shared isthmus in postinfarction patients with pleomorphic, hemodynamically tolerated ventricular tachycardias. J Cardiovasc Electrophysiol 13: 237–241

9. Brunckhorst C, Delacretaz E, Soejima K, Maisel WH, Friedman PL, Stevenson WG (2004) Identification of the ventricular tachycardia isthmus after infarction by pacemapping. Circulation 110:652–659

10. Buyon JP, Waltuck J, Kleinman C, Copel J (1995) In utero identification and therapy of congenital heart block. Lupus 4:116–121

11. Callans DJ, Ren JF, Michele J, Marchlinski FE, Dillon SM (1999) Electroanatomic left ventricular mapping in the porcine model of healed anterior myocardial infarction. Correlation with intracardiac echocardiography and pathological analysis. Circulation 100:1744–1750

12. Callans DJ, Zado E, Sarter BH, Schwartzman D, Gottlieb CD, Marchlinski FE (1998) Procedural efficacy of radiofrequency ablation of ventricular tachycardia in patients with healed myocardial infarction: an intention to treat analysis. Am J Cardiol 82:429–432

13. Callans D, Menz V, Schwartzman D, Gottlieb CD, Marchlinski FE (1997) Repetitive monomorphic tachycardia from the left ventricular outflow tract: electrocardiographic patterns consistent with a left ventricular site of origin. J Am Coll Cardiol 29:1023–1027

14. Cohen TJ, Chien WW, Lurie KG, Young C, Goldberg HR, Wang YS, Langberg JJ, Lesh MD, Lee MA, Griffin JC et al (1991) Radiofrequency catheter ablation for treatment of bundle branch reentrant ventricular tachycardia: results and long-term follow-up. J Am Coll Cardiol 18: 1767–1773

15. Delacretaz E, Ganz LI, Soejima K, Friedman PL, Walsh EP, Triedman JK, Sloss LJ, Landzberg MJ, Stevenson WG (2001) Multi atrial macro-reentry circuits in adults with repaired congenital heart disease: entrainment mapping combined

with three-dimensional electroanatomic mapping. J Am Coll Cardiol 37:1665–1676

16. El-Shalakany A, Hadjis T, Papageorgiou P, Monahan K, Epstein L, Josephson ME (1999) Entrainment/mapping criteria for the prediction of termination of ventricular tachycardia by single radiofrequency lesion in patients with coronary artery disease. Circulation 99:2283–2289

17. Furniss S, Anil-Kumar R, Bourke JP, Behulova R, Simeonidou E (2000) Radiofrequency ablation of haemodynamically unstable ventricular tachycardia after myocardial infarction. Heart 84:648–652

18. Gerstenfeld E, Dixit S, Callans DJ, Rajawat Y, Rho R, Marchlinski FE (2003) Quantitative comparison of spontaneous and paced 12-lead electrocardiogram during right ventricular outflow tract ventricular tachycardia. J Am Coll Cardiol 41:2046–2053

19. Hachiya H, Aonuma K, Yamauchi Y, Harady T, Igawa M, Nogami A, Iseka Y, Hiroe M, Marumo F (2000) Electrocardiographic characteristics of left ventricular outflow tract tachycardia. Pacing Clin Electrophysiol 23:1930–1934

20. Hachiya H, Aonuma K, Yamauchi Y, Igawa M, Nogami A, Iesaka Y (2002) How to diagnose, locate, and ablate coronary cusp ventricular tachycardia. J Cardiovasc Electrophysiol 13:551–556

21. Hadjis TA, Stevenson WG, Harada T, Friedman PL, Sager P, Saxon LA (1997) Preferential locations for critical reentry circuit sites causing ventricular tachycardia after inferior wall myocardial infarction. J Cardiovasc Electrophysiol 8:363–370

22. Haissaguerre M, Extramiana F, Hocini M, Cauchemez B, Jais P, Cabrera JA, Farre J, Leenhardt A, Sanders P, Scavee C, Hsu LF, Weerasooriya R, Shah DC, Frank R, Maury P, Delay M, Garrigue S, Clementy J (2003) Mapping and ablation of ventricular fibrillation associated with long-QT and Brugada syndromes. Circulation 108:925–928

23. Haissaguerre M, Shah DC, Jais P, Shoda M, Kautzner J, Arentz T, Kalushe D, Kadish A, Griffith M, Gaita F, Yamane T, Garrigue S, Hocini M, Clementy J (2002) Role of Purkinje conducting system in triggering of idiopathic ventricular fibrillation. Lancet 359:677–678

24. Haissaguerre M, Shoda M, Jais P, Nogami A, Shah DC, Kautzner J, Arentz T, Kalushe D, Lamaison D, Griffith M, Cruz F, de Paola A, Gaita F, Hocini M, Garrigue S, Macle L, Weerasooriya R, Clementy J (2002) Mapping and ablation of idiopathic ventricular fibrillation. Circulation 106:962–967

25. Hsia H, Marchlinski FE (2002) Characterization of the electroanatomic substrate for monomorphic ventricular tachycardia in patients with nonischemic cardiomyopathy. Pacing Clin Electrophysiol 25:1114–1127

26. Jadonath R, Schwartzman D, Preminger MW, Gottlieb CD, Marchlinski FE (1995) The utility of the 12 lead electrocardiogram in localizing the site of origin of right ventricular outflow tract tachycardia. Am Heart J 130:1107–1113

27. Kamakura S, Shimizu W, Matsuo K, Taguchi A, Suyama K, Kurita T, Aihara N, Ohe T, Shimomura K (1998) Localization of optimal ablation site of idiopathic ventricular tachycardia from right and left ventricular outflow tract by body surface ECG. Circulation 98:1525–1533

28. Kanagaratnam L, Tomassoni G, Schweikert R, Pavia S, Bash D, Beheiry S, Niebauer M, Saliba W, Chung M, Tchou P, Natale A (2001) Ventricular tachycardia arising from the aortic sinus of valsalva: an under-recognized variant of left outflow tract ventricular tachycardia. J Am Coll Cardiol 37:1408–1414

29. Kornowski R, Hong MK, Gepstein L, Goldstein S, Ellahham S, Ben-Haim SA, Leon MB (1998) Preliminary animal and clinical experience using an electromechanical endocardial mapping procedure to distinguish infarcted from healthy myocardium. Circulation 98:1116–1124

30. Krebs ME, Krause PC, Engelstein ED, Zipes DP, Miles WM (2000) Ventricular tachycardias minicking those arising from the right ventricular outflow tract. J Cardiovasc Electrophysiol 11:45–51

31. Kumagai K, Yamauchi Y, Takahashi A, Yokoyama Y, Sekiguchi Y, Watanabe J, Iesaka Y, Shirato K, Aonuma K (2005) Idiopathic left ventricular tachycardia originating from the mitral annulus. J Cardiovasc Electrophysiol 16:1029–1036

32. Li YG, Gronefeld G, Israel C, Bogun F, Hohnloser SH (2002) Bundle branch reentrant tachycardia in patients with apparent normal His-Purkinje conduction: the role of functional conduction impairment. J Cardiovasc Electrophysiol 13:1233–1239

33. Lin D, Hsia HH, Gerstenfeld EP, Dixit S, Callans DJ, Nayak H, Russo A, Marchlinski FE (2005) Idiopathic fascicular left ventricular tachycardia: linear ablation lesion strategy for noninducible or nonsustained tachycardia. Heart Rhythm 2:934–939

34. Marchlinski FE, Callans DJ, Gottlieb CD, Zado ES (2000) Linear ablation lesions for control of unmappable ventricular tachycardia in patients with ischemia and nonischemic cardiomyopathy. Circulation 101:1288–1296

35. Marrouche NF, Verma A, Wazni O, Schweikert R, Martin DO, Saliba W, Kilicaslan F, Cummings J, Burkhardt JD, Bhargava M, Bash D, Brachmann J, Guenther J, Hao S, Beheiry S, Rossillo A, Raviele A, Themistoclakis S, Natale A (2004) Mode of initiation and ablation of ventricular

fibrillation storms in patients with ischemic cardiomyopathy. J Am Coll Cardiol 43:1715–1720

36. Movsowitz C, Schwartzman D, Callans DJ, Preminger M, Zado E, Gottlieb CD, Marchlinski FE (1996) Idiopathic right ventricular outflow tract tachycardia: Narrowing the anatomical location for successful ablation. Am Heart J 131:930–936

37. Nakagawa H, Beckman KJ, McClelland JH, Wang X, Arruda M, Santoro I, Hazlitt HA, Abdalla I, Singh A, Gossinger H et al (1993) Radiofrequency catheter ablation of idiopathic left ventricular tachycardia guided by a Purkinje potential. Circulation 88:2607–2617

38. Nogami A, Naito S, Tada H, Taniguchi K, Okamoto Y, Nishimura S, Yamauchi Y, Aonuma K, Goya M, Iesaka Y, Hiroe M (2000) Demonstration of diastolic and presystolic Purkinje potentials as critical potentials in a macroreentry circuit of verapamil-sensitive idiopathic left ventricular tachycardia. J Am Coll Cardiol 36:811–823

39. Ouyang F, Bänsch D, Schaumann A, Ernst S, Linder C, Falk P, Hachiya H, Kuck KH, Antz M (2003) Catheter ablation of subepicardial ventricular tachycardia using electroanatomic mapping. Herz 28:591–597

40. Ouyang F, Fotuhi P, Ho SY, Hebe J, Volkmer M, Gova M, Burns M, Antz M, Ernst S, Cappato R, Kuck KH (2002) Repetitive monomorphic ventricular tachycardia originating from the aortic sinus cusp: electrocardiographic characterization for guiding catheter ablation. J Am Coll Cardiol 39:500–508

41. Posada Rodriguez IJ, Gutierrez-Rivas E, Cabello A (1997) [Cardiac involvement in neuromuscular diseases]. Rev Esp Cardiol 50:882–901

42. Sadanaga T, Saeki K, Yoshimoto T, Funatsu Y, Miyazaki T (1999) Repetitive monomorphic ventricular tachycardia of the left coronary cusp origin. Pacing Clin Electrophysiol 22:1553–1556

43. Schreieck J, Zrenner B, Deisenhofer I, Schmitt C (2005) Rescue ablation of electrical storm in patients with ischemic cardiomyopathy: A potential-guided ablation approach by modifying substrate of intractable, unmappable ventricular tachycardia. Heart Rhythm 2:10–14

44. Schreieck J, Zrenner B, Deisenhofer I, Schneider M, Karch MR, Kolb C, Schmitt C (2005) Recurrence rate of ventricular tachycardia after radiofrequency current ablation in post infarction patients. Comparison of focal ablation with linear isthmus ablation and potential-guided substrate ablation. Circulation 112 (suppl):II-520

45. Schreieck J, Zrenner B, Dong J, Deisenhofer I, Schneider MA, Kolb C, Schmitt C (2004) Ablation of post infarction ventricular tachycardia targeting delayed local potentials guided by electroanatomical mapping (abstract). J Am Coll Cardiol 43 (suppl A):154A

46. Schweikert R, Saliba WI, Tomassoni G, Marrouche NF, Cole CR, Dresing TJ, Tchou PJ, Bash D, Beheiry S, Lam C, Kanagaratnam L, Natale A (2003) Percutaneous pericardial instrumentation for endo-epicardial mapping of previously failed ablations. Circulation 108:1329–1335

47. Shimoike E, Ohnishi Y, Ueda N, Maruyama T, Kaji Y (1999) Radiofrequency catheter ablation of the left ventricular outflow tachycardia from the coronary cusp: a new approach to the tachycardia focus. J Cardiovasc Electrophysiol 10:1005–1009

48. Soejima K, Stevenson WG, Sapp JL, Selwyn AP, Couper G, Epstein LM (2004) Endocardial and epicardial radiofrequency ablation of ventricular tachycardia associated with dilated cardiomyopathy: importance of low-voltage scars. J Am Coll Cardiol 19:1834–1842

49. Soejima K, Stevenson WG, Maisel WH, Sapp JL, Epstein LM (2002) Electrically unexcitable scar mapping based on pacing threshold for identification of the reentry circuit isthmus: Feasibility for guiding ventricular tachycardia ablation. Circulation 106:1678–1683

50. Stevenson WG, Kahn H, Sager P, Saxon LA, Middlekauff HR, Natterson PD, Wiener I (1993) Identification of reentry circuit sites during catheter mapping and radiofrequency ablation of ventricular tachycardia late after myocardial infarction. Circulation 88:1647–1670

51. Stevenson WG, Friedman PL, Sager PT, Saxon LA, Kocovic D, Harada T, Wiener I, Khan H (1997) Exploring postinfarction reentrant ventricular tachycardia with entrainment mapping. J Am Coll Cardiol 29:1180–1189

52. Szumowski L, Sanders P, Walczak F, Hocini M, Jais P, Kepski R, Szufladowicz E, Urbanek P, Derejko P, Bodalski R, Haissaguerre M (2004) Mapping and ablation of polymorphic ventricular tachycardia after myocardial infarction. J Am Coll Cardiol 44:1700–1706

53. Tada H, Ohe T, Yutani C, Shimizu W, Kurita T, Aihara N, Kamakura S, Shimomura K (1996) Sudden death in a patient with apparent idiopathic ventricular tachycardia. Jpn Circ J 60:133–136

54. Tadokoro T, Ikeda K, Sudo K, Mizuno A, Ohbayashi T, Morita H, Unno T, Hayashi N, Noguchi K (1989) [Pacemaker implantation in 7 days or less old of early neonates]. Rinsho Kyobu Geka 9:490–493

55. Timmermans C, Rodriguez LM, Crijns HJGM, Moorman AFM, Wellens HJJ (2003) Idiopathic left bundle-branch block-shaped ventricular tachycardia may originate above the pulmonary valve. Circulation 108:1960–1967

56. Tsuchiya T, Okumura K, Honda T, Honda T, Iwasa A, Yasue H, Tabuchi T (1999) Significance of late diastolic potential preceding Purkinje po-

tential in verapamil-sensitive idiopathic left ventricular tachycardia. Circulation 99:2408–2413

57. Van Dessel PFHM, De Bakker JM, Van Hemel NM, Linnenbank AC, Jessurun ER, Defauw JA (2001) Pacemapping of postinfarction scar to detect ventricular tachycardia exit sites and zones of slow conduction. J Cardiovasc Electrophysiol 12:662–670

58. Wen MS, Yeh SJ, Wang CC, Lin FC, Wu D (1997) Successful radiofrequency ablation of idiopathic left ventricular tachycardia at a site away from the tachycardia exit. J Am Coll Cardiol 30:1024–1031

59. Wetzel U, Hindricks G, Dorszewski A, Schirdewahn P, Gerds-Li JH, Piorkowski C, Kobza R, Tanner H, Kottkamp H (2003) Electroanatomic mapping of the endocardium. Implication for catheter ablation of ventricular tachycardia. Herz 28:583–590

10 Catheter ablation of atrial fibrillation

Isabel Deisenhofer, Heidi Estner, Alexander Pustowoit

▌Introduction

Catheter ablation has become an accepted option in the therapeutic spectrum for the treatment of atrial fibrillation (AF) [12, 17, 44]. However, debate about the optimal ablation strategy is ongoing and will probably be the prevailing issue in EP for the next few years if not decades. Some definitions and mechanistic concepts regarding the genesis of atrial fibrillation are helpful when planning the ablation [8].

▌Definitions

▌**Paroxysmal AF.** Episodes of AF which do not last longer than 7 days and terminate spontaneously. Typically, paroxysms of AF last from seconds up to several hours and are initiated by atrial runs or very frequent atrial ectopic beats. The "initiating trigger" is the characteristic feature of this AF type. Ablating or isolating the trigger is the most common treatment strategy. If the focal activity is monomorphic, it is sometimes called focal AF.

▌**Persistent AF.** The episodes of AF last longer than in paroxysmal AF (from 7 days up to several months) and do not terminate spontaneously. Pharmacological or electric cardioversion is necessary for termination. After cardioversion, sinus rhythm can be maintained for several days to months.

▌**Permanent (chronic) AF.** AF is present for several months to years and neither pharmacological nor electrical cardioversion is successful anymore (immediate relapse or primary failure).

▌10.1 Basic concepts of atrial fibrillation

Many theories exist about the genesis and perpetuation of AF. However, we will focus on a few of them which seem to be important if AF ablation is intended. The results of bench and clinical studies investigating AF (and the electrophysiological alterations occurring while AF initiates, persists and becomes permanent) are summarized below.

10.1.1 Multiple wavelets

This concept was first presented by Moe in the 1960s [30, 31]. During AF, multiple reentrant

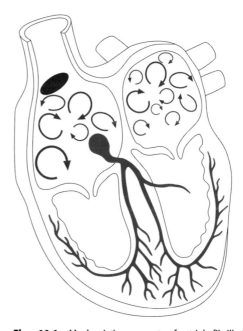

Fig. 10.1. Mechanistic concept of atrial fibrillation (after Moe): multiple reentrant wavelets (red arrows) circulate in both atria, constantly changing their direction, wave length and location. The conduction of electric activation to the ventricles takes its normal course (via the AV node)

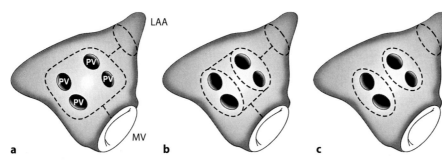

Fig. 10.2. Surgical ablation of atrial fibrillation: left atrial line designs. The original left atrial linear lesion set of Cox et al. is shown in **a**. Current surgical lesion schemes are shown in **b** and **c**. All concepts shown include an isolation of the pulmonary vein orifices. There are, however, surgical approaches connecting only the pulmonary vein ostia with linear lesions, without an isolation attempt. Most commonly, a line connecting the pulmonary vein area to the mitral annulus is added. *LAA* left atrial appendage, *MV* mitral valve, *PV* pulmonary vein

wavelets which change constantly in number, location and cycle length co-exist in the left and right atrium (LA and RA) (Figure 10.1).

The multiple wavelet theory implies that a critical mass large enough for longer wavefronts and several circuits is necessary for maintenance of AF. Consequently, long linear lesions cutting the LA and RA into smaller areas of conducting tissue could make AF nonsustained or completely suppress it [2, 9, 23]. This concept has been put into practice by surgeons with the so-called Maze procedure [4, 9]. Lines of complete conduction block, initially achieved with a "cut and sew" surgical technique, aim to segment both atria into areas too small to offer enough place for more than two or three circuits (Figure 10.2).

These circuits will organize to one reentry which will eventually stop because of a lack of space. Currently, the cut-and-sew lines are replaced by intraoperatively applied ablation lines created with various tools like cryo and microwave probes [9].

10.1.2 The triggering foci

The initiating trigger for paroxysms of AF is very often repetitive atrial activity (e.g., atrial runs) (Figure 10.3).

Discussion is ongoing about the exact percentage, but it seems to be clear that about 60–90% of the triggering foci are located inside or at the ostium of pulmonary veins (PV) [3, 5, 12, 25, 34, 52, 53, 62]. Direct ablation of the foci is often laborious. Triggers might not be active at the moment of the EP study or they may initiate AF immediately (requiring cardioversion). Triggers might be present in more than one PV and multiple triggers might be present in one PV. Electrical isolation of the entire PV during sinus rhythm overcomes the limitations of focus ablation and significantly reduces the risk of PV stenosis. A less frequent source of triggering foci besides the PV are other great thoracic veins [10, 19, 20, 25]: in decreasing frequency the coronary sinus (CS) and its tributaries (e.g., the vein of Marshall) and the superior vena cava (SVC). Anatomic variants (e.g., persistent left SVC) are also reported to have arrhythmogenic potential [19]. Up to 40% (4–40%) of the trig-

Fig. 10.3. Telemetric strip recording (**a** 25 mm/s), surface ECG at rest (**b** 50 mm/s) and intracardiac recording (**c** 100 mm/s) from the right superior PV during EP study of a patient with paroxysmal atrial fibrillation with marked focal activity ("focal AF"). In **a**, only a few sinus beats occur while atrial runs prevail. The 12-lead surface ECG in **b** allows the analysis of P wave morphology of these very monomorphic atrial runs. To correctly judge the P wave polarity and amplitude, the T wave of the preceding beat has to be subtracted (use your imagination or use the specially created software, e.g., from Bard Inc). In the presented case, the P wave is positive in I, II, III and aVF; aVL shows an isoelectric P and P in V1 is short and positive. This suggests a focus in the right superior pulmonary vein. In **c**, the 10 overlapping bipolar recordings of the circular 10-polar Lasso catheter (Biosense-Webster) placed in the right superior pulmonary veins are shown (PV 1/2 to 10/1). In sinus rhythm, the (small) atrial far field potential (**a**) precedes a typical, sharp local pulmonary vein potential (PVP). In the second and the following beats, the sequence of atrial far field to pulmonary vein potential is inverted, the activation occurs from inside the vein

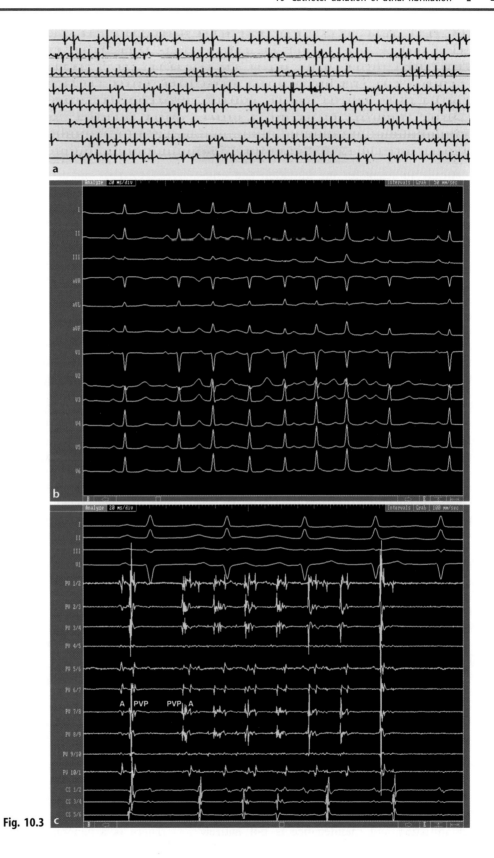

Fig. 10.3

gering foci are reported to be of extravenous location, most commonly located in various regions of the LA [5, 25, 52, 53].

10.1.3 Electrical remodeling and the "trigger and substrate" discussion

Repetitive focal atrial activity alone is not automatically sufficient for the initiation and especially for the maintenance of atrial fibrillation. Considering this, the role of the myocardial substrate maintaining AF has come more and more into the focus of interest. It has been shown in multiple studies that AF is a self-sustaining process: Once started, AF induces changes in the action potential, ionic channels expression and eventually changes in atrial refractoriness, thus, facilitating the maintenance and the relapse of AF [2, 23, 44, 55, 63]. As a consequence, episodes of AF will increase in frequency and duration the more frequent and the longer the atria are fibrillating ("AF begets AF") [2, 23, 55, 63]. Therefore, ablation or modification of the substrate seems another attractive concept in the ablative therapy for AF. However, the importance of the substrate compared to the trigger probably varies depending on the type of AF described above. While initiating triggers are of crucial importance in focal AF, the maintaining substrate is of primary importance in permanent AF which has been ongoing for several months or years [34, 63].

There are different techniques for substrate ablation or modification. Linear lesions, especially in the posterior wall of the LA which is considered to harbor "rotors", i.e., areas with high frequency atrial activity, are part of several substrate modification approaches. Extending ablation lesions to the peri-PV located LA tissue by linear lesions placed outside the PV ostia or ablating areas of fractionated electrograms which could represent areas of fibrillatory conduction is another possibility of substrate modification [14, 23, 32, 44, 47].

10.1.4 The modulating effect of vegetative nerval inputs

The importance of vegetative neural inputs in AF initiation and maintenance is not entirely clear. It has been assumed that the propensity for atrial fibrillation in the same person is to some extent dependent on vegetative tone. Physical or emotional stress may increase the probability for AF. Similarly, the so-called "vagal" AF can be regarded as a result of an imbalance of parasympathetic and sympathetic cardiac neural input [3, 10, 35, 50, 51]. In experimental studies, parasympathetic stimulation has been used for the induction and maintenance of AF. Vagal stimulation leads to shortening of atrial refractoriness and action potential duration and to an increase of refractoriness dispersion [50, 51]. It has been shown that the extent of focal activity in PV can be modulated by drugs affecting the sympathetic activity such as isoproterenol and esmolol [3, 35, 50, 51]. Similarly, an AF suppressing effect with inhibition of cardiac autonomic nerves has been demonstrated [50].

10.2 General remarks to the ablation procedure

Ablation of AF is still a challenging and new approach and should be performed only in selected, experienced centers. The minimal requirement is some experience with left atrial procedures using a transseptal approach. Operators should be familiar with 3D mapping systems and interpretation of complex intracardiac electrograms. The learning curve for ablation of AF can be long and tedious as procedures might last several hours and reduction of procedure and fluoroscopy time is achieved only after 20–30 patients.

10.2.1 Selection of patients and pre-/postablation management

In our opinion, only patients with symptoms clearly related to AF (such as palpitations or dyspnea) and cardiomyopathy or heart failure related to the tachyarrhythmia should be considered for ablation. AF occurrence should not be due to a reversible cause and at least one antiarrhythmic drug therapy should have failed. It seems reasonable to start with ablation of paroxysmal AF in relatively healthy younger patients, ideally with "lone atrial fibrillation".

There is a general consensus that transesophageal echocardiography (TEE) should be performed during the week prior to the procedure to rule out intracardiac thrombi. Prior oral anticoagulation or heparin administration is still being discussed [8], but we strongly recommend performing AF ablation only if an effective oral anticoagulation during at least 4 weeks prior to ablation has been documented. Monitoring of the activated clotting time (ACT) during ablation as well as postablation effective oral anticoagulation (INR = 2–3) during a minimum of 3–6 months is essential to minimize the risks for thromboembolic complications, even in patients with lone atrial fibrillation [5, 8, 13, 17, 20, 36, 44, 60].

In most centers, pre- and postablation assessment of PV diameter by a 3D reconstructive imaging technique (CT scan or MRI) is routinely performed to screen for postinterventional PV stenosis [1, 17, 24, 40, 42, 60].

10.2.2 Evaluation of ablation effect

The evaluation of the success rate after AF ablation is discussed controversially. There is consensus that outcome should be evaluated preferably by a combination of symptom evaluation (e.g., quality of life scores) and ECG monitoring. Recent studies demonstrated that up to 30% of initially highly symptomatic patients have only asymptomatic episodes of AF after ablation [17, 24]. Therefore, we prefer sequential continuous 7 day Holter ECG recordings (1, 3 and subsequently every three months) to event-recorder monitoring. In our opinion it is mandatory to follow the patients closely and intensively to screen for late occurring complications [1, 5, 17, 24, 42, 60]. Temporary, supportive administration of antiarrhythmic drugs is under discussion and some groups evaluate the ablation success only after a blanking period of variable duration (e.g., the first month after ablation procedure), since it is known that the propensity for AF is high in the first few weeks after AF ablation [1, 3, 10, 28, 32, 38, 44, 60].

Regarding the above mentioned issues, the methods of follow-up have to be considered when comparing success rates of AF ablation in different studies and centers (Tables 10.1 and 10.2).

10.3 Ablation techniques – description, endpoints and pitfalls

We will try to focus on the currently used AF ablation approaches and their technical aspects, procedural endpoints and pitfalls. Tables 10.1 and 10.2 give an overview of the success rates in selected studies with special regard to the different ablation techniques, the follow-up methods, duration and major complications.

10.3.1 Targeting the triggers

▪ The focal approach

This approach has almost been abandoned due to its poor outcome, the high incidence of PV stenosis and the time-consuming procedure [3, 12, 25, 52, 53]. The ablation target is the elimination of atrial foci inducing AF. It is presumed that arrhythmogenic foci can be located anywhere in the right and left atrium with preferential locations, such as the pulmonary veins.

▪ **Procedural approach.** Simultaneous multisite mapping in the RA and LA during sinus rhythm is used to identify the earliest site of activation in atrial extrasystoles (ideally initiating AF). The ideal tool for multisite mapping and single beat analysis of activation should 1) cover both atria, 2) have a spatial resolution making ablation possible with the analysis of only one beat and 3) not mechanically produce atrial extrasystoles.

Unfortunately, none of the existing mapping tools fulfills all requirements: Multiple catheters in the RA/LA provide simultaneous recordings, but the spatial resolution is poor and atrial extrasystoles can be induced mechanically. A variant of this technique has been described by Haissaguerre et al. [12]. Their group used two ablation catheters placed inside two different PV. This enabled a rather precise mapping of PV foci, but the technique is not suitable for non-PV foci. Our group performed several studies using multipolar (64-electrodes) basket catheters to map one or both atria [34, 52]. This approach provides a good spatial resolution in the RA which has an optimal shape for the basket to fit in. A single beat analysis of atrial extrasystole is also possible. For the LA, the bas-

Table 10.1. Ablation of AF targeting the initiating triggers

Publication	Ablation approach	Success			Follow-up		Complications	
		Success/total n of patients (percentage)	Success in paroxysmal AF	Success in persistent AF	Follow-up technique	mean FU (months) ±SD	PV stenosis ≥50%	TIA/stroke
Haissaguerre et al. NEJM 1998 [12]	"focal approach" inside the PV, no isolation attempted	28/45 (62%)	28/45 (62%)	–	Holter (every 3 months); any symptom	8±6	N/A	N/A
Chen SA et al. Circulation 1999 [3]	"focal approach" inside the PV, no isolation attempted	68/79 (81%)	68/79 (81%)	–	Holter (every 2 months) ± event recorder	6±2	25/59 PV(42%) (serial TEE)	2/0
Haissaguerre et al. Circulation 2000 [13]	PVI First description of PV isolation	51/70 (73%)	51/70 (73%)	–	N/A	4±5	0 (angiography and CT scan)	0
Oral et al. Circulation 2002 [36]	PVI during AF	34/40 (85%)	N/A	–	Symptoms (± event recorder)	N/A	0 (N/A)	0
Marrouch et al. Circulation 2002 [28]	PVI ICE-guided energy titration	137/152 (91%)	N/A	N/A	Blanking period (80 days), symptoms ± event recorder	9±2	12/586 PV (2.5%) (CT scan)	0
Deisenhofer et al. Am J Cardiol 2003 [5]	PVI	38/75 (51%)	–	–	7-day Holter ECG (every 3 months)	8±4	6/75 patients (8%)	0
Arentz et al. Circulation 2003 [1]	PVI Basket mapping of the PV	34/55 (62%)	26/37 (70%)	8/18 (44%)	Holter at 12 months ± event recorder	12±0	1/55 patients (1.8%) (MRA)	0
Vasamreddy et al. Heart Rhythm 2004 [59]	PVI Irrigated tip catheter for PV isolation	39/75 (52%)	32/42 (76%)	7/33 (21%)	Telephonic contact (every 3 months) ± event recorder	11±8	3/75 patients (4%) MRI	2/75 patients (2.7%) with stroke
Karch et al. Circulation 2005 [24]	PVI Randomization: Circumferential versus segmental PV ablation	33/50 (66%)	–	–	7-day Holter ECGs		6/50 patients (12%) serial CT and MRI	2/50 patients (4%) with TIA

Table 10.2. AF ablation targeting the maintaining substrate

Publication	Ablation approach	Success				Follow-up		Complications	
		Success/total n of patients (percentage)	Success in paroxysmal AF	Success in persistent AF	Follow-up technique	mean FU (months) ±SD		PV stenosis ≥50%	TIA/stroke
Haissaguerre et al. J Cardiovasc Electrophysiol 1996 [11]	Right and left atrial lines	15/45 (33%) with right atrial lines only 6/10 (60%) with right + left atrial lines + foci ablation	15/45 (33%)	–	Symptoms + Holter at 3 and 6 months	11±4		N/A	0
Ernst et al. Circulation 1999 [7]	Carto-controlled right and left atrial linear lesion set	total 2/45 (4%); 2/32 (6%) with right atrial lines only; 0/12 with biatrial lines	2/45 (4%)	–	Holter and symptoms at 1, 3 and 6 months	N/A		N/A	1 stroke
Pappone et al. Circulation 2001 [44]	CPVA, second description, large cohort	188/251 (75%)	148/179 (83%)	40/72 (56%)	Holter (monthly ≥3 months)	10±5		0 (TEE)	0
Oral et al. Circulation 2003 [38]	Randomization: CPVA versus PV isolation	34/40 (85%)	34/40 (85%)	–	Symptoms (± event recorder)	5±3		0 (CT scan)	0
Hocini et al. Eur Heart J 2004 [18]	CPVA and evaluation of PV isolation	13/20 (65%) patients (55% of PV isolated during circumferential ablation)	13/20 (65%)	–	Hospitalization with monitoring/ stress test at 1, 3, 6 and 12 months + symptoms	13±8		0 (serial CT at 12 months)	0
Vasamreddy et al. Heart Rhythm 2005 [60]	CPVA + left atrial lines	39/70 (56%)	13/21 (62%)	26/49 (53%)	8-week follow-up in hospital, then referring physician (every 3 months) ± event recorder	6±3		2/70 patients (3%) with PV occlusion; serial MRI	1 stroke
Karch et al. Circulation 2005 [24]	Randomization: CPVA versus PV isolation	21/50 (42%)	N/A	N/A	7-day-Holter ECGs	6±0		3/50 patients 6%) serial CT + MRI	1 stroke and 2 TIA (2 and 4%)

Table 10.2 (continued)

Publication	Ablation approach	Success			Follow-up		Complications	
		Success/total n of patients (percentage)	Success in paroxysmal AF	Success in persistent AF	Follow-up technique	mean FU (months) ±SD	PV stenosis ≥50%	TIA/stroke
Nademanee et al. J Am Coll Cardiol 2004 [32]	Electrogram-guided (focal) ablation in LA and RA	110/121 (91%); 8 patients with amiodarone therapy, 18 patients with 2 ablations	54/57 (95%)	56/64 (88%)	Holter ± event recorder (every 3 months)	12±0	N/A (not evaluated)	1 stroke
Ouyang et al. Circulation 2004 [40]	Circumferential lines with mandatory and assessed PV isolation	39/41 (95%) 9 patients with 2 ablations	39/41 (95%)	–	Holter 1, 3, 6 months + event recorder (weekly + if symptoms)	5±1	0 (TEE)	0

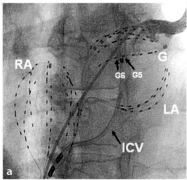

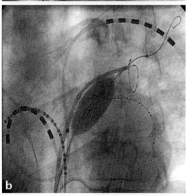

Fig. 10.4. Examples of catheter settings for mapping of AF (focal approach): **a** shows a biatrial basket mapping setting (LAO 45° view). The two basket catheters are deployed in the right (RA) and left atrium (LA). Spline G with its electrode G5 and G6 is marked. In addition to the two basket catheters, an internal cardioversion catheter (ICV) is placed via the V. femoralis with the proximal shocking electrodes in the RA (two of these are visible in the lower left corner of the figure) and its distal shocking electrodes in the pulmonary artery (not visible). A ventricular sensing electrode between the two shocking poles is placed in the right ventricle (and is in the presented image superimposed on electrode G5 and G6 of the left atrial basket catheter). With a multipurpose catheter, angiography of the left superior PV is performed. In **b**, an Ensite Array balloon catheter is deployed in the LA (filled with contrast dye; positioned over the wire). In addition, a 16-polar 2.5 F catheter is placed in the coronary sinus via an Amplatz angiography catheter, a 20-polar Halo catheter is placed along the tricuspid valve and an internal cardioversion catheter is placed via RA and RV in the left pulmonary artery. For PV mapping, a 10-polar Lasso catheter is placed at the ostium of the left superior PV (no electrical PV isolation but direct ablation of the focus intended)

ket shape does not correspond very well to the complex anatomy and essential parts of the LA, the interatrial septum and the ostia of the right PV are not covered (Figure 10.4).

The noncontact mapping system (Ensite Array, endocardial solutions) seems to respond to all requirements previously mentioned. However, the displayed electrograms are "noncontact" electrograms, i.e., computed "virtual electrograms" and not locally recorded true "contact" electrograms. Thus, the accuracy of the system to reflect all morphologic features of the local electrograms, which are characteristic in focal activity, is limited. Furthermore, the spatial resolution at the ostia of PV is limited, and the filter settings substantially influence the delineation of earliest activation as detected by the system [48, 49].

Finally, the electroanatomic 3D Carto system has a high spatial resolution and records true local ("contact") electrograms. It has the disadvantage that it requires repetitive or ongoing monomorphic activity since a single beat analysis is not possible.

Regarding the limitations of the available mapping tools and considering that an acute "firing" of foci during the EP study is rather a fortuity than the rule, the focal approach has not been used in many studies. However, it still has its place in the case of atrial (non-PV) foci or repeat ablation procedure after failure of standard AF ablation approaches [23].

▌ Pulmonary vein isolation

In recent years, the electric isolation of all accessible PV has become the cornerstone of any AF ablation approach. The reported success rates vary between 60–82% (see Table 10.1) [1, 5, 13, 24, 26, 28, 34, 56, 58, 59].

The target of the "conventional" PV-isolation approach is to ablate all muscular sleeves extending from the LA into the PV at the atrial interface of the PV-LA junction. The additional ablation of fragmented or complex ostial potentials has been introduced recently to perform a limited substrate modification besides the trigger isolation [1, 14, 18, 28, 39]. This concept corresponds to findings that the special decremental conduction properties of this PV-LA "junctional area" are the substrate for reentry and fibrillatory conduction [3, 22].

▌ **Standard equipment.** Includes a multipolar mapping catheter in the coronary sinus (CS), a multipolar, circular mapping catheter for the circumferential mapping of the PV and an ablation catheter (preferentially an open irrigated tip ablation catheter).

■ Transseptal approach and PV angiography

For PV isolation, access to the LA has to be obtained with at least one long sheath (for the circumferential mapping catheter) and the ablation catheter. This can be achieved by single transseptal puncture with double access to the LA or with a double transseptal puncture technique.

■ Transseptal puncture technique

The transseptal puncture itself bears risks and can result in considerable complications such as pericardial tamponade, aortic dissection and even death. Risks can be minimized by following a step-by-step procedure. We will describe the technique used in our EP lab, but are, of course, aware that different techniques might be used successfully and without complications in other centers.

A multipolar catheter is placed in the coronary sinus (CS, see Chapter 4) and a standard pigtail angiography catheter is advanced via the aortic arch to the aortic root. These two catheters provide information about the location of the aorta and (approximately) of the posterior mitral annulus in relation to the interatrial septum.

Then, a long sheath large enough for the ablation catheter (in general 8F or larger) is advanced over the wire to the superior vena cava (SVC). Of note, the long sheath should have a curve of about 30–60° to allow a stable positioning on the interatrial septum. We use the Preface® transseptal sheath (Cordis). The transseptal puncture needle (with the so-called Brockenbrough curve) is advanced into the introducer of the sheath as far as 2–4 mm to the tip of the introducer. Local pressure (via the long sheath) and arterial blood pressure (via the pigtail catheter in the aorta) are monitored throughout the procedure.

In the LAO (45–55°) projection, the long sheath with the needle inside the introducer should be turned to the septum, with the needle curve pointing posteriorly, to 4–6 o'clock with 12 o'clock being the sternum and 6 o'clock the spine. Then, the long sheath and needle are slowly withdrawn on the septum without changing the angle of the tip direction. At a given moment, slightly caudally to the position of the pigtail and cranially to the CS catheter, the sheath/needle should "jump" into the fossa ovalis (see Figure 10.5). Of note, pressure monitor-

ing first shows RA pressure, then a constant (high) pressure will be observed if the tip of the sheath is pressing hard against the septum. If no such jump is seen, the whole sheath should be replaced (again over the wire) in the SVC and slowly withdrawn again in a slightly different angle (e.g., 6 o'clock instead of 5 o'clock).

The sheath is held in the position it jumped to and the correct orientation of the sheath/needle is checked in a second fluoroscopic projection (see Figure 10.5). We do this in a RAO (30°) view. The tip should point in the same direction as

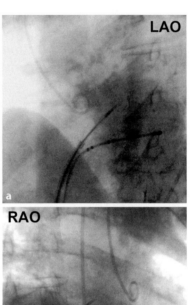

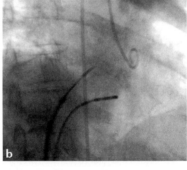

Fig. 10.5. Position of the transseptal sheath and introducer with the needle slightly withdrawn inside the introducer just before successful transseptal puncture. In LAO (**a**) the curve of the needle/sheath points posteriorly and the tip is located in the middle between the pigtail (placed in the aortic root) and the coronary sinus catheter. In RAO (**b**), the curve of the sheath/needle is pointing in the same direction as the CS catheter and the tip of the introducer is at almost half the distance between the pigtail and the spine. If the curve is pointing in direction of the pigtail catheter or if the tip is placed very close to the pigtail, the site and orientation of the needle should be changed to avoid puncturing the aorta. Inversely, if the curve is pointing to the spine or the tip is placed very posteriorly, a risk of perforation of the posterior RA or LA exists

the CS catheter and should not point too anteriorly (i.e., to the pigtail placed in the aortic root). Ideally, it is placed in the middle of the distance between pigtail catheter and spine.

If the position of the sheath/needle is found to be correct in two fluoroscopic views, puncture of the septum can be performed by pushing the needle completely into the sheath. Ideally, a jump of the whole sheath/needle system can be felt the moment the needle crosses the membranous part of the septum in the fossa ovalis. Along with this, the sudden appearance of the typical left atrial pressure curve can be observed in the pressure monitoring over the needle. Under fluoroscopic guidance, the introducer is now pushed over the needle into the LA. Of note, the pressure monitoring should still show left atrial pressure. If one feels comfortable with the puncture, the whole sheath can be advanced into the LA by pushing it over the introducer. Another possibility is the insertion of a guide wire over the introducer into the left superior PV (which points in the same direction as the transseptal puncture). Over this wire, the whole sheath can now be advanced securely to the LA.

Intracardiac echocardiography (ICE) is sometimes helpful for the transseptal puncture and the placement of the circular mapping catheter at the ostium of the PV. Some groups also use ICE to titrate the power delivery during ablation [26]. As soon as transseptal access is obtained, heparin (first a bolus, then continuously) must be administered intravenously and the dosage adjusted according to the activated clotting time (ACT; levels should be between 250–350 s) [1, 5, 13, 37].

In our experience, angiography of the PV (by hand injection of 10 ml of contrast dye for each) is extremely useful to localize the PV and their respective ostia. For optimal visualization of the PV in a more perpendicular view, we recommend the following: 1) LAO projection (e.g., 45°) for the left-sided PV, 2) AP view (right superior PV), and 3) RAO (30°; right inferior PV) projection.

The distance of the PV ostium to a fluoroscopic landmark, e.g., the border of the spine or the heart silhouette can be used in the following for correct placement of the circular mapping catheter (Figure 10.6).

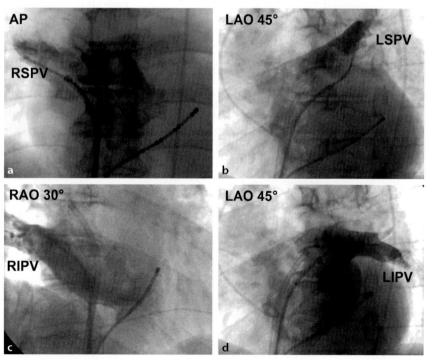

Fig. 10.6. Angiographies of all four pulmonary veins. The angiograms were performed by hand-injection of 10 ml contrast medium directly into the ostium of the PV. Note the different fluoroscopic views for the different PV. It is of use to memorize some anatomic structures and their respective distance to the ostium of the PV in the given projection. *RSPV* right superior PV, *LSPV* left superior PV, *RIPV* right inferior PV, *LIPV* left inferior PV

▌ Circumferential PV mapping

Most commonly, several muscular sleeves that cover a variable percentage of the whole ostial circumference extend from the LA to the PV [1, 3, 13, 22, 28, 33, 37, 62]. Interestingly, these muscular sleeves advance into the PV in spirals, like coils of a spring, overlap in some parts of the PV ostium and create an area with "criss-cross" conductive fibers at the ostium of the PV. The circumferential mapping of a PV is performed with a circular shaped mapping catheter which can be of simple circular shape (e.g., the Lasso catheter). Overlapping bipolar tracings (e.g., 1–2, 2–3, 3–4) with high resolution recording settings should be chosen to guarantee a high density complete mapping of the PV ostial perimeter (Figure 10.7) [5, 13, 24, 37].

In some studies, "mini" basket catheters have been used for PV mapping (for more details

about basket catheter structure, see Chapter 3). They provide circular mapping of the PV at different levels and offer by this not only cross-sectional information of electrical PV activation but also information about the longitudinal course of electrical conduction inside a PV [1]. In Figures 10.8 and 10.9, the concept of basket catheter mapping and a basket recording inside a right superior PV is shown and explained. Distally inside the PV, clearly distinguishable (roundly formed) low-amplitude LA far-field potentials (first deflection in sinus rhythm) and sharp ("blade-like") higher-amplitude local PV potentials will be recorded. When the mapping catheter is withdrawn towards the PV ostium, these two potentials will fuse and finally cannot be distinguished (Figure 10.9).

In the left-sided PV, the ostially fused LA far-field potential and the PV potentials can be further separated by pacing from the (distal) CS catheter (Figure 10.10).

Deep inside the PV, the number of bipoles on the mapping catheter showing sharp PV potentials will decrease. This reflects the decreasing amount of myocardial tissue covering the PV wall deep inside the vein. The atrial far-field signals will also decline dramatically in amplitude the further inside the PV the mapping catheter is advanced (see Figure 10.9).

▌ Special features of right- and left-sided PV electrogram recordings

In left-sided PV, it is sometimes difficult to distinguish the relatively discrete and high-amplitude far-field potentials of the closely located left atrial appendage from local sharp PVP. This

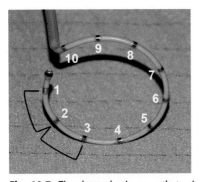

Fig. 10.7. The decapolar Lasso catheter is one example of a circular shaped mapping catheter for circumferential mapping of the PV. The electric activity should be recorded with overlapping electrodes (1–2, 2–3,…, 10–1; as indicated with the black brackets), to guarantee a complete circular mapping

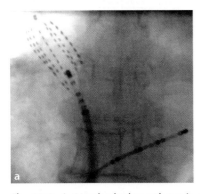
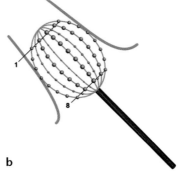

Fig. 10.8. A 64-polar basket catheter is placed in the right superior PV (**a**). It consists of eight flexible splines (named A to H). On each spline, eight electrodes are mounted, and the electrodes are named according to the spline and the

position on the spline they are mounted (e.g., A1 or H8). Overlapping bipolar recordings are obtained from each electrode (e.g., A2/3) and displayed on the pages of the EP recording system (see Figure 10.9)

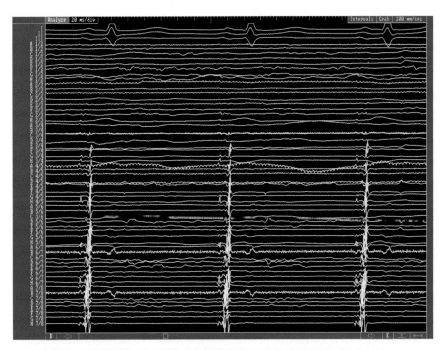

Fig. 10.9. Recordings from the right superior PV: All 64 bipolar recordings of the basket catheter are shown and aligned from the very ostially placed electrodes (A-H 7/8; on the bottom) to the very distally placed electrodes (A-H 1/2, top). In the most ostially obtained electrograms (electrode 7/8 recordings), a fusion of low amplitude and low slope atrial far-field signals with very sharp, higher amplitude PV potentials can be seen. In more distally located electrograms (A-H 6/7 and 5/6), the left atrial signal is more separated from the PV potential. In even more distally recorded electrograms, a gradual decrease in overall amplitude can be observed (in A-H 4/5 to 3/4) as well as a gradual increase in the distance between the (now tiny) LA far-field signal and local PV potentials (e.g., in A4/5 and H3/4). A total loss of recordable electrograms can be stated in the most distally placed bipoles 1/2 and 2/3. This loss of electrograms corresponds to the ending of the muscular sleeves extending from the LA to the PV

is particularly true for the anterior aspect of the left PV which is located extremely close to the left atrial appendage (especially true for the left superior PV). Pacing inside the left atrial appendage while recording in the PV can help to differentiate true PV potentials from left atrial appendage activity [57]. A ventricular far-field signal can often be recorded more distally inside the left inferior PV due to the close anatomical relation with the mitral annulus. In the right-sided PV, a right atrial far-field potential can be recorded at the anterior aspect of the right superior PV preceding the left atrial far-field potential. Following these two far-field potentials, the near-field local PV potential – if present – will be recorded.

▊ Placing the circular mapping catheter correctly

The correct positioning of the circular mapping catheter in the PV is of crucial importance in PV isolation. If the catheter is placed too ostially, it may dislocate frequently into the LA. If it is placed too distally, the risk of PV stenosis due to radiofrequency delivery inside the PV may increase. To assess the actual position of the mapping catheter in relation to the PV ostium, the following features are helpful:

▊ Comparison of the angiographic ostium localization and the relationship of fluoroscopic landmarks to the actual fluoroscopic position of the mapping catheter (using the same projection!) (Figure 10.11)

▊ Analysis of the recorded potentials: if the mapping catheter is just distal to the ostium, LA far-field potentials should still have approximately the same amplitude as PVP and the two potentials should not be separated by more than 20–30 ms. Ideally, complex potentials are recorded on the mapping catheter with both potentials still fused, indicating a truly ostial position.

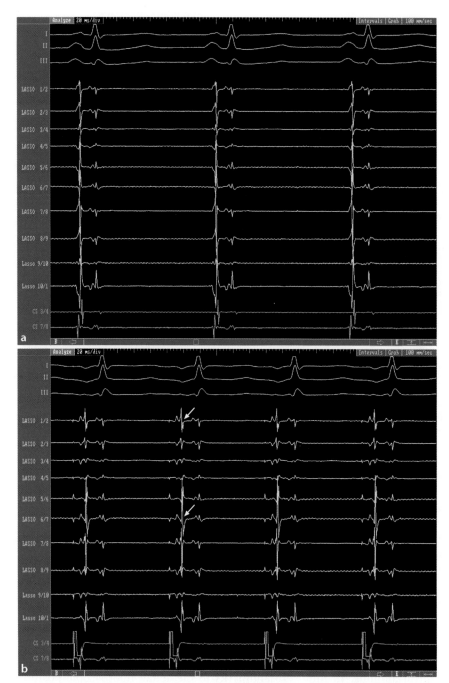

Fig. 10.10. Lasso is placed in the left superior PV. In sinus rhythm (**a**), a fusion of LA far-field signals and (relatively large) sharply deflecting PV potentials (arrows) can be seen in all bipoles. During CS pacing (**b**), these two potentials become more separated, thus, allowing to distinguish both

▌ The movement of the mapping catheter: if it is not moving with the heart beat it might be placed relatively deep inside the PV.

▌ Placing the ablation catheter at the same level as the circular mapping catheter in the PV: is the recorded impedance more than 10–20 Ohms higher than the impedance measured in the LA? If yes, the position is too distally in the vein.

▌ The fluoroscopic position of the mapping catheter: if it is positioned outside the fluoroscopic heart silhouette (in LAO for left PV, in

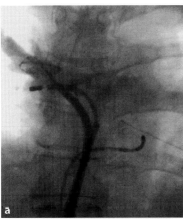

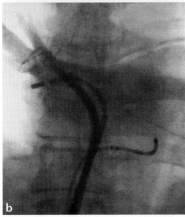

Fig. 10.11. AP fluoroscopic view of the right superior PV during angiography. An 8-polar reference catheter is placed in the CS and a Lasso and ablation catheter are placed transseptally in the right superior PV. The Lasso catheter is advanced into the LA and the right superior PV with the help of a long steerable sheath with an inner diameter of 12 F (Agilis®, St. Jude). With dye injection into the right superior PV, it becomes clear that the Lasso is placed in an oblique angle inside the PV and not – as shown in the **b** – in a perpendicular to the PV diameter. Although the positioning of the Lasso in **b** is better than in **a**, the Lasso is in both instances advanced deep into the vein – neither position is ostial enough to securely avoid energy delivery inside the PV. In this example, the PV ostium is located fluoroscopically slightly left of the right border of the spine – the Lasso should be withdrawn. This kind of "misplacement" of the Lasso catheter is a very frequent observation. It might lead to misinterpretation of the intracardiac and especially the intra-PV activation sequence and can, thereby lead to erroneous ablation

AP for right superior PV and in RAO for right inferior PV), it is usually far beyond the ostium!

The electric PV isolation

The endpoint of PV isolation is the complete abolition or dissociation of all PV potentials from the left atrial activation [1, 5, 13, 37, 56]. This can be achieved by sequentially targeting the earliest electrical input into the PV, i.e., the earliest ostially recorded PV potential (Figure 10.12, p. 226).

Due to several inputs into the PV, ablation of one input does not abolish all PV potentials. It leads to a change in PV potential sequence with an increased delay of PV potentials and a different bipole leading the intra-PV activation cascade since another input "takes over" (Figure 10.13, p. 227, 228).

In most instances, simultaneous delay or disappearance of the PV potentials on several bipoles during ablation is observed, although RF energy is delivered only at one small segment of the PV perimeter. Both observations could be explained by the described spiral course of the muscular strings entering the PV.

If during the initial mapping, the recorded PV potentials occur simultaneously on all bipoles of the circular mapping catheter (which indicates a broad input into the PV), one should start ablating at the roof of the PV since this is a preferential input point. By abolition of this input, a more distinct activation sequence of the PV potentials will appear and the earliest electrical input can now be targeted (Figure 10.14, p. 229).

Very commonly, interconnections between ipsilateral PV at more distal levels (extra LA) occur. Therefore, it is sometimes impossible to isolate only one PV because it is still activated via the ipsilateral PV [1, 24, 56]. In these cases, rather than ablating only one PV, operators should alternate between the two (or more) ipsilateral PV and try to isolate them together.

PV rhythms

After successful PV isolation, dissociated PV rhythms are commonly observed inside the PV distal to the ablation level [1, 5, 24, 26, 38, 61, 62]. These rhythms prove the achievement of electric PV isolation (Figures 10.15 and 10.16).

Moreover, these rhythms can be interpreted as additional evidence for the arrhythmogenic nature of PV myocardium. Intra-PV foci, as well as small reentrant circuits with the PV ostium being a constituent part of the reentry might be observed [22, 62]. Various electric phenomena

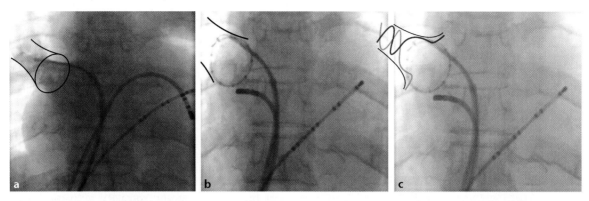

Fig. 10.12. Schematic to explain the rationale of PV isolation. **a–c** are in AP view, with a multipolar catheter in the CS and two transseptally placed catheters. An angiogram of the right superior PV is shown in the left panel (using a standard multi-purpose angiographic catheter; the ablation catheter is in the "waiting position" at the lateral mitral annulus). In the next fluoroscopic view, the Lasso catheter is placed at the ostium of the right superior PV, with the approximate position of the PV traced with the drawn lines. In the right panel, the potential course of two myocardial fibers extending from the LA into the PV is demonstrated with two spiral lines (orange and red) extending from the ostium deep inside the vein. The ablation catheter is placed closely to one of these LA-PV connections. In this schematic, the isolation of the PV could be achieved with only two very discrete radiofrequency ablation lesions

inside isolated PV including ongoing AF while the rest of the LA is in stable sinus rhythm have been described (Figure 10.16). These findings contributed significantly to the understanding of the role of the PV in AF initiation and maintenance.

▮ PV isolation during AF

AF ablation aiming at PV isolation is performed during sinus rhythm or AF. Ablation during AF is technically more demanding [27, 36] as it requires a longer fluoroscopy time, more RF ablation pulses and a longer overall procedure time even in the hands of experienced operators [27]. The principle of PVP disappearance is the same as in sinus rhythm, but the differentiation of the electrograms into "far-field LA" or "PV potential" is much more difficult (Figures 10.16 and 10.17). One advantage of ablation during AF is less movement of the catheters with the beating heart due to the lack of atrial systole. However, it is necessary to recheck the completeness of electrical isolation in sinus rhythm.

▮ 3D mapping systems in PV isolation

Although it can be performed with conventional mapping techniques, PV isolation using 3D mapping systems has advantages, especially with regard to fluoroscopy duration and dosage. In our experience, the electroanatomic Carto system (especially with integrated 3D anatomy; CartoMerge) currently offers the best visualization of the LA. The NavX System has the advantage of displaying all intracardially placed catheters in real time, including catheter displacement due to deep breathing and heart beat (Figure 10.18). Using this system, the display of the circular mapping catheter orientation and shape is extremely helpful when starting PV isolation.

▮ Complications in PV isolation

The most feared but frequently encountered complication of PV isolation is the occurrence of PV stenosis (Figure 10.19 and Table 10.1) [5, 42, 48]. The development of PV stenosis is related to the position and to the amount of radiofrequency energy delivered. Radiofrequency energy delivered too far distally can lead to dramatic PV diameter reduction with severe stenosis or even PV occlusion. The power delivery should be limited to a maximum of 30–35 W and preferably open irrigated tip catheters should be used to avoid local charring [26, 59]. The avoidance of PV stenosis should have first priority when performing PV isolation as the long-term outcome of this complication is not known (Figure 10.19). It has been shown that at least some of these stenoses might aggravate over time (even 12 months after the procedure) and also progression of a stenosis to an occlusion has been reported [1, 5].

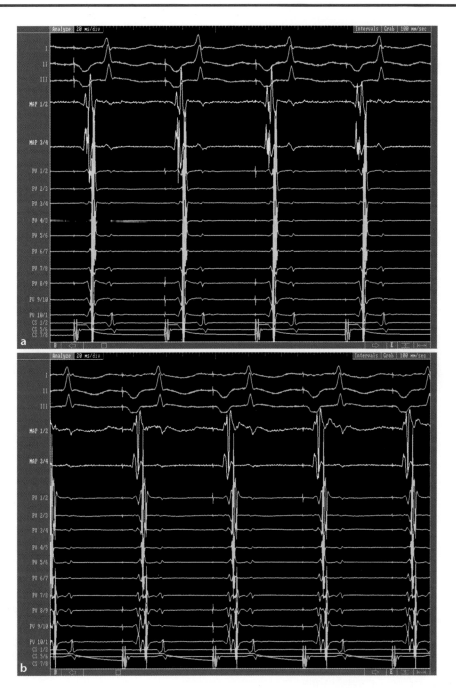

Fig. 10.13. Stepwise electric isolation of the left superior PV (during CS pacing). At the beginning (**a**), the LA far field potentials and the PV potentials are completely fused and even CS pacing cannot separate them. This leads to almost synchronous potentials in all Lasso bipoles. We started ablating at the roof of the PV (bipole 1/2 and 10/1) at a location with a promising fractionated ostial potential (see local potential on MAP 1/2 = ablation catheter). After three radiofrequency applications (**b**), a more distinct activation cascade of the PV potentials emerges, with the earliest PV potential now in Lasso 3/4 and 4/5, which corresponds to the anterior-inferior aspect of the PV perimeter. Ablation here leads to a second shift of PV potential cascade and an even more pronounced separation of LA and PV potentials (**c**): now, the electric input in the PV as assessed by the earliest PV potential, is seen in Lasso bipoles 6/7 and 7/8, which will be the posterior-inferior segment of the PV. Finally, ablation at this site results in complete isolation of the PV (**d**), with no PV potentials visible anymore and solely LA far field potentials remain

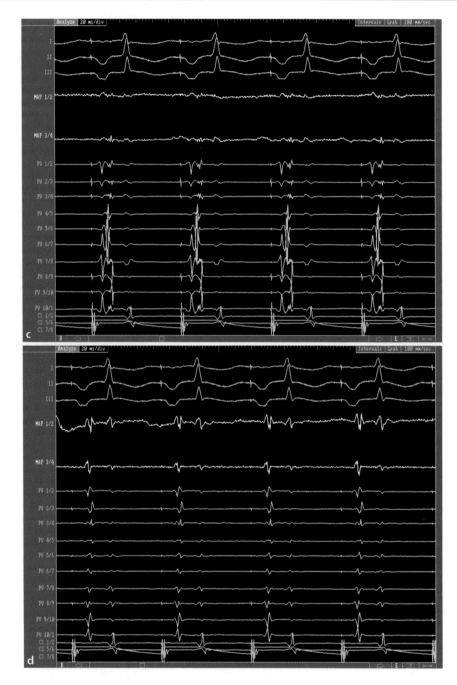

Fig. 10.13 c, d

Perforation of the heart has been a frequent complication in PV isolation. Pericardial effusion with subsequent pericardial tamponade is a life-threatening complication which is sometimes difficult to overcome [5, 59]. The occurrence of this complication is often linked to the experience of the operator: when trying to enter the left superior PV, the catheter is often misplaced into the left atrial appendage (Figure 10.20, p. 236).

If it is advanced further, (unnoticed) perforation of the thin tissue in this area might occur. Some hints help to avoid this complication: 1) the catheter will move with the beating heart when misplaced inside the left atrial appendage, 2) the orientation is more anteriorly than posteriorly (e.g., in RAO projection) and 3) the intracardiac potentials markedly *increase in amplitude* if the catheter is advanced further into the

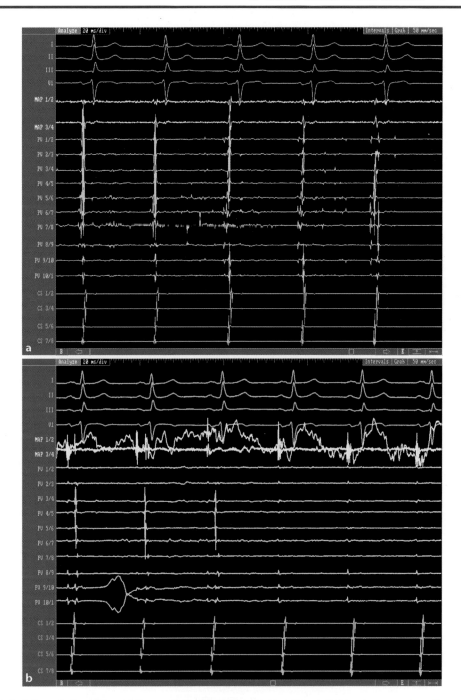

Fig. 10.14. Complete electric isolation of the right superior PV (in sinus rhythm). The same catheter setting as in Figure 10.13 is shown. In (**a**), sharp PV potentials are already slightly delayed compared to the LA far field potentials. In the lower panel (**b**), PV potentials which are already distinc- tively delayed by four previous radiofrequency energy applications disappear during ablation at pole 10/1 completely, thus, confirming complete electric isolation of the PV. The artifact on the ablation catheter (Map 1/2) is due to radiofrequency delivery

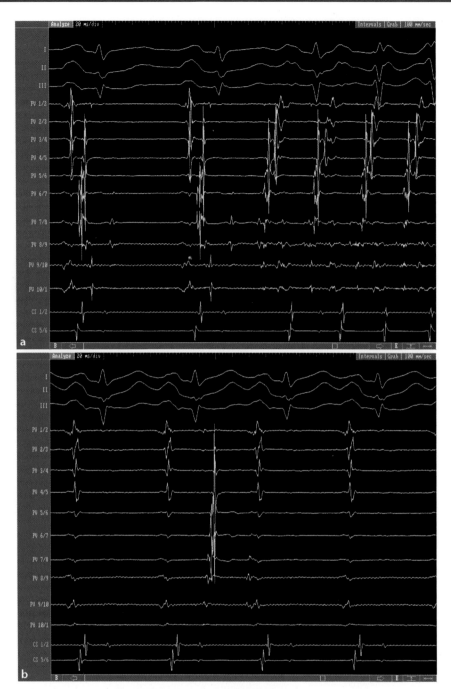

Fig. 10.15. Intracardiac recordings of a patient with atrial runs 2 years after PV isolation for AF. The Lasso is placed in the right superior PV, as well as the ablation catheter. The first two beats in **a** show normal sinus rhythm. Due to the previous PV isolation, the PV potentials occur only late after the left atrial far field signals, and a clear activation sequence of the PV potentials, with bipole 6/7 and 7/8 leading, is visible. It is very interesting to note that in bipole 9/10 and 10/1, very late PV potentials and in 7/8 and 8/9, even further delayed small PV potentials can be observed. The latter are recorded even after the ventricular far field signals in the CS catheter. The third beat in **a** is an extra-systole arising distally in the PV. A characteristic inversion of potential sequence with leading PV potential, followed by LA far field (and not, as in sinus, LA to PV potential sequence) can be observed in this beat. In the following beats, there is a focal firing from inside this vein which leads to a focal atrial tachycardia-like pattern. During focal firing, the leading PV potentials occur in the bipoles 7/8 and 8/9, i.e., the two bipoles which show very late PV potentials during sinus rhythm. In **b**, the same PV with unchanged Lasso position is shown after successful isolation. The previously recorded focal firing from inside the PV is still present with the same PV potential sequence, but electric activity remains "entrapped"

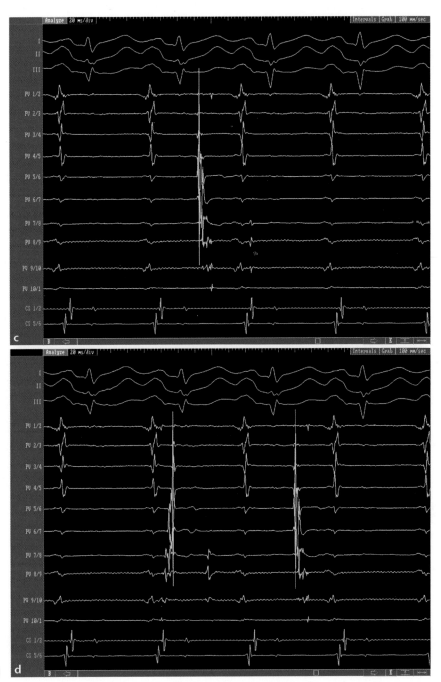

Fig. 10.15 c, d

inside the PV and is not conducted to the LA ("blocked PV potentials" or "intrinsic, isolated PV rhythm"). Interestingly, in this patient, a second, also blocked PV focus could be observed (see **c**). This focus shows a clearly different PV potentials activation sequence with bipole 3/4 and 4/5 leading the activation cascade. In **d**, both foci, exhibiting different PV potential sequences (the first one is the "clinically active" focus, the second activation sequence was found only after isolation of the PV), are both dissociated from LA activity. In a focal approach ablation, the existence of two foci in the same PV could have caused considerable problems

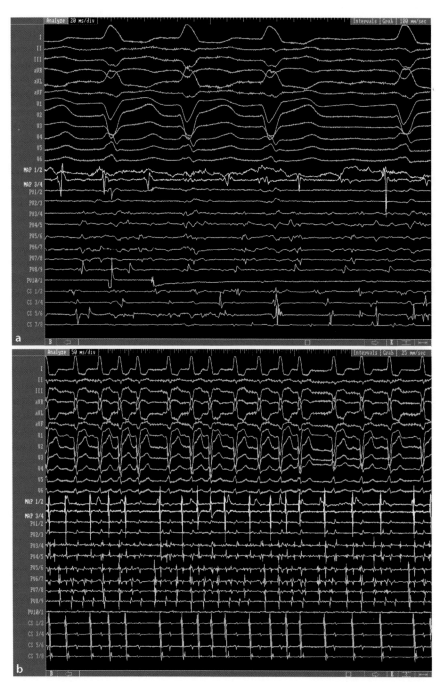

Fig. 10.16. Complete PV isolation stops AF in the left atrium but not in the PV. Tracings from a patient with a common left PV ostium and episodes of AF lasting several hours to days. The Lasso catheter is placed in the common left PV. Of note, different speeds are used for optimal visualization (speed is displayed in the upper right corner of the recordings). At the beginning (**a**), AF is recorded in the Lasso and the CS catheter. After some ablations (**b**), AF persists unchanged in the PV (as seen in the Lasso recordings), but CS recordings show a considerably regularized rhythm, mimicking atypical atrial flutter or focal activity. During further ablation (**c**), the atrial rate as recorded in the CS and ablation catheter slows down even more, and reaches a rate which is typical for fast sinus rhythm rather than AF, but the CS activation sequence (CS distal to CS proximal) clearly indicates a left atrial origin of this rhythm and the rhythm itself is not regular. Of note, singular P waves can be distinguished in the surface ECG tracings. In the same panel, due to further ablation, the intra-PV ongoing AF is not conducted anymore to the LA and DDD pacing of an implanted pacemaker initiates. After two bifocally stimulated complexes, normal sinus rhythm with physiologic AV conduction occurs. In **d**, the intra-PV ongoing AF (Lasso recordings) together with the normal sinus rhythm in the atrium (CS and Map recordings) can

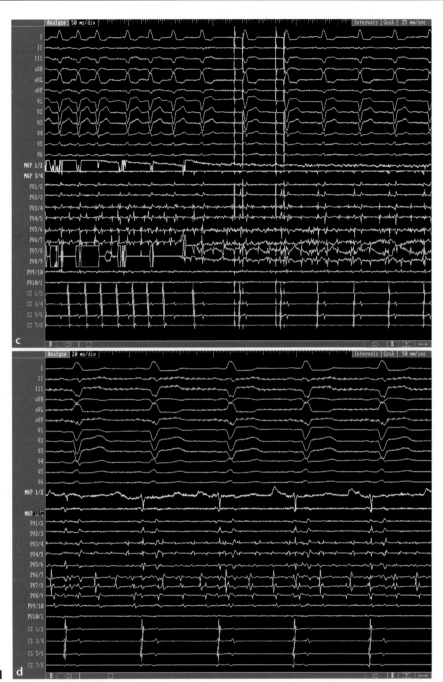

Fig. 10.16 c, d

be seen. Most probably, the left common PV is in this patient an important maintainer of AF rather than solely initia-
tor of AF. With successive ablation of all electrical PV–LA
connections, the ratio of conduction of AF ongoing inside

the PV to the LA decreases. Interestingly, the LA itself in this
special patient does not seem to have a propensity to fibril-
late, as soon as the maintaining substrate (= left common
PV) is isolated from the LA by PV isolation

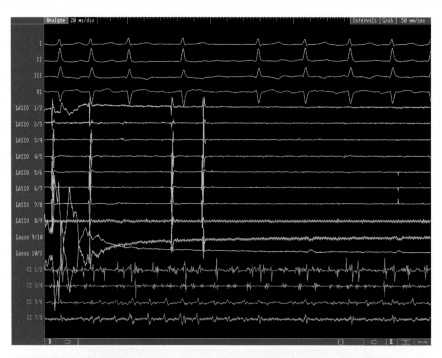

Fig. 10.17. PV isolation during ongoing AF in the LA. In this patient with persistent AF, the first step of ablation consisted in isolation of the PV. The Lasso catheter is placed in the right inferior PV. A complete electric isolation of the vein is achieved (right part of the panel) after the conduction to the vein had already been extremely slowed down by abla-tion (four spikes in the PV recordings PV 1/2 to 10/1 in the left part of the panel). Of note, in this patient, the right inferior PV does not contribute to the maintenance of AF, since, as recorded in the CS catheter, AF is ongoing in the LA with unchanged rate

appendage, whereas they *decrease in amplitude* when advanced into a PV.

∎ Alternative approaches to PV isolation

Since PV isolation with a circular mapping catheter and an additional ablation catheter is technically demanding, attempts have been made to simplify this approach. Models of bal-loon-shaped catheters ablating with different energy sources, e.g., microwave, ultrasound or laser have been developed [33]. However, only a few techniques came to use in humans and up to now none of them has received official ap-proval. There are still considerable technical problems to create a safe and practicable device providing circular energy delivery. The device has to be placed safely and in a stable manner in the PV ostium without increasing the risk for PV stenosis, occlusion of side branches or col-lateral damage to extracardiac structures (e.g., the phrenic nerve). Apart from this, there is also a conceptual problem to this approach. It remains questionable if circumferential energy

application to the whole perimeter of the PV os-tium is desirable when only some sectors of the circumference contain conducting fibers con-necting the LA and the PV.

10.3.2 Substrate modification/ablation techniques

∎ Linear lesions ("modified Maze" procedures)

After reports of high curing rates for AF by sur-gically created compartments of the RA and LA with long lines of block achieved with a "cut-and-sew" technique, interventional electrophy-siologists tried to imitate this approach by drawing long ablation lines. Numerous schemes of lesions in the right atrium, left atrium and biatrial approaches have been suggested with variable success rates [7, 11]. The most com-mon reason for failure of these approaches was the inability to create impervious lines of block with the means of point-by-point lesions [7]. The concept of copying surgical linear schemes has been widely abandoned in EP due to disap-

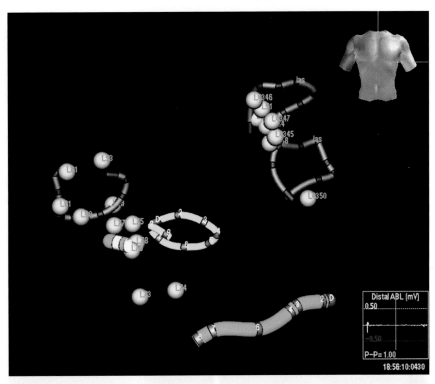

Fig. 10.18. PV isolation using the 3D NavX catheter navigation system. An AP view is presented. The geometry of the LA was not reconstructed, but instead, "shadows" of the Lasso catheter placed in the respective PV were taken and are displayed during the ablation procedure. The "actual" Lasso catheter (and not its shadow) is displayed in bright yellow and is placed in the right inferior PV. Grey dots represent sites of ablation and the ablation catheter (short green catheter) is placed between the right superior and inferior PV. The CS catheter is displayed in green

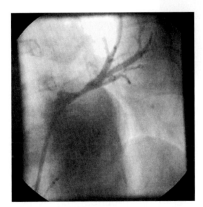

Fig. 10.19. PV angiogram immediately after PV isolation of the left inferior PV is displayed. The patient had a subtotal occlusion of the left inferior PV caused by RF applications

pointing results in conjunction with laborious and long-lasting procedures.

▮ Circumferential pulmonary vein ablation

The circumferential pulmonary vein ablation (CPVA) approach was first described by Pappone et al. [43, 44]. With this approach, wide encircling lesions placed outside the ostia of the ipsilateral PV (0.5–1 cm away from the ostium) aim to modify the substrate for AF and to delay the LA-PV conduction (Figure 10.21). There are limited data suggesting that CPVA modulates vegetative cardiac nervous inputs, since the so-called fat pads (containing the mixed ganglionated vegetative plexus) are often located on or directly adjacent to the deployed circular lines [43, 60].

▮ **Electroanatomic LA map.** The first step after a single transseptal puncture is the 3D reconstruction of the LA with the help of the electroanatomic Carto mapping system. The area of the PV ostia should be mapped extensively to allow optimal placement of the linear lesion [18, 60]. An extensive PV ostial mapping is espe-

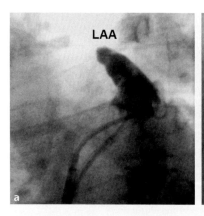
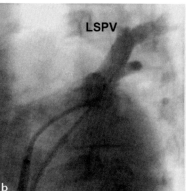
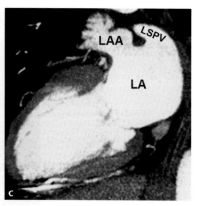

Fig. 10.20. Anatomical relationship between the left atrial appendage (LAA) and the left superior PV. In **a**, a contrast dye injection of the left superior PV was attempted, with the Lasso catheter placed in this PV. Instead of the PV, the LAA was injected, and its finger-like aspect can be seen nicely (left panel). Later on, in the same fluoroscopic view and with unchanged Lasso catheter position, an angiogram of the left superior PV was obtained (**b**). In a left posterior oblique (LPO) open cut view of the LA as obtained with a contrast-enhanced CT scan (**c**), the close anatomic relationship of these two anatomic structures can be appreciated

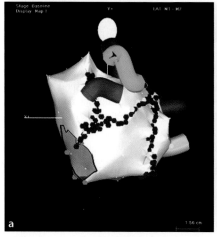
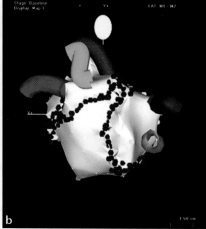

Fig. 10.21. Electroanatomic map of the LA in a modified left posterior oblique and PA view. The ablation lines are represented by red ablation points, the PV are displayed as colored tubes (in this patient, three left PV can be seen). Of note, due to the wide distance of the linear lesions to the PV ostia, the two encircling lesions are almost touching in the posterior superior LA

cially important as the PV are visualized as "tubes" of a constant diameter in the Carto system, irrespective of their "true" diameter. This limitation has been overcome with the newly developed CartoMerge system, integrating a 3D reconstructed model of the patient's LA anatomy into the electroanatomic map and thereby offering a more realistic image of the PV ostia. Other parts of the LA which should be mapped thoroughly are the mitral annulus (especially its lateral part for the left isthmus line) and the left atrial appendage (since the left encircling lesion is placed in between the left superior PV and the posterior aspect of the appendage).

▮ **Deployment of linear lesions.** We recommend marking the planned ablation lines in the 3D map of the LA prior to ablation in order to have a template to follow during linear ablation (at least in the first 50 patients). If the line is too distant to the PV ostium, it tends to be very long which implies the risk of being incomplete. If it is placed too close to the ostium, PV stenosis can occur even with this approach [18, 24,

60]. Some parts of the lesion are technically demanding such as the line between left atrial appendage and left superior pulmonary vein, since there is only a small myocardial "rim" on which the ablation line must be drawn. Therefore, the deployment of these lines is almost impossible without the use of a long, stabilizing sheath. Different sheaths with varying curves are commercially available. However, exchanging a long transseptal sheath is always a possible source for complications (e.g., air embolism) and we, therefore, recommend using the same sheath for transseptal puncture and left atrial mapping/ablation.

A reduction of local bipolar electrogram amplitude of ≥80% or ≤0.1 mV and a conduction delay over the ablation line is the endpoint of this technique. Both can be checked by a "remap" after the ablation. A remap should be performed especially when starting with this approach [43]. It is important to note that the complete electric isolation of the PV is not a requirement for ablation and is not checked routinely. In fact, it has been demonstrated that 45% to 80% of the encircled PV are electrically not isolated [18, 24]. In addition to the two encircling lesions at least one line connecting the inferior-posterior part of the left circle with the posterolateral mitral annulus should be deployed (the so-called left isthmus line or mitral isthmus line). To avoid postablation macroreentry and to further modify the posterior wall of the LA (thought to contribute substantially to the maintenance of AF), two lines connecting both circles posteriorly have been added to the initially suggested lesion set [45]. In the first descriptions, an 8 mm tip ablation catheter and a power setting of up to 100 W/65 °C were used [38, 44]. For reasons explained below, open irrigated tip catheters with a maximum energy and temperature delivery of 50 W and 48 °C are currently preferred [18, 24, 60].

▮ **Pitfalls of CPVA.** It is essential for this technique to create a reliable, exactly reconstructed anatomy of the LA with – even more importantly – a careful reconstruction of the PV ostial region. The new CartoMerge system does certainly offer advantages for the mapping of the complex PV ostial region. The ablation catheter should be dragged and pushed along the planned ablation lines in very small movements to avoid the creation of a multitude of unconnected point lesions. As mentioned above, drawing "line models" in the electroanatomic map has proven to be very helpful.

The most serious complication of CPVA is the occurrence of an atrioesophageal fistula. There is a close anatomical relationship of the posterior LA and the esophagus and in some patients only a thin layer of fatty and connective tissue separates both (Figure 10.22).

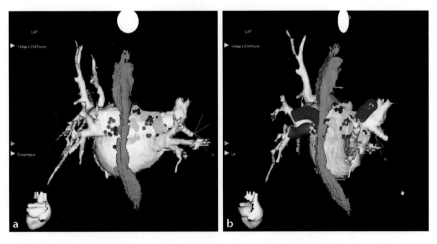

Fig. 10.22. CartoMerge mapping of the LA and display of the esophagus (in blue). The electroanatomical LA map (with red ablation tags) and the 3D reconstructed CT anatomy of the LA (displayed in grey) are fused into one. The close anatomical relationship of LA and esophagus is shown in PA (**a**) and modified right posterior oblique (**b**) view. Of note, the course of the esophagus in this patient is closer to the left PV than to the right PV and consequently, ablation targeting the ostia of the left PV carries a higher risk of esophageal injury

There have been four reported cases of atrioesophageal fistula to date, all of them occurring with the use of an 8 mm tip ablation catheter [46]. Most operators have now moved to lower ablation energy and/or irrigated tip catheters. Nevertheless, staying too long on the same ablation point or delivering energy repetitively in an area where two lines are intersecting, especially in the posterior LA, should be avoided [18, 60].

The most frequent "complication" of CPVA, in our experience, is the development of atypical left atrial flutter. Incidence rates from 4–25% with varying arrhythmia mechanisms have been reported. Reentries facilitated by discontinuous lesions play a major role in the genesis of these arrhythmias [6, 18, 24, 29, 38, 60]. Patients tend to have more symptoms than in AF because of a fast AV conduction ratio (e.g., 2:1 with a ventricular rate of 150 bmp) and the arrhythmia often persists for weeks or even months.

The ablation procedures for atypical flutter after CPVA are long-lasting and often not completely successful [6]. This is due to multiple forms of flutter during the procedure, unstable arrhythmias and reentrant circuits of very small size which are extremely difficult to map. The slow conduction zones of the reentrant circuits seem to be located close to or on the previously deployed lesions (for more details see Chapter 7) [6].

PV stenosis has been reported after CPVA and is a potential complication [24, 60]. This complication should not be underestimated, especially if lines between the ipsilateral PV are added to the linear lesion set.

The risk for pericardial effusion or tamponade requiring pericardiocentesis is similar to that during PV isolation and the same is true for the risk of embolic events such as stroke. It has to be remembered, however, that long lesions are deployed in CPVA and that the mean ablation delivery time is considerably longer than in PV isolation [24, 38]. We prefer to maintain ACT levels of >300 s throughout the procedure to minimize the risk for embolic events.

▮ **Observations during CPVA.** Very frequently, a progressive regularization of atrial activation is observed in the CS while ablating in the LA (namely in posterior and septal LA) [18, 38, 49]. In some cases, AF will organize to atrial macroreentry or will even stop completely.

Slowing of the ventricular rate is also reported, sometimes even with long asystolic pauses which are probably due to vagal effects transmitted through the vegetative ganglionated plexus [38, 43, 44, 60]. It has been suggested to place a backup pacing catheter in the RV before starting the ablation [43].

As this ablation approach might require extensive radiofrequency application with long ablation times and high power ablation, a moderate reactive (noninfectious) pericardial effusion (in general <1 cm of width in echocardiography) is observed in approximately 30–50% of patients after the ablation without need for specific treatment [24].

▮ Electrogram-guided substrate modification

This approach differs fundamentally from the AF ablation techniques mentioned above. It aims neither at creating linear lesions nor at modifying or isolating the initiating triggers.

The basis of this approach is the hypothesis that atrial regions exhibiting very fragmented, low voltage electrical activity represent preferred areas of slow conduction for the small, changing microreentries present during AF [32]. An area of relative slow conduction is necessary for the existence and persistence of a given reentry. Therefore, it is assumed that the multiple microreentries during AF cannot persist if all areas of slow conduction have been ablated (Figures 10.23 and 10.24). Another hypothesis is that rotors, drivers or generators of AF, which are characterized by fragmented potentials, are eliminated with this ablation technique. The endpoint of this approach is either termination of AF during ablation (in persistent and permanent AF) or termination of AF during ablation and noninducibility thereafter (in paroxysmal AF). Nademanee et al., the first to describe this technique, could achieve sinus rhythm during ablation even in patients who had been suffering from chronic AF for years (Table 10.2) [32]. To date, few publications describe this technique, most of them in conjunction with other ablation approaches. There is not much information about preferential ablation sites or percentage of targeted atrial locations [14, 32, 47]. Findings in our own center suggest that areas with fragmented, complex potentials are often located at the PV ostia, the roof of the LA, the interatrial septum (from both atria), the root of the left atrial appendage

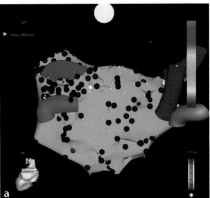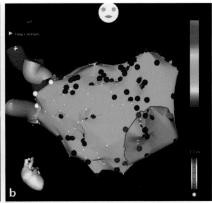

Fig. 10.23. Electrogram-guided substrate modification. AP (**a**) and PA (**b**) view of the electroanatomic map ("anatomical map" with uniform color display) of the LA. The PV are shown with their respective branches. Ablation sites are marked with red tags. The nonlinear ablation strategy in the electrogram-guided substrate modification approach is obvious looking at the dispersion of ablation tags all over the LA. Of note, some areas, e.g., the PV ostia, were ablated more intensively than others

and the CS ostium. The decision where to ablate is sometimes difficult and is most commonly based on the morphology of signals as well as on the intuition of the operator. There are currently attempts to develop a "fragmentation index" helping the operator to decide about the ablation placement [47].

∎ **Pitfalls.** Although experience with this approach is limited, some features seem to be important: since local potentials vary over time in their morphology during AF (e.g., from "sharp" to "soft"), electrograms should be evaluated over a time period of 10 to 20 s or more [47]. Atrial activity recorded in the CS should regularize during ablation and slow down. If no further change in atrial rate or organization after some regularization is observed, additional mapping of the right atrium should be performed. The CS activation sometimes shows a higher rate of atrial depolarization in the more proximal located electrodes. This indicates that a "fibrillatory" region is located in the proximity of these electrodes. It is helpful to have a multipolar catheter placed inside the right atrium to have a better "overview" over the electrical activity of both atria. If paroxysmal AF stops during ablation, reinduction with decremental atrial burst pacing should be performed. This maneuver is not necessary in persistent or permanent forms of AF since AF will not stop by coincidence in these patients.

∎ Circular linear lesions isolating the PV

This approach aims at isolating the PV completely by deploying circular linear lesions in the atrial tissue located close to the PV ostia (Table 10.2) [40]. In some respect, it is a conjunction of PV isolation and CPVA. A controlled complete isolation of PV is achieved with lesions placed in the LA, thus minimizing the risk for PV stenosis. A 3D reconstruction of the LA with the electroanatomic mapping system is used in the same manner as in CPVA to place the ablation lines. To monitor the complete PV isolation, two circular mapping catheters are placed in the ostia of the ipsilateral PV. Disappearance of all PV potentials is the endpoint for ablation (Figure 10.25). This approach has been shown to be effective in both paroxysmal and persistent AF [41], although the data in persistent AF (95% of success) rely on relatively short-term follow-up results and a considerable percentage of patients were still under the effects of amiodarone treatment. More studies with a longer follow-up and less interference of drug treatment for AF have to be awaited to finally judge the value of this approach. At least two transseptal punctures are required since in addition to the two long sheaths (for the circular catheters), an ablation catheter has to be introduced into the LA [40]. It seems even more important than in CPVA to move the ablation catheter carefully with small movements and delicate rotation.

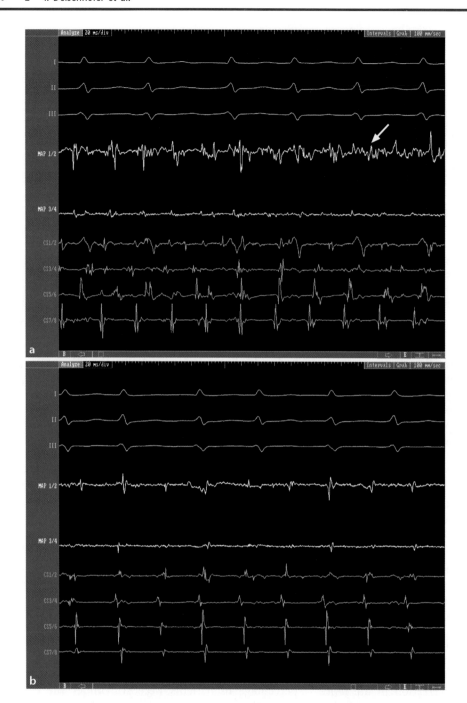

Fig. 10.24. Patient with persistent AF for 2 years. The intra-cardiac recordings at the beginning (**a**) show ongoing AF with the typical, very fast and variable atrial rate and a poly-morphic aspect of electrograms in the CS (recordings CS 1/2 to 7/8) and ablation catheter (Map 1/2 and 3/4). With the progressive ablation of complex fractionated electrograms (an example is shown in the first panel in the Map catheter, see arrow), a stepwise organization and regularization of the atri-al signals occurs (**b**) and a more atrial flutter like pattern can be sometimes observed. Finally, after further deceleration of the atrial rate, AF stops under ablation (**c**)

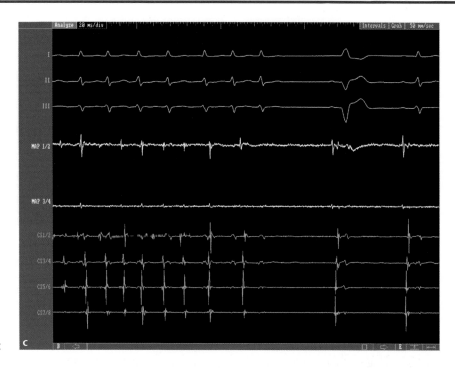

Fig. 10.24 c

∎ **Pitfalls.** There is evidence that relapse of AF using this approach is almost always linked to recurrent PV–LA conduction despite previously completed lines. It is essential to test the completeness of the deployed lines before stopping the procedure. Small recurrent gaps or still conducting but momentary "stunned" myocardial fibers can be detected by the administration of 6–18 mg of adenosine [1, 40]. It is of utmost importance for this procedure (which usually lasts 4–9 hours) that patients do not move because the technique relies heavily on the correctness of the 3D reconstruction. If the position reference has moved, a completely new anatomic reconstruction has to be generated and information about the linear lesions already deployed is completely lost. Remapping is time-consuming and cumbersome, especially if the lines were not completed yet. There are not enough data to prove that PV stenosis is avoided completely with this technique. Therefore, a final judgement of this approach regarding possible complications cannot be made at this point.

∎ **Similar approaches.** A wide range of approaches similar to the one described by Ouyang [40] have been published. Most commonly, PV isolation is achieved by applying wide encircling linear lesions, thus, avoiding PV stenosis and modifying the substrate as well.

The terms used to describe these techniques are similar (wide area circumferential ablation [WACA], left atrial circumferential ablation [LACA]) and so are the ablation techniques: using a 3D reconstructive mapping system, circumferential ablation of PV is performed. In a second step, isolation of PV is controlled (sometimes with a conventional ablation catheter, sometimes with a circular mapping catheter) and completed if necessary. As it is time-consuming and sometimes just impossible to locate the conducting gaps in the previous deployed lines, the so-called "touch-up" ablations to complete the isolation of PV are very frequently applied close to the ostium of the PV.

10.3.3 Catheter ablation of cardiac autonomic nerves – targeting the "fat pads"

This is a more experimental approach which has not yet been commonly used. In fact, the data published up to now are only experimental regarding the effect of this technique. The targets of this ablation approach are the so-called "fat pads", which contain mixed vegetative ganglionated plexus. The localization of the fat pads in humans is slightly variable. Most commonly, four of the fat pads are located close to the four ostia of the PV. The ganglionated

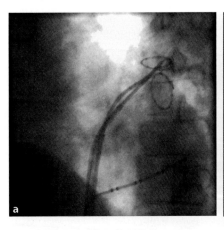
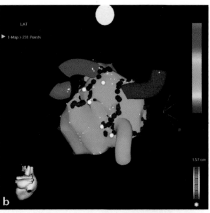

Fig. 10.25. Circular linear lesions isolating the PV. Fluoroscopic view (LAO) of the two Lasso catheters placed in both left PV. Modified right posterior oblique view of the left atrial electroanatomic map (anatomical map displayed). The left and right ipsilateral PV were isolated by long encircling lesions (red ablation tags). Of note, the circular lesions are drawn guided by electrograms and some parts of the lines were ablated more intensively than others. This is due to the fact that during ablation in these parts of the line, a change in the LA-PV conduction ratio was observed and consequently ablation was prolonged and intensified to consolidate this desired ablation effect

plexus are thought to influence the heart (especially the atrial myocardial refractoriness and the activity of arrhythmogenic foci) by both sympathetic and parasympathetic inputs.

The description of the current ablation techniques is divided into two steps: first, the identification of the location of fat pads and second, the control of ablation effect. To identify the fat pad location, an ablation catheter is advanced endocardially to the assumed fat pad location and high frequency (> 50 Hz) burst pacing with high output is performed. If the fat pad is located in proximity to the pacing site, the activation of vagal inputs in the ganglionated plexus by this test pacing will lead to a dramatic prolongation of AV conduction, provoking higher degree AV block or longer RR intervals (> 1.5 s) [50, 51].

In case of a positive testing, ablation is performed at these sites and the ablation effect is controlled using the same provocative pacing maneuver. If ablation was successful, no decrease in ventricular rate is observed anymore [50]. Overall, there is not much clinical experience with this approach and further studies have to be undertaken to clarify its importance in the setting of AF ablation.

10.3.4 Combination of AF ablation techniques – the individualized AF ablation approach, tailored to a specific patient

To further increase the success rate in AF ablation, the combination of two or more ablation approaches in a single patient has been proposed [14, 15, 16, 21, 39]. It is important to identify patients who would profit from such an extended procedure as opposed to a standard therapy scheme. Interestingly, the ablation endpoints of the electrogram-guided substrate-modification [32] in terms of AF termination or regularization of AF (in patients with persistent AF) or non-inducibility of AF after ablation-induced termination (in paroxysmal AF) have become the best accepted criteria to decide whether to extend the ablation procedure to another approach or whether to stop after one ablation approach.

■ The inducibility of AF as endpoint in paroxysmal AF

In patients with paroxysmal AF, the testing of the inducibility of sustained AF episodes was proposed to identify the subset of patients who may benefit from an additional ablation approach [14, 39]. Various combinations have been suggested, e.g. the ablation of complex, fractionated atrial electrograms (CFAE) after electric isolation of the PV or circumferential PV ablation, as well as adding linear lesions in the left atrium (left isthmus line or roof line between both superior PV) to the PV isolation or circumferential PV ablation [14, 21, 39]. In the published data, the individualized approach seems to offer advantages over a single method in most patients with paroxysmal AF and can increase the success rates in these patients (see Table 10.2).

On the other hand, the resulting procedure times might be extensively long. Testing the inducibility might easily be biased since there are many factors influencing the propensity for AF during the EP procedure (e.g. drugs) and the inducibility manoeuvres might be more or less aggressive depending on the stimulation protocol.

▮ Regularization or termination of AF in persistent AF

Persistent AF will most probably not stop by chance during ablation. Regularization of AF (to more organized forms of AF or to an atrial tachycardia) or termination of AF has become a surrogate for (at least partially) successful ablation [14, 15, 16, 32]. The phenomenon of regularization or termination of AF has been described in some ablation approaches and can occasionally be observed in the circumferential PV ablation and the PV isolation as stand-alone therapy (although in the latter it seems to be rather rare) [7, 13, 18, 27, 39, 43, 44]. However, the regularization or termination of AF as the formal procedural endpoint requires a combination of at least two ablation approaches in most patients. Recently the group from Bordeaux presented a "step-by-step" protocol with the endpoint of acute restoration of sinus rhythm [15, 16]. In patients with persistent AF, they performed in a randomized sequence (1) PV isolation, (2) isolation of other great thoracic veins (SVC and CS) and (3) ablation of complex electrical activity as expressed by fractionated electrograms in various atrial sites. The final step always consisted of linear lesions, first the roof line connecting both superior PV and then the mitral isthmus line [15]. Independent of the sequence in which steps 1–3 were taken, each additional step increased the probability of termination of AF by approximately 30%, resulting in a final termination rate of 87% (52/60 patients). During a follow-up period of 3 months, 24 pa-

tients experienced regular atrial tachycardia. After ablation of atrial tachycardias in a repeat procedure, the overwhelming majority of patients (95%) were in stable sinus rhythm during a mean follow-up time of 11 months [16].

This complex and individualized approach has the limitation that a sequence of relatively complex ablation approaches is applied, resulting in long procedure times even in experienced centres [16]. Secondly, the subsequent arrhythmias (i.e. the atrial tachycardias after the first ablation procedure) are – at least in our experience – difficult to map and ablate, especially if more than one type occurs [6]. Probably this approach can only be performed in high volume centres, which are able to complete AF ablation with one of the described approaches in less than 1–1.5 hours of procedure time.

▮ Conclusion

AF differs from all other arrhythmias treated with catheter ablation in several aspects. There are multiple methods and techniques to ablate AF based on specific electrophysiologic features of this intriguing arrhythmia. The possible benefit of each approach must be judged on reported success rates (which sometimes might be too enthusiastic or based on incomplete follow-up data) as well as possible complications.

It is still unclear which ablation approach offers the best results, but it is slowly emerging that the isolation of pulmonary veins seems to offer reasonable and reproducible curing rates in paroxysmal AF. For persistent and chronic AF (and to increase success rates in paroxysmal AF), a combination of several approaches seems to be reasonable. It is almost impossible to predict future directions of AF ablation, since this is a very fast evolving field with a multitude of theoretical and practical approaches currently under investigation.

▮ References

1. Arentz T, von Rosenthal J, Blum T, Stockinger J, Burkle G, Weber R, Jander N, Neumann FJ, Kalusche D (2003) Feasibility and safety of pulmonary vein isolation using a new mapping and navigation system in patients with refractory atrial fibrillation. Circulation 108:2484–2490
2. Chen J, Mandapati R, Berenfeld O, Skanes AC, Gray RA, Jalife J (2000) Dynamics of wavelets and their role in atrial fibrillation in the isolated sheep heart. Cardiovasc Res 48:220–232

3. Chen SA, Hsieh MH, Tai CT, Tsai CF, Prakash VS, Yu WC, Hsu TL, Ding YA, Chang MS (1999) Initiation of atrial fibrillation by ectopic beats originating from the pulmonary veins: electrophysiological characteristics, pharmacological responses, and effects of radiofrequency ablation. Circulation 100:1879–1886

4. Cox JL, Boineau JP, Schuessler RB, Kater KM, Lappas DG (1993) Five-year experience with the maze procedure for atrial fibrillation. Ann Thorac Surg 56:814–823; discussion 823–814

5. Deisenhofer I, Schneider MA, Bohlen-Knauf M, Zrenner B, Ndrepepa G, Schmieder S, Weber S, Schreieck J, Weyerbrock S, Schmitt C (2003) Circumferential mapping and electric isolation of pulmonary veins in patients with atrial fibrillation. Am J Cardiol 91:159–163

6. Deisenhofer I, Estner H, Zrenner B, Schreieck J, Weyerbrock S, Hessling G, Scharf K, Konietzko A, Karch MR, Schmitt C (2006) Left atrial tachycardia after circumferential pulmonary vein ablation for atrial fibrillation – incidence, electrophysiologic characteristics and results of radiofrequency ablation. Europace in press

7. Ernst S, Schluter M, Ouyang F, Khanedani A, Cappato R, Hebe J, Volkmer M, Antz M, Kuck KH (1999) Modification of the substrate for maintenance of idiopathic human atrial fibrillation: efficacy of radiofrequency ablation using nonfluoroscopic catheter guidance. Circulation 100:2085–2092

8. Fuster V, Ryden LE, Asinger RW, Cannom DS, Crijns HJ, Frye RL, Halperin JL, Kay GN, Klein WW, Levy S, McNamara RL, Prystowsky EN, Wann LS, Wyse DG, Gibbons RJ, Antman EM, Alpert JS, Faxon DP, Fuster V, Gregoratos G, Hiratzka LF, Jacobs AK, Russell RO, Smith SC, Jr., Klein WW, Alonso-Garcia A, Blomstrom-Lundqvist C, de Backer G, Flather M, Hradec J, Oto A, Parkhomenko A, Silber S, Torbicki A (2001) ACC/AHA/ESC Guidelines for the Management of Patients With Atrial Fibrillation: Executive Summary A Report of the American College of Cardiology/American Heart Association Task Force on Practice Guidelines and the European Society of Cardiology Committee for Practice Guidelines and Policy Conferences (Committee to Develop Guidelines for the Management of Patients With Atrial Fibrillation) Developed in Collaboration With the North American Society of Pacing and Electrophysiology. Circulation 104:2118–2150

9. Gillinov AM, McCarthy PM, Blackstone EH, Rajeswaran J, Pettersson G, Sabik JF, Svensson LG, Cosgrove DM, Hill KM, Gonzalez-Stawinski GV, Marrouche N, Natale A (2005) Surgical ablation of atrial fibrillation with bipolar radiofrequency as the primary modality. J Thorac Cardiovasc Surg 129:1322–1329

10. Goya M, Ouyang F, Ernst S, Volkmer M, Antz M, Kuck KH (2002) Electroanatomic mapping and catheter ablation of breakthroughs from the right atrium to the superior vena cava in patients with atrial fibrillation. Circulation 106: 1317–1320

11. Haissaguerre M, Jais P, Shah DC, Gencel L, Pradeau V, Garrigues S, Chouairi S, Hocini M, Le Metayer P, Roudaut R, Clementy J (1996) Right and left atrial radiofrequency catheter therapy of paroxysmal atrial fibrillation. J Cardiovasc Electrophysiol 7:1132–1144

12. Haissaguerre M, Jais P, Shah DC, Takahashi A, Hocini M, Quiniou G, Garrigue S, LeMouroux A, Le Metayer P, Clementy J (1998) Spontaneous initiation of atrial fibrillation by ectopic beats originating in the pulmonary veins. N Engl J Med 339:659–666

13. Haissaguerre M, Shah DC, Jais P, Hocini M, Yamane T, Deisenhofer I, Chauvin M, Garrigue S, Clementy J (2000) Electrophysiological breakthroughs from the left atrium to the pulmonary veins. Circulation 102:2462–2465

14. Haissaguerre M, Sanders P, Hocini M, Hsu LF, Shah DC, Scavee C, Takahashi Y, Rotter M, Pasquie JL, Garrigue S, Clementy J, Jais P (2004) Changes in atrial fibrillation cycle length and inducibility during catheter ablation and their relation to outcome. Circulation 109:3007–3013

15. Haissaguerre M, Hocini M, Sanders P, Sacher F, Rotter M, Takahashi Y, Rostock T, Hsu LF, Bordachar P, Reuter S, Roudaut R, Clementy J, Jais P (2005) Catheter ablation of long-lasting persistent atrial fibrillation: Clinical outcome and mechanisms of subsequent arrhythmias. J Cardiovasc Electrophysiol 16:1138–1147

16. Haissaguerre M, Sanders P, Hocini M, Takahashi Y, Rotter M, Sacher F, Rostock T, Hsu LF, Bordachar P, Reuter S, Roudaut R, Clementy J, Jais P (2005) Catheter ablation of long-lasting persistent atrial fibrillation: critical structures for termination. J Cardiovasc Electrophysiol 16: 1125–1137

17. Hindricks G, Piorkowski C, Tanner H, Kobza R, Gerds-Li JH, Carbucicchio C, Kottkamp H (2005) Perception of atrial fibrillation before and after radiofrequency catheter ablation: relevance of asymptomatic arrhythmia recurrence. Circulation 112:307–313

18. Hocini M, Sanders P, Jais P, Hsu L-F, Weerasoriya R, Scavée C, Takahashi Y, Rotter M, Raybaud F, Macle L, Clémenty J, Haissaguerre M (2004) Prevalence of pulmonary vein disconnection after anatomical ablation for atrial fibrillation: consequences of wide atrial encircling of the pulmonary veins. European Heart Journal 26(7):696–704

19. Hsu LF, Jais P, Keane D, Wharton JM, Deisenhofer I, Hocini M, Shah DC, Sanders P, Scavee C, Weerasooriya R, Clementy J, Haissaguerre M (2004) Atrial fibrillation originating from persistent left superior vena cava. Circulation 109:828–832

20. Hwang C, Wu TJ, Doshi RN, Peter CT, Chen PS (2000) Vein of marshall cannulation for the analysis of electrical activity in patients with focal atrial fibrillation. Circulation 101:1503–1505

21. Jais P, Hocini M, Hsu LF, Sanders P, Scavee C, Weerasooriya R, Macle L, Raybaud F, Garrigue S, Shah DC, Le Metayer P, Clementy J, Haissaguerre

M (2004) Technique and results of linear ablation at the mitral isthmus. Circulation 110:2996–3002

22. Jais P, Hocini M, Macle L, Choi KJ, Deisenhofer I, Weerasooriya R, Shah DC, Garrigue S, Raybaud F, Scavee C, Le Metayer P, Clementy J, Haissaguerre M (2002) Distinctive electrophysiological properties of pulmonary veins in patients with atrial fibrillation. Circulation 106: 2479–2485

23. Jalife J (2003) Rotors and spiral waves in atrial fibrillation. J Cardiovasc Electrophysiol 14:776–780

24. Karch MR, Zrenner B, Deisenhofer I, Schreieck J, Ndrepepa G, Dong J, Lamprecht K, Barthel P, Luciani E, Schomig A, Schmitt C (2005) Freedom from atrial tachyarrhythmias after catheter ablation of atrial fibrillation: a randomized comparison between 2 current ablation strategies. Circulation 111:2875–2880

25. Lee SH, Tai CT, Hsieh MH, Tsao HM, Lin YJ, Chang SL, Huang JL, Lee KT, Chen YJ, Cheng JJ, Chen SA (2005) Predictors of non-pulmonary vein ectopic beats initiating paroxysmal atrial fibrillation: implication for catheter ablation. J Am Coll Cardiol 46:1054–1059

26. Macle L, Jais P, Weerasooriya R, Hocini M, Shah DC, Choi KJ, Scavee C, Raybaud F, Clementy J, Haissaguerre M (2002) Irrigated-tip catheter ablation of pulmonary veins for treatment of atrial fibrillation. J Cardiovasc Electrophysiol 13: 1067–1073

27. Macle L, Jais P, Scavee C, Weerasooriya R, Shah DC, Hocini M, Choi KJ, Raybaud F, Clementy J, Haissaguerre M (2003) Electrophysiologically guided pulmonary vein isolation during sustained atrial fibrillation. J Cardiovasc Electrophysiol 14:255–260

28. Marrouche NF, Martin DO, Wazni O, Gillinov AM, Klein A, Bhargava M, Saad E, Bash D, Yamada H, Jaber W, Schweikert R, Tchou P, AbdulKarim A, Saliba W, Natale A (2003) Phased-array intracardiac echocardiography monitoring during pulmonary vein isolation in patients with atrial fibrillation: impact on outcome and complications. Circulation 107:2710–2716

29. Mesas CE, Pappone C, Lang CC, Gugliotta F, Tomita T, Vicedomini G, Sala S, Paglino G, Gulletta S, Ferro A, Santinelli V (2004) Left atrial tachycardia after circumferential pulmonary vein ablation for atrial fibrillation: electroanatomic characterization and treatment. J Am Coll Cardiol 44:1071–1079

30. Moe GK (1962) On the multiple wavelet hypothesis of AF. Arch Int Pharmacodyn Ther. 140:183–188

31. Moe GK, Rheinboldt WC, Abildskov JA (1964) A Computer Model of Atrial Fibrillation. Am Heart J 67:200–220

32. Nademanee K, McKenzie J, Kosar E, Schwab M, Sunsaneewitayakul B, Vasavakul T, Khunnawat C, Ngarmukos T (2004) A new approach for catheter ablation of atrial fibrillation: mapping of the electrophysiologic substrate. J Am Coll Cardiol 43:2044–2053

33. Natale A, Pisano E, Shewchik J, Bash D, Fanelli R, Potenza D, Santarelli P, Schweikert R, White R, Saliba W, Kanagaratnam L, Tchou P, Lesh M (2000) First human experience with pulmonary vein isolation using a through-the-balloon circumferential ultrasound ablation system for recurrent atrial fibrillation. Circulation 102:1879–1882

34. Ndrepepa G, Karch MR, Schneider MA, Weyerbrock S, Schreieck J, Deisenhofer I, Zrenner B, Schomig A, Schmitt C (2002) Characterization of paroxysmal and persistent atrial fibrillation in the human left atrium during initiation and sustained episodes. J Cardiovasc Electrophysiol 13:525–532

35. Olshansky B (2005) Interrelationships between the autonomic nervous system and atrial fibrillation. Prog Cardiovasc Dis 48:57–78

36. Oral H, Knight BP, Ozaydin M, Chugh A, Lai SW, Scharf C, Hassan S, Greenstein R, Han JD, Pelosi F, Jr., Strickberger SA, Morady F (2002) Segmental ostial ablation to isolate the pulmonary veins during atrial fibrillation: feasibility and mechanistic insights. Circulation 106:1256–1262

37. Oral H, Knight BP, Tada H, Ozaydin M, Chugh A, Hassan S, Scharf C, Lai SW, Greenstein R, Pelosi F, Jr., Strickberger SA, Morady F (2002) Pulmonary vein isolation for paroxysmal and persistent atrial fibrillation. Circulation 105: 1077–1081

38. Oral H, Scharf C, Chugh A, Hall B, Cheung P, Good E, Veerareddy S, Pelosi F, Jr., Morady F (2003) Catheter ablation for paroxysmal atrial fibrillation: segmental pulmonary vein ostial ablation versus left atrial ablation. Circulation 108:2355–2360

39. Oral H, Chugh A, Lemola K, Cheung P, Hall B, Good E, Han J, Tamirisa K, Bogun F, Pelosi F, Jr., Morady F (2004) Noninducibility of atrial fibrillation as an end point of left atrial circumferential ablation for paroxysmal atrial fibrillation. A randomized study. Circulation 110:2797–2801

40. Ouyang F, Antz M, Ernst S, Hachiya H, Mavrakis H, Deger FT, Schaumann A, Chun J, Falk P, Hennig D, Liu X, Bansch D, Kuck KH (2005) Recovered pulmonary vein conduction as a dominant factor for recurrent atrial tachyarrhythmias after complete circular isolation of the pulmonary veins: lessons from double Lasso technique. Circulation 111:127–135

41. Ouyang F, Ernst S, Chun J, Bansch D, Li Y, Schaumann A, Mavrakis H, Liu X, Deger FT, Schmidt B, Xue Y, Cao J, Hennig D, Huang H, Kuck KH, Antz M (2005) Electrophysiological findings during ablation of persistent atrial fibrillation with electroanatomic mapping and double Lasso catheter technique. Circulation 112:3038–3048

42. Packer DL, Keelan P, Munger TM, Breen JF, Asirvatham S, Peterson LA, Monahan KH, Hauser

MF, Chandrasekaran K, Sinak LJ, Holmes DR, Jr. (2005) Clinical presentation, investigation, and management of pulmonary vein stenosis complicating ablation for atrial fibrillation. Circulation 111:546–554

43. Pappone C, Rosanio S, Oreto G, Tocchi M, Gugliotta F, Vicedomini G, Salvati A, Dicandia C, Mazzone P, Santinelli V, Gulletta S, Chierchia S (2000) Circumferential radiofrequency ablation of pulmonary vein ostia: A new anatomic approach for curing atrial fibrillation. Circulation 102:2619–2628

44. Pappone C, Oreto G, Rosanio S, Vicedomini G, Tocchi M, Gugliotta F, Salvati A, Dicandia C, Calabro MP, Mazzone P, Ficarra E, Di Gioia C, Gulletta S, Nardi S, Santinelli V, Benussi S, Alfieri O (2001) Atrial electroanatomic remodeling after circumferential radiofrequency pulmonary vein ablation: efficacy of an anatomic approach in a large cohort of patients with atrial fibrillation. Circulation 104:2539–2544

45. Pappone C, Manguso F, Vicedomini G, Gugliotta F, Santinelli O, Ferro A, Gulletta S, Sala S, Sora N, Paglino G, Augello G, Agricola E, Zangrillo A, Alfieri O, Santinelli V (2004) Prevention of iatrogenic atrial tachycardia after ablation of atrial fibrillation: A prospective randomized study comparing circumferential pulmonary vein ablation with a modified approach. Circulation 110:3036–3042

46. Pappone C, Oral H, Santinelli V, Vicedomini G, Lang CC, Manguso F, Torracca L, Benussi S, Alfieri O, Hong R, Lau W, Hirata K, Shikuma N, Hall B, Morady F (2004) Atrio-esophageal fistula as a complication of percutaneous transcatheter ablation of atrial fibrillation. Circulation 109:2724–2726

47. Sanders P, Berenfeld O, Hocini M, Jais P, Vaidyanathan R, Hsu LF, Garrigue S, Takahashi Y, Rotter M, Sacher F, Scavee C, Ploutz-Snyder R, Jalife J, Haissaguerre M (2005) Spectral analysis identifies sites of high-frequency activity maintaining atrial fibrillation in humans. Circulation 112:789–797

48. Scanavacca MI, Kajita LJ, Vieira M, Sosa EA (2000) Pulmonary vein stenosis complicating catheter ablation of focal atrial fibrillation. J Cardiovasc Electrophysiol 11:677–681

49. Scharf C, Oral H, Chugh A, Hall B, Good E, Cheung P, Pelosi F, Jr., Morady F (2004) Acute effects of left atrial radiofrequency ablation on atrial fibrillation. J Cardiovasc Electrophysiol 15:515–521

50. Schauerte P, Scherlag BJ, Pitha J, Scherlag MA, Reynolds D, Lazzara R, Jackman WM (2000) Catheter ablation of cardiac autonomic nerves for prevention of vagal atrial fibrillation. Circulation 102:2774–2780

51. Scherlag BJ, Yamanashi W, Patel U, Lazzara R, Jackman WM (2005) Autonomically induced conversion of pulmonary vein focal firing into atrial fibrillation. J Am Coll Cardiol 45:1878–1886

52. Schmitt C, Ndrepepa G, Weber S, Schmieder S, Weyerbrock S, Schneider M, Karch MR, Deisen-

hofer I, Schreieck J, Zrenner B, Schomig A (2002) Biatrial multisite mapping of atrial premature complexes triggering onset of atrial fibrillation. Am J Cardiol 89:1381–1387

53. Schneider MA, Ndrepepa G, Zrenner B, Karch MR, Schreieck J, Deisenhofer I, Schmitt C (2000) Noncontact mapping-guided catheter ablation of atrial fibrillation associated with left atrial ectopy. J Cardiovasc Electrophysiol 11:475–479

54. Schneider MA, Ndrepepa G, Weber S, Deisenhofer I, Schomig A, Schmitt C (2004) Influence of high-pass filtering on noncontact mapping and ablation of atrial tachycardias. Pacing Clin Electrophysiol 27:38–46

55. Schotten U, Duytschaever M, Ausma J, Eijsbouts S, Neuberger HR, Allessie M (2003) Electrical and contractile remodeling during the first days of atrial fibrillation go hand in hand. Circulation 107:1433–1439

56. Seshadri N, Marrouche NF, Wilber D, Packer D, Natale A (2003) Pulmonary vein isolation for treatment of atrial fibrillation: recent updates. Pacing Clin Electrophysiol 26:1636–1640

57. Shah D, Haissaguerre M, Jais P, Hocini M, Yamane T, Macle L, Choi KJ, Clementy J (2002) Left atrial appendage activity masquerading as pulmonary vein potentials. Circulation 105:2821–2825

58. Tse HF, Reek S, Timmermans C, Lee KL, Geller JC, Rodriguez LM, Ghaye B, Ayers GM, Crijns HJ, Klein HU, Lau CP (2003) Pulmonary vein isolation using transvenous catheter cryoablation for treatment of atrial fibrillation without risk of pulmonary vein stenosis. J Am Coll Cardiol 42:752–758

59. Vasamreddy CR, Lickfett L, Jayam VK, Nasir K, Bradley DJ, Eldadah Z, Dickfeld T, Berger R, Calkins H (2004) Predictors of recurrence following catheter ablation of atrial fibrillation using an irrigated-tip ablation catheter. J Cardiovasc Electrophysiol 15:692–697

60. Vasamreddy CR, Dalal D, Eldadah Z, Dickfeld T, Jayam VK, Henrickson C, Meininger G, Dong J, Lickfett L, Berger R, Calkins H (2005) Safety and efficacy of circumferential pulmonary vein catheter ablation of atrial fibrillation. Heart Rhythm 2:42–48

61. Weber S, Ndrepepa G, Schneider M, Schmitt C (2004) Two-to-one conduction block between left atrium and right lower pulmonary vein preceding complete vein isolation during radiofrequency current ablation. Pacing Clin Electrophysiol 27:829–830

62. Weerasooriya R, Jais P, Scavee C, Macle L, Shah DC, Arentz T, Salerno JA, Raybaud F, Choi KJ, Hocini M, Clementy J, Haissaguerre M (2003) Dissociated pulmonary vein arrhythmia: incidence and characteristics. J Cardiovasc Electrophysiol 14:1173–1179

63. Wijffels MC, Kirchhof CJ, Dorland R, Allessie MA (1995) Atrial fibrillation begets atrial fibrillation. A study in awake chronically instrumented goats. Circulation 92:1954–1968

11 Mapping and ablation in the pediatric population

Andreas Pflaumer, Gabriele Hessling, Bernhard Zrenner

11.1 Introduction

Cardiac arrhythmias in the pediatric population have been recognized since the 18th century, but treatment was limited to vagal stimulation and digitalis for a long time. Medical treatment (often based on the experience in the adult population) has improved mortality and morbidity but is often associated with side effects especially during long-term treatment. Cardiac surgery as a therapeutic approach for the definitive treatment of arrhythmias was introduced in 1968 [18], but had the limitation of a very invasive procedure. In 1979, the concept of catheter ablation was inspired by accidental His-ablation with DC cardioversion [87]. Four years later, Gillette [3] reported the first DC His-ablation in children as an emergency procedure for life-threatening junctional ectopic tachycardia (JET). The introduction of RF current in adults in 1986 [45, 54] was soon followed by the first ablations in pediatric patients [10, 86]. Since then, numerous improvements and further developments like cryoablation and electroanatomical mapping systems have led to the application of catheter ablation for almost all types of cardiac arrhythmias.

It is quite obvious that smaller vessel and heart size hampers ablation in the pediatric population. Differences in rate, duration and severity of arrhythmias in childhood demand special knowledge of the physiology and pathophysiology of the heart and its conduction system. Defining the appropriate indication and the adequate performance of ablation therapy is derived from this knowledge.

This chapter offers a general overview of catheter ablation in the pediatric age group with a focus on features especially differing between children and adults. Special considerations in patients with congenital heart disease are addressed in Chapter 12 of this book.

11.2 General considerations

11.2.1 Anatomy and physiology of the heart and conduction system

It is obvious that the substantial difference in heart size of a newborn compared with an adult requires different strategies. The knowledge of the expected size of vessels and valves is important in order to choose the appropriate access and catheters. For example, the access to a left lateral accessory pathway in a newborn via the fragile aortic valve (diameter of about 9 mm) carries a substantial risk of valve damage Table 11.1 shows a selection of normal values of echocardiographic [47] and anatomic measurements [38] from neonates to adolescents.

Not only the size, but also the physiology of the conduction system is changing with age. During infancy a significant change in ECG morphology and baseline conduction intervals occurs. Normal values for baseline ECG intervals and their changes with age have been described [23]. Their consideration is crucial for the further assessment of arrhythmias. In general, it is important to remember that conduction intervals or refractory periods are shorter the smaller the child is. Table 11.2 summarizes the normal EP values measured in pediatric patients.

11.2.2 Indications, contraindications, complications and patient education

The indication for the ablation of an arrhythmia in the adult group is based on the decision of the patient in many instances. With the exception of life-threatening arrhythmias, this decision depends on the physical and psychological burden caused by the arrhythmia which are weighed against the risks of ablation.

Table 11.1. Normal values of M-mode echocardiography measurements in healthy infants and children (in mm, modified data from Kampmann et al. [47] and Goldberg et al. [38])

Body surface area (m²)	Right ventricle end-diastolic	Inter-ventricular septum	Left ventricle end-diastolic	Left ventricular posterior wall	Pulmonary artery diameter	Aortic diameter	Left atrium	Distance from CS to TV	Length of triangle of Koch
0.25	8.7	3.8	20.0	3.6	12.8	10.4	14.0	3.0	3.0
0.4	8.9	4.1	26.0	4.2	15.4	12.9	16.8	4.0	5.0
0.5	9.3	4.3	29.0	4.6	18.3	14.9	18.7	5.0	7.0
0.8	10.5	5.2	35.8	5.7	20.8	17.9	22.5	6.0	9.5
1.0	11.2	5.8	38.5	5.9	24.0	19.9	25.0	8.0	14.0
1.4	14.0	6.7	43.3	6.9	26.8	22.7	28.2	N/A	N/A
2.0	17.5	9.3	53.4	8.1	29.5	27.4	32.5	N/A	N/A

Table 11.2. Normal electrophysiology values in children (in ms, modified data from Park [23], Lau et al. [44] and Beerman [4])

Age in years	PR interval (mean)	QRS (mean)	AH (range)	HV (range)
0–2	100	50	49–94	17–49
2–5	110	60	43–98	23–52
6–10	130	70	43–116	25–52
11–15	140	70	47–111	24–56
15+	150	80	47–127	22–52

In pediatric catheter ablation – especially in infants – neither the burden nor the risks of the procedure can be assessed easily. Sometimes the arrhythmia tends to influence the parents' quality of life more than the infant's. Data are sparse regarding the natural history of arrhythmias presenting in childhood, different treatment strategies and the long-term effects of ablation. As evidence-based treatment is not available, a careful individualized approach, based on the available data and personal experience, seems to be justified.

After diagnosing an arrhythmia which is amenable for catheter ablation, its natural history has to be addressed. No treatment might be an option if there are only minor symptoms or a self-limiting course of the arrhythmia is expected. The side effects and risks of medical treatment have to be considered. Success rates, risks of arrhythmia recurrence [55], contraindications and complications of the ablation procedure for the specific arrhythmia and age group have to be addressed. Before making an individual decision, additional diagnostic procedures like Holter, stress ECG, and echocardiography should be performed.

According to the NASPE Position Statement, there are only a few arrhythmias specified as a Class I indication for ablation in pediatric patients: 1) supraventricular tachycardia leading to ventricular dysfunction or carrying a risk of sudden death or 2) hemodynamic relevant, recurrent ventricular tachycardia.

This restrictive approach correlates to the available data material and the risk of potential complications. Number and kind of complications of RF ablation are reported in the Pediatric Radiofrequency Registry [52]. Both depend on the type of arrhythmia and the body height and weight (best described as the body surface area = BSA).

According to the current recommendations of the Heart Rhythm Society, ablation in children with an BSA < 0.6 m² or less than 15 kg should only be performed if medical treatment has failed and the arrhythmia presents a serious health threat [7, 52]. The most recent data from the Pediatric Ablation Registry [6] support the use of ablation by experienced physicians in selected cases of infants less than 18 months of age. According to Campbell et al. [11, 12], some centers advocate the use of ablation as a pri-

Table 11.3. Indications for RFCA procedures in pediatric patients, NASPE Position Statement 2002 [33]

∎ **Class I**	1.	WPW syndrome following an episode of aborted sudden cardiac death
	2.	The presence of WPW syndrome associated with syncope when there is a short preexcited RR interval during atrial fibrillation (preexcited R-R interval < 250 ms) or the antegrade effective refractory period of the AP measured during programmed electrical stimulation is < 250 ms
	3.	Chronic or recurrent SVT associated with ventricular dysfunction
	4.	Recurrent VT that is associated with hemodynamic compromise and is amenable to catheter ablation
∎ **Class II A**	1.	Recurrent and/or symptomatic SVT refractory to conventional medical therapy and age > 4 years
	2.	Impending congenital heart surgery when vascular or chamber access may be restricted following surgery
	3.	Chronic (occurring for > 6 12 months following an initial event) or incessant SVT in the presence of normal ventricular function
	4.	Chronic or frequent recurrences of intraatrial reentrant tachycardia
	5.	Palpitations with inducible sustained SVT during electrophysiological testing
∎ **Class II B**	1.	Asymptomatic preexcitation (WPW pattern on an electrocardiogram [ECG]), age > 5 years, with no recognized tachycardia, when the risks and benefits of the procedure and arrhythmia have been clearly explained
	2.	SVT, age > 5 years, as an alternative to chronic antiarrhythmic therapy which has been effective in control of the arrhythmia
	3.	SVT, age < 5 years (including infants) when antiarrhythmic medications, including sotalol and amiodarone, are not effective or are associated with intolerable side effects
	4.	IART, one to three episodes per year, requiring medical intervention
	5.	AVN ablation and pacemaker insertion as an alternative therapy for recurrent or intractable intraatrial reentrant tachycardia
	6.	One episode of VT associated with hemodynamic compromise and which is amenable to catheter ablation
∎ **Class III**	1.	Asymptomatic WPW syndrome, age < 5 years
	2.	SVT controlled with conventional antiarrhythmic medications, age < 5 years
	3.	Nonsustained, paroxysmal VT which is not considered incessant (i.e., present on monitoring for hours at a time or on nearly all strips recorded during any 1-hour period of time) and where no concomitant ventricular dysfunction exists
	4.	Episodes of nonsustained SVT that do not require other therapy and/or are minimally symptomatic

mary treatment for SVT even in children younger than 4 years despite the still unknown long-term outcome.

All the issues mentioned above have to be discussed with the parents before performing an ablation. Depending on age and development, the pediatric patient should participate in the preprocedural talks. The better the preablation diagnostics, risk-benefit analysis and preparation of the procedure is, the easier the handling of parents and the child will be even with the occurrence of complications.

∎ **Classification of recommendations**

∎ **Class I:** Evidence or general agreement that given procedure or intervention is useful or effective.

∎ **Class II:** Conflicting evidence exists about the usefulness of an intervention or procedure.

IIA: Weight of evidence favors intervention or procedure

IIB: Usefulness of intervention or procedure is less well established

∎ **Class III:** Evidence exists that intervention/ procedure is not useful and/or is possibly harmful.

11.2.3 Technical considerations

▌ **Setting in the EP lab.** To achieve the best results, the setting in the EP lab should be optimized including a dedicated EP lab team to avoid technical problems. Depending on the patient's age and cooperation, appropriate local anesthesia, sedation, analgesia or general anesthesia (in the small child) is necessary. A multidisciplinary team of anesthesiologists, pediatric cardiologists and electrophysiologists is mandatory to handle all possible problems. According to the NASPE Position Statement, ablation procedures should only be performed if cardiac surgery is available to deal with possible serious complications (e.g., perforation) [33]. The nursing personnel should be familiar with sedation and monitoring and should have training in basic and pediatric life support.

For managing complex arrhythmias and to decrease the amount of fluoroscopy, a biplane X-ray device and a 3D electroanatomical mapping system (e.g., Carto® or NavX®) should be available. Pulsed fluoroscopy should be used at the lowest frame-rate possible; the field of view should be minimized by adjusting the shutter. Capture of fluoroscopy images should be used rather than cine angiography. The image intensifier should be as close as possible, the X-ray source as far away as possible from the patient. The RF ablation system has to monitor temperature of the ablation electrode and automatically adjust power output. All monitoring and treatment facilities should be appropriate for children (like external pads and paddles for the defibrillator). A description of all necessary details for the setting in the EP lab is found in the literature [33, 72, 73].

▌ **Vascular access, anticoagulation and catheter choice.** Vascular access is achieved via the modified percutaneous Seldinger technique using guide wires to introduce a sheath into the vessel and the catheter being inserted through the sheath. Access is preferably in the groin (femoral vessels), which is more comfortable for the examiner and the child. The cubital veins tend to be too small especially in infants. Internal jugular access can be achieved in most children and even small infants under deep sedation or general anesthesia with a small risk of pneumothorax or bleeding.

The size of the sheath(s) depends on the number and type of catheters required for the procedure. The use of more than one sheath in a vessel should be avoided in children less than 15 kg, whereas a single 7 French sheath is possible even in a newborn. Special designs (Figure 11.1) allow to position up to three 2F diagnostic catheters through one sheath for a complete diagnostic procedure. If an arterial puncture is necessary for retrograde access, the smallest possible sheath size should be chosen to avoid spasm and/or thrombosis of the femoral artery. Often a transseptal access is preferable to prevent damage to the aortic valve or femoral artery. Access to the left atrium can be achieved either by using a persistent foramen ovale (PFO) or by transseptal puncture using a Brockenbrough needle. In the hands of an experienced examiner, a transseptal procedure carries minimal risk [56].

Anticoagulation with heparin should be started prior to the procedure, if there is low flow or another condition with a high risk for thrombosis. Otherwise anticoagulation with heparin (50 units/kg) is started after insertion of the sheaths. Heparinization throughout the

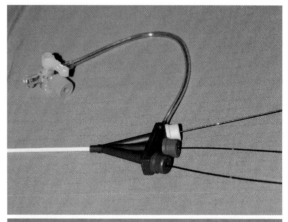

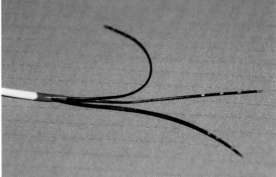

Fig. 11.1. 7F guiding catheter, which allows delivery of up to 3 nonsteerable 2F quadripolar catheters

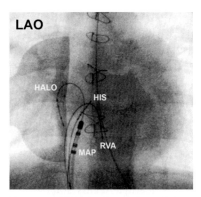

Fig. 11.2. Ablation of cavotricuspid-dependent atrial flutter in a 2-year old child (after surgical ASD closure) with a 4 mm tip catheter (MAP). 2F quadripolar catheters are positioned in the lateral right atrial wall (HALO) in the His position (HIS) and in the right ventricular apex (RVA)

procedure is only necessary, if there is a high risk of thrombosis or a procedure duration over 4 hours. There are no large studies that address this issue but the risk of embolism in patients without congenital heart defects seems to be very small [85]. Postprocedural anticoagulation with low dose acetylsalicylic acid is recommended after left-sided procedures. Oral anticoagulation with vitamin K antagonists is only reasonable in high-risk patients.

Catheter choice is a mixture of personal experience and preference but limited by vascular access and vessel size. Advancing a 6F steerable catheter in the coronary sinus of infants is not always possible and correct placement of the tiny 2F catheters (Figures 11.1 and 11.2) is sometimes difficult to achieve.

11.2.4 Ablation techniques

One of the most debated issues in pediatric ablation is the unknown mid- and long-term effect of the lesions created. The extent of the lesion is responsible for the efficacy of the ablation. That means the lesion has to be large enough for permanent tissue damage but small enough not to damage other structures (as the coronary arteries). Most of the experience with lesion growth is derived from animal models or pathology specimen of adult patients and limited to radiofrequency current. The application of RF energy with a standard 4 mm tip electrode seems to be safe and effective in adults, but there are concerns regarding smaller children and infants. The le-

sion size with these catheters varies between 4 and 8 mm depending on contact pressure and duration of energy delivery [2].

Case reports in the pediatric age group reporting a narrowing or occlusion of the right coronary artery [7, 21, 48, 76] or the left coronary artery [20, 24] have been published. Coronary artery injury in animal models can be produced by RF energy applied from the endocardial surface and is likely to be a relevant risk in small hearts [77]. Another concern is the possible growth of the fibrous lesions created by ablation as demonstrated in an animal model by Saul et al. [71]. Possible late complications like proarrhythmia, late AV block, coronary artery disease and altered vagal tone are not addressed sufficiently yet. The retrospective analysis of ablation in small children hints to a relationship between the occurrence of complications and the application dose [7, 52].

As shown in an animal model, using a smaller tip catheter in children could decrease the maximum lesion size [78] but clinical data are lacking. "Test" RF applications with lower temperature and shorter duration were also suggested [6] but again this technique lacks clinical validation. Cryoablation seems to be a promising new technique especially in decreasing the risk of AV block [49, 60]. Long-term data concerning the recurrence rate have to be generated. All these observations support the restrictive use of catheter ablation in infants and small children. The number and duration of RF lesions during the ablation should be guided by patient size.

11.3 Specific arrhythmias in the pediatric population

11.3.1 Focal atrial tachycardia (FAT)

▪ **Indications.** Focal atrial tachycardia accounts for only 4–8% of all SVT cases in pediatric patients with no age preference [13, 37]. It rarely occurs in association with structural heart defects or other diseases in infancy. In young adults after surgery for congenital heart disease (especially after the Fontan procedure), FAT is a known entity. Frequent episodes or incessant FAT is an important cause of ventricular dysfunction in children [15]. The atrial rates may vary from 130 up to 280 bpm. Analysis of the P wave axis and morphology from the surface ECG (see Figure 8.4) can help to differentiate sinus tachycardia from focal activity and to locate the focus [79] which has implications for therapy. Drug treatment is often difficult, but patients with successful medical treatment have a higher rate of spontaneous resolution during follow-up [59]. In children over three years of age, FAT is unlikely to resolve (spontaneously or with medication) and ablation can be considered in selected cases [68]. Incessant FAT with ventricular dysfunction not responding to medical treatment is an indication for catheter ablation at any age and ventricular function shows fast recovery after the ablation (Figure 11.3) [53, 64, 69].

Multifocal or chaotic atrial tachycardia (MAT) with at least three different, distinct, nonsinus P wave morphologies and varying PR intervals is a rare arrhythmia in childhood. The ECG shows atrial rates from 100 up to 280 bpm. The first presentation of this type of tachycardia is usually in the neonatal period and structural heart disease is identified in approximately half of patients [25]. Medical treatment is sometimes difficult but in most cases, control of heart rate is possible. The spontaneous resolution rate is high (over 75% within one year). A few ablation cases [39, 83] are described and it seems that ablation of one focus might cure the patient.

▮ **Mapping and ablation.** In general the proceeding and technique are the same as described in Chapter 8. FAT suppression under sedation or anesthesia can be a problem. To reduce fluoroscopy time, 3D-mapping techniques are helpful in the pediatric age group [92]. As mentioned before, P wave axis and morphology on the surface ECG give important hints for the location of the focus. Distribution of location seems to be similar in children and adults.

Right-sided and left-sided foci are equal in distribution and this feature seems unchanged with age. Within the left atrium the most prevalent locations of foci are close to the mitral valve, in the left atrial appendage, and in and around the pulmonary veins [79, 82]. Foci in pulmonary veins play an important role in the genesis of atrial fibrillation (see Chapter 10) and may present in rare cases in the young as multifocal atrial tachycardia with reduced ventricular function. Primary success rate of FAT ablation seems to depend on age and location of the focus and is estimated between 80% and 90%. The recurrence rate is up to 30%, but repetitive ablation can finally cure most of the patients. Surgical therapy after repetitive ablation in desperate cases may be possible with an acceptable risk [14, 67].

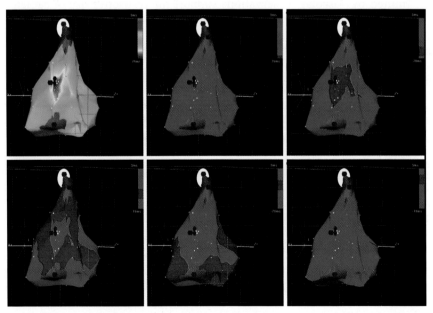

Fig. 11.3. Electroanatomical map (CARTO®) of focal atrial tachycardia (incessant) originating from the posterolateral right atrium in a 3-year old boy with severe ventricular dysfunction. The left upper panel shows an activation map during tachycardia with the earliest activation in red; the red dots represent ablation points. The other panels show a propagation map of excitation spreading from the focus all over the right atrium

11.3.2 Atrial flutter and intraatrial reentrant tachycardia (IART)

▌ **Indications.** The prevalence of typical atrial flutter is highest in the fetal and neonatal age group. Whereas drug treatment seems to be the best choice during fetal life, cardioversion or overdrive pacing is preferable in the newborn [57]. Recurrence is very rare and therefore ablation is not indicated in this age group. In adolescents, typical atrial flutter has a higher recurrence rate. Catheter ablation is performed with a high success rate in this age group and should be the treatment of choice in patients with recurrent flutter episodes.

Intraatrial reentrant tachycardia (IART) is very rare in children without structural heart disease [88] and will be discussed in Chapter 12.

▌ **Mapping and ablation.** In typical atrial flutter, the surface ECG shows the well-known sawtooth pattern. Before starting the ablation, entrainment mapping from the cavotricuspid isthmus should be performed to prove isthmus-dependent peritricuspid flutter (see Figure 6.10). Electroanatomical mapping is usually performed in cases with structural heart disease (see Chapter 12). After the ablation, one or two diagnostic catheters are used to check the created isthmus block line in order to improve the long-term success rate. The ablation should not be performed with an 8 mm tip catheter in small children (Figure 11.2). RF energy and time of ablation should be reduced as the right coronary artery is running close to the isthmus and can be potentially injured [63, 70].

11.3.3 Accessory pathways

▌ **Wolff-Parkinson-White syndrome (WPW)**

▌ **Indications.** Atrioventricular reentrant tachycardia (AVRT) with an accessory pathway as part of the reentrant circuit often presents within the first months of life, followed by peaks of presentation in children between 8–10 years and once again between 15–18 years [66]. AVRT without overt preexcitation ("concealed WPW") is present in about 25% of patients diagnosed [62].

Spontaneous resolution of AVRT or preexcitation diagnosed within the first year of life is reported in up to 90% of cases until the age of 18

months, but there seems to be a recurrence later in life in up to 30%. Persistence of AVRT beyond the age of 5 indicates that there is less than a 25% chance of spontaneous resolution [66]. Considering the natural history of WPW syndrome, the treatment of choice during the first year of life is antiarrhythmic medication, which is able to control the arrhythmia in the vast majority of patients. Catheter ablation does not play a significant role in neonates and infants with accessory pathways.

Much has been written about the potential risk of sudden death from a rapid ventricular response in response to fast antegrade conduction over an accessory pathway. Population-based studies suggest a very low risk of sudden death in young and asymptomatic patients [46, 62]. Specialized cardiac centers are often biased due to a much higher prevalence of severe symptoms in their patient population. The risk of sudden death is significantly increased in studies from these patient populations and ablation therapy is often advocated after risk stratification [11, 17, 65]. In the pediatric population, a reliable risk stratification has not yet been established. Villain et al. report that low risk is associated more with the absence of atrial vulnerability than with the electrophysiological properties of the accessory pathway [89]. Other authors propose risk stratification using exactly these electrophysiological parameters [65], but data analysis shows that risk stratification developed for adults can not simply be transferred to pediatric patients [29]. The proposed parameter of the antegrade effective refractory period (AERP) of the accessory pathway (AP) as a risk marker depends on the age of the child and the adrenergic state (which might be altered with sedation or anesthesia). Nevertheless, the determination of the AERP of the AP is implemented in the decision-making process in many institutions and the Heart Rhythm Society recommendations. In these recommendations, an AERP less than 250 ms is used as the cut-off for a class I indication of ablation, but only in patients with a prior syncope.

Another class I indication for ablation of an accessory pathway is an episode of aborted sudden death. Ablation is recommended also in drug refractory cases or in patients with severe side effects from medication, even if they are younger than five years of age. In symptomatic patients older than five years, ablation of the accessory pathway appears to be justified. The optimal management of asymptomatic children with an accessory pathway is still controversial. As mentioned above, the risk of sudden death in childhood seems to be very low and risk stratification has not been established yet. So the decision for catheter ablation in these cases has to be made on an individualized basis.

∎ **Mapping and ablation.** Prior assessment of the approximate location of an accessory pathway is possible from the surface ECG [8] and can help to minimize the necessary vascular access. Advancing a small catheter into the coronary sinus helps to distinguish right-sided from left-sided pathways and facilitates mapping and ablation (Figure 11.4). Transseptal access should be considered in small patients with a left-sided pathway to avoid aortic valve injury (Figure 11.5).

Success and recurrence rates depend mainly on the location of the pathway [12, 55, 85]. Primary success rates using radiofrequency ablation are highest in left lateral pathways with up to 98% and lowest in right anteroseptal pathways with 81%. The overall risk of AV block is about 1.2%, being especially high with septal pathways [85]. Cryoablation has been used especially with septal pathways with a high success rate without heart block but with a higher recurrence rate of about 20% [27, 35].

The specific mapping and ablation techniques do not differ significantly from these in the adult population, but shorter refractory periods require very exact and distinct signal processing and evaluation. In small children, energy delivery should be reduced because of the risk of damaging the coronary arteries [20, 24].

In children the occurrence of multiple pathways is reported in up to 10% of cases [91]. Therefore, a careful electrophysiological evaluation has to be performed after a successful ablation to exclude the existence of a second accessory pathway.

∎ **Mahaim fibers**

The so-called Mahaim tachycardia, which is characterized by an ECG pattern resembling LBBB, was thought to be due to a nodal-fascicular connection. Klein and Tchou showed that these accessory pathways are atriofascicular connections that conduct only antegradely and insert into the distal right bundles branch [50, 80]. The surface ECG in sinus rhythm shows only discrete preexcitation with a narrow QRS with rS pattern in lead III and absence of the Q wave in lead I [75]. The Mahaim type of accessory pathway is very rare and there are no sufficient data concerning incidence and treatment

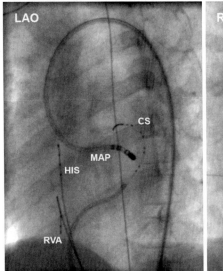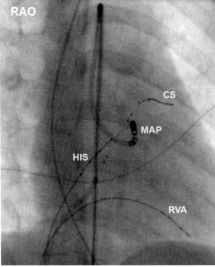

Fig. 11.4. Left anterior oblique (LAO) and right anterior oblique (RAO) views: ablation of a left lateral accessory pathway in a 10-year old girl. The ablation catheter (MAP) is positioned through the aortic valve into the left ventricle below the mitral annulus. 2F quadripolar catheters are in the His and right ventricular apex (RVA) position, a 1.4F octapolar catheter is guided by an Amplatz catheter and positioned in the coronary sinus (CS)

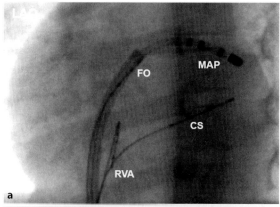

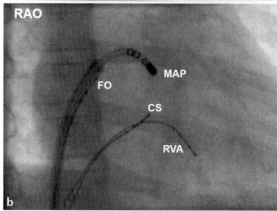

Fig. 11.5. The LAO and RAO views of a transseptal ablation of a left lateral accessory pathway of a 5-year old boy. 2F quadripolar catheters are positioned in fossa ovalis, coronary sinus and right ventricular apex. The transseptal sheath with the ablation catheter (MAP) is positioned in the left atrium at the lateral mitral ring

success. Mahaim fibers have a high prevalence in the setting of Ebstein's anomaly of the tricuspid valve. Association with other accessory pathways or AVNRT is common, even without structural heart disease.

Medical treatment strategies are similar to WPW syndrome and ablation is possible and feasible if medical treatment fails. Two strategies have been proposed:

▌ Activation mapping of the earliest local ventricular potential and ablation at the right ventricular free wall [58]. Two problems should be kept in mind with this approach: Inadvertent RBBB due to ablation close to the right bundle and incessant tachycardia after incomplete ablation.

▌ Searching for the "M" (= Mahaim) potential (see Figure 4.34) along the tricuspid annulus.

This technique seems to be superior to the one mentioned previously [41] but mechanical suppression can anticipate ablation [22].

Examples of an ablation of a Mahaim fiber are found in Chapter 4.

▌ Permanent junctional reciprocating tachycardia (PJRT)

▌ **Indications.** This tachycardia is another special type of accessory pathway-dependent orthodromic tachycardia with the RP interval being longer than the PR interval. Usually tachycardia is incessant and is presenting as cardiac failure in about one third of patients. Structural heart disease is very uncommon, onset of symptoms is usually early in childhood [26]. Medical treatment is reported to be successful in 50% up to 80% [28, 84] of cases leading to resolution of congestive heart failure. If rate control with drug treatment is not easily achieved, ablation should also be performed in smaller children with a minimal risk of AV block. Spontaneous resolution of tachycardia is described in up to 20% of patients [84].

▌ **Mapping and ablation.** The accessory pathways in PJRT have only retrograde decremental conduction properties with a long VA time (Figure 11.6) [82]. The tachycardia circuit involves the AV node antegradely and the accessory pathway retrogradely. Conventional mapping in the right atrioventricular groove usually reveals an early atrial potential in the posteroseptal region during tachycardia. Variable locations on the right, but also on the left side have been described [82]. A positive P wave in lead I and negative P waves in the inferior leads during tachycardia are suggestive of a location right posteroseptally [34]. Differential diagnosis includes focal atrial tachycardia with an inferior vector and atypical AVNRT. Multiple accessory pathways have been described in PJRT [74]. The primary success rate of radiofrequency ablation (intention to treat) is between 75% and 90%, depending on age and pathway location [1, 9, 28, 84]. Cryoablation seems to be promising especially in septal pathways [36]. There is no sufficient data on long-term outcome in small children but in older children and adults the long-term success rate is excellent with a recurrence rate of less than 5% [34].

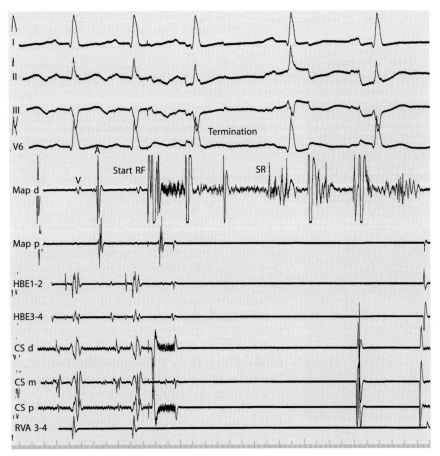

Fig. 11.6. Permanent junctional reentrant tachycardia. Tachycardia termination during RF ablation at the right posteroseptal AV junction. Note the long RP interval with negative P waves in the inferior leads (II, III). The atrial signal (A) on the ablation catheter (MAP) precedes P wave onset (long VA interval at the ablation site). *HBE* His bundle electrogram, *CS* coronary sinus, *RVA* right ventricular apex, *d* distal, *m* middle, *p* proximal

11.3.4 Atrioventricular nodal reentry tachycardia (AVNRT)

∎ **Indications.** Whereas AVNRT is the most common form of SVT in the adult population, the incidence in the pediatric population varies with age [19, 40, 51]. There are only very few descriptions of neonates presenting with AVNRT. After the age of four to five, the incidence of AVNRT increases gradually. The course and outcome of AVNRT is generally benign. Episodes presenting in infancy tend to have a low risk of recurrence [40]. If documentation of paroxysmal supraventricular tachycardia fails or is not sufficient to differentiate an AVNRT from an AVRT, a transesophageal study may be useful for differentiating the mechanisms. First-line drug treatment with beta-blocking agents seems to be most appropriate.

From an anatomical standpoint, the size of the triangle of Koch limits the use of ablation therapy in the pediatric population. As dimensions of the triangle of Koch are related to the dimensions of the tricuspid valve and the body surface area (BSA) [32, 38], ablation should be avoided in children with BSA < 0.6 m² unless there is a life-threatening situation. Considering the benign clinical course of this tachycardia, we would limit catheter ablation to children with a BSA > 0.8 m². In this group ablation seems to be safe, but coronary artery stenosis or AV block has been described.

■ **Mapping and ablation.** Induction of the tachycardia during the EP study is possible in over 90% of the cases [81], but in nearly half of the patients an isoproterenol infusion is necessary [85]. If the procedure is performed under general anesthesia, tachycardia induction might be more laborious. Mapping and ablation of the slow pathway region is performed as in adults (see Chapter 5). An advanced navigation system as the NavX® or LocaLisa® system helps in locating standard catheters nonfluoroscopically which is especially useful in younger patients to reduce fluoroscopy time. Electroanatomical mapping is helpful in patients with congenital heart disease. In children without structural heart disease, the success rate of radiofrequency ablation of the slow pathway is over 95% [85] with a recurrence rate of less than 5% [55]. The risk of AV block in the Multicenter Prospective Pediatric Cardiac Ablation Study (including data from the beginning of the radiofrequency ablation era) was about 2% [85].

As complete AV block in children is a serious event, ablation using cryoenergy was introduced to further reduce this risk. First studies show promising data with a risk of AV block approaching 0%, but the number of ablations is still too low to draw a final conclusion. Recurrence rates seem to be slightly higher [49, 60] with cryoenergy as compared to RF ablation.

11.3.5 Junctional ectopic tachycardia (JET)

JET as a rare tachycardia form that occurs most commonly in two settings: 1) during the fetal or newborn period or 2) after surgery for congenital heart disease. JET in the fetal or newborn period is usually incessant, often refractory to drugs and leads to ventricular dysfunction in most cases [13]. An association between congenital JET and congenital complete AV block has recently been suggested [30].

The assumed mechanism of JET is focal activity of perinodal tissue due to abnormally enhanced automaticity. Drug treatment can decrease the heart rate, but sinus rhythm is rarely established for a longer period [16, 90]. If control of the heart rate cannot be achieved, the mortality is as high as 30% [90]. Ablation treatment was first reported in 1983 [3], but at that time creation of complete AV block was the only available choice.

Ablation is usually performed during tachycardia, targeting the earliest atrial activation [43]. Newer ablation techniques include using controlled energy delivery, 3D techniques to tag the conduction system and cryoenergy to avoid complete AV block [31, 43]. There are case reports on successful ablation treatment even in newborns [5]. Despite these advances, the risk of AV block with ablation is still high, but also without ablation there seems to be a significant risk of AV block [30, 90]. There are no evidence-based recommendations on the treatment, and ablation should only be performed if drug treatment fails to control the heart rate.

11.3.6 Ventricular tachycardia (VT)

■ **Indications.** Compared with the adult population, VT is rare in pediatric patients. Premature ventricular contractions (PVCs) are commonly found in healthy newborns, infants, children and adolescents and are considered benign if not associated with structural heart disease. Ventricular escape beats are also benign in the absence of AV nodal disease. Another type of benign ventricular arrhythmia in children is the accelerated ventricular rhythm (ventricular rhythm slightly faster than sinus rhythm) which varies in rate with patient activity.

According to the different mechanisms present in children, VT can be divided into five groups:
1. In idiopathic VT (usually with structural normal hearts), the risk of sudden death seems low, the time course is not well defined and ablation seems to be a promising therapy with success rates up to 95%. Well-known entities are nonreentrant VT from the right or left ventricular outflow tract or idiopathic verapamil-sensitive VT. Morwood et al. showed [61] that ablation success is lower if all intention-to-treat procedures are included in the data analysis. Acute success with ablation in the right ventricle was achieved in only about 60% of cases, in the left ventricle in about 80% of cases. Reasons for the low success rates are inability to induce stable VT, hemodynamic instability of the patient and high-risk locations of the presumed target. A recurrence rate of about 30% is reported after a median follow-up of four years. Nevertheless, catheter ablation in this VT group is feasible and might

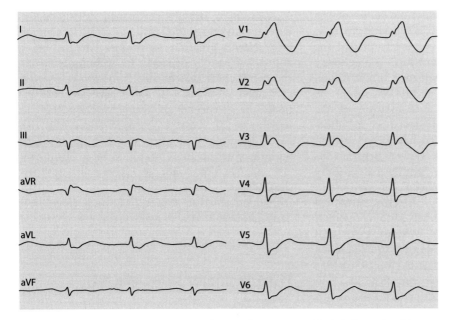

Fig. 11.7. Surface ECG from a patient with Brugada type 1 syndrome. The elevated ST segment (<2 mm in leads V1–V3) descends with an upward convexity to an inverted T wave. This is referred to as the "coved type" Brugada pattern

be an alternative to drug treatment. The exact mapping and ablation techniques are discussed in Chapter 9 of this book.
2. VT caused by ion channel disease (e.g., long QT syndrome, Brugada syndrome; Figure 11.7). These channelopathies are associated with a significant risk of sudden death depending on age, genetics, clinical and ECG findings. An implantable cardioverter defibrillator (ICD) might be indicated as no definitive treatment is available. Ablation of ventricular tachycardia or ventricular fibrillation in these diseases is still experimental [42].
3. The association of VT with hypertrophic or dilated cardiomyopathy. As the disease is rare in children, no sufficient data and (as in channelopathies) no definitive treatment strategy is available. Here also the implantation of an ICD might be the therapy of choice depending on risk analysis in the individual patient.
4. Myocarditis may be associated with VT, especially if congestive heart failure is present. The role of ablation is uncertain, as symptoms may improve with successful treatment of heart failure.

5. The presence of structural heart disease with VT is critical, as there is a high risk for further deterioration. Catheter ablation or the implantation of an ICD might be indicated (see Chapter 12).

∎ **Mapping and ablation.** An arterial access with invasive blood pressure measurement online is helpful to estimate the hemodynamic impact of the tachycardia. Most centers favor a light level of conscious sedation to avoid VT suppression, but patient age or hemodynamic status can require deeper levels of anesthesia. The ventricular stimulation protocol often demands up to four extrastimuli, burst pacing or isoproterenol infusion to induce tachycardia. As in adults, biplane angiograms to exclude structural heart disease should be performed. 3D mapping systems are helpful in reducing fluoroscopy time, mapping and tagging of the conduction system and constructing ablation lines.

The use of irrigated tip electrodes is generally not recommended in smaller children to avoid coronary injury due to deeper range of energy delivery. Late scar expansion is possibly a consequence of RF lesions [71], so VT ablation in small children should be undertaken with caution. Future developments of 3D mapping, cryoablation and the growing knowledge of underlying (genetic) mechanisms of VT will hopefully lead to individualized therapeutic concepts as well as improve the success rate of VT ablation to avoid the lifetime burden of an ICD.

▌ References

1. Aguinaga L, Primo J, Anguera I, Mont L, Valentino M, Brugada P, Brugada J (1998) Long-term follow-up in patients with the permanent form of junctional reciprocating tachycardia treated with radiofrequency ablation. Pacing Clin Electrophysiol 21:2073–2078

2. Akar JG, Kok LC, Haines DE, DiMarco JP, Mounsey JP (2001) Coexistence of type I atrial flutter and intra-atrial re-entrant tachycardia in patients with surgically corrected congenital heart disease. J Am Coll Cardiol 38:377–384

3. Beder SD, Gillette PC, Garson A Jr, Porter CB, McNamara DG (1983) Symptomatic sick sinus syndrome in children and adolescents as the only manifestation of cardiac abnormality or associated with unoperated congenital heart disease. Am J Cardiol 51:1133–1136

4. Beerman LB (1991) Intracardiac Electrophysiology. In: Neches WH, Park SC, Zuberbuhler JR (eds) Pediatric cardiac catheterization. Futura Inc, Mount Kisco, pp 121–139

5. Berul CI, Hill SL, Wang PJ, Marx GR, Fulton DR, Estes NA, 3rd (1998) Neonatal radiofrequency catheter ablation of junctional tachycardias. J Interv Card Electrophysiol 2:91–100

6. Blaufox AD, Numan M, Knick BJ, Saul JP (2001) Sinoatrial node reentrant tachycardia in infants with congenital heart disease. Am J Cardiol 88:1050–1054

7. Blaufox AD, Paul T, Saul JP (2004) Radiofrequency catheter ablation in small children: relationship of complications to application dose. Pacing Clin Electrophysiol 27:224–229

8. Boersma L, Garcia-Moran E, Mont L, Brugada J (2002) Accessory pathway localization by QRS polarity in children with Wolff-Parkinson-White syndrome. J Cardiovasc Electrophysiol 13:1222–1226

9. Bokenkamp R, Bertram H, Trappe HJ, Luhmer I, Paul T (1998) [High frequency catheter ablation in young patients with permanent junctional reentry tachycardia and ectopic atrial tachycardia]. Z Kardiol 87:364–371

10. Bolling SF, Morady F, Calkins H, Kadish A, de Buitleir M, Langberg J, Dick M, Lupinetti FM, Bove EL (1991) Current treatment for Wolff-Parkinson-White syndrome: results and surgical implications. Ann Thorac Surg 52:461–468

11. Campbell RM, Strieper MJ, Frias PA, Collins KK, Van Hare GF, Dubin AM (2003) Survey of current practice of pediatric electrophysiologists for asymptomatic Wolff-Parkinson-White syndrome. Pediatrics 111:e245–247

12. Campbell RM, Strieper MJ, Frias PA, Danford DA, Kugler JD (2002) Current status of radiofrequency ablation for common pediatric supraventricular tachycardias. J Pediatr 140:150–155

13. Case CL, Gillette PC (1993) Automatic atrial and junctional tachycardias in the pediatric patient: strategies for diagnosis and management. Pacing Clin Electrophysiol 16:1323–1335

14. Cecconi M, Renzi R, Bettuzzi MG, Colonna P, Cuccaroni G, Ricciotti R, Pozzato E, Berrettini U, Sgarbi E, Sparvieri F et al (1993) [Congenital isolated complete atrioventricular block: longterm experience with 38 patients]. G Ital Cardiol 23:39–53

15. Chiladakis JA, Vassilikos VP, Maounis TN, Cokkinos DV, Manolis AS (1997) Successful radiofrequency catheter ablation of automatic atrial tachycardia with regression of the cardiomyopathy picture. Pacing Clin Electrophysiol 20:953–959

16. Cilliers AM, du Plessis JP, Clur S-AB, Dateling F, Levin SE (1997) Junctional ectopic tachycardia in six paediatric patients. Heart 78:413–415

17. Clancy RM, Buyon JP, Tamargo I, Caballero R, et al (2004) More to death than dying: apoptosis in the pathogenesis of SSA/Ro-SSB/La-associated congenital heart block. Rheum Dis Clin North Am 30:589–602

18. Cobb FR, Blumenschein SD, Sealy WC, Boineau JP, Wagner GS, Wallace AG (1968) Successful surgical interruption of the bundle of Kent in a patient with Wolff-Parkinson-White syndrome. Circulation 38:1018–1029

19. Crosson JE, Hesslein PS, Thilenius OG, Dunnigan A (1995) AV node reentry tachycardia in infants. Pacing Clin Electrophysiol 18:2144–2149

20. Davy JM, Pons M, Raczka F, Piot C (1999) [Electrocardiographic aspects of the pathology of the bundle of His]. Arch Mal Coeur Vaiss 92 Spec No 1:37–45

21. de Paola AA, Leite LR, Arfelli E (2003) Mechanical reperfusion of acute right coronary artery occlusion after radiofrequency catheter ablation and long-term follow-up angiography. J Invasive Cardiol 15:173–175

22. De Ponti R, Storti C, Stanke A, Ferrari AA, Longobardi M, Salerno-Uriarte JA (1994) [Radiofrequency catheter ablation in patients with Mahaim-type slow-conduction accessory right atrioventricular pathway]. Cardiologia 39:169–180

23. Deanfield J, Thaulow E, Warnes C, Webb G, Kolbel F, Hoffman A, Sorenson K, Kaemmer H, Thilen U, Bink-Boelkens M, Iserin L, Daliento L, Silove E, Redington A, Vouhe P, Priori S, Alonso

MA, Blanc JJ, Budaj A, Cowie M, Deckers J, Fernandez Burgos E, Lekakis J, Lindahl B, Mazzotta G, Morais J, Oto A, Smiseth O, Trappe HJ, Klein W, Blomstrom-Lundqvist C, de Backer G, Hradec J, Parkhomenko A, Presbitero P, Torbicki A (2003) Management of grown up congenital heart disease. Eur Heart J 24:1035–1084

24. Dinckal H, Yucel O, Kirilmaz A, Karaca M, Kilicaslan F, Dokumaci B (2003) Left anterior descending coronary artery occlusion after left lateral free wall accessory pathway ablation: what is the possible mechanism? Europace 5:263–266

25. Dodo H, Gow RM, Hamilton RM, Freedom RM (1995) Chaotic atrial rhythm in children. Am Heart J 129:990–995

26. Dorostkar PC, Silka MJ, Morady F, Dick M, 2nd (1999) Clinical course of persistent junctional reciprocating tachycardia. J Am Coll Cardiol 33:366–375

27. Drago F, De Santis A, Grutter G, Silvetti MS (2005) Transvenous cryothermal catheter ablation of re-entry circuit located near the atrioventricular junction in pediatric patients: efficacy, safety, and midterm follow-up. J Am Coll Cardiol 45:1096–1103

28. Drago F, Silvetti MS, Mazza A, Anaclerio S, Pino AD, Grutter G, Bevilacqua M (2001) Permanent junctional reciprocating tachycardia in infants and children: effectiveness of medical and nonmedical treatment. Ital Heart J 2:456–461

29. Dubin AM, Collins KK, Chiesa N, Hanisch D, Van Hare GF (2002) Use of electrophysiologic testing to assess risk in children with Wolff-Parkinson-White syndrome. Cardiol Young 12:248–252

30. Dubin AM, Cuneo BF, Strasburger JF, Wakai RT, Van Hare GF, Rosenthal DN (2005) Congenital junctional ectopic tachycardia and congenital complete atrioventricular block: a shared etiology? Heart Rhythm 2:313–315

31. Fishberger SB, Rossi AF, Messina JJ, Saul JP (1998) Successful radiofrequency catheter ablation of congenital junctional ectopic tachycardia with preservation of atrioventricular conduction in a 9-month-old infant. Pacing Clin Electrophysiol 21:2132–2135

32. Francalanci P, Drago F, Agostino DA, Di Liso G, Di Ciommo V, Boldrini R, Ragonese P, Bosman C (1998) Koch's triangle in pediatric age: correlation with extra- and intracardiac parameters. Pacing Clin Electrophysiol 21:1576–1579

33. Friedman RA, Walsh EP, Silka MJ, Calkins H, Stevenson WG, Rhodes LA, Deal BJ, Wolff GS, Demaso DR, Hanisch D, Van Hare GF (2002) NASPE Expert Consensus Conference: Radiofrequency catheter ablation in children with and without congenital heart disease. Report of the writing committee. North American Society of Pacing and Electrophysiology. Pacing Clin Electrophysiol 25:1000–1017

34. Gaita F, Haissaguerre M, Giustetto C, Fischer B, Riccardi R, Richiardi E, Scaglione M, Lamberti F, Warin JF (1995) Catheter ablation of permanent junctional reciprocating tachycardia with radiofrequency current. J Am Coll Cardiol 25:648–654

35. Gaita F, Haissaguerre M, Giustetto C, Grossi S, Caruzzo E, Bianchi F, Richiardi E, Riccardi R, Hocini M, Jais P (2003) Safety and efficacy of cryoablation of accessory pathways adjacent to the normal conduction system. J Cardiovasc Electrophysiol 14:825–829

36. Gaita F, Montefusco A, Riccardi R, Giustetto C, Grossi S, Caruzzo E, Bianchi F, Vivalda L, Gabbarini F, Calabro R (2004) Cryoenergy catheter ablation: a new technique for treatment of permanent junctional reciprocating tachycardia in children. J Cardiovasc Electrophysiol 15:263–268

37. Gillette PC, Garson A Jr (1977) Electrophysiologic and pharmacologic characteristics of automatic ectopic atrial tachycardia. Circulation 56:571–575

38. Goldberg CS, Caplan MJ, Heidelberger KP, Dick M, 2nd (1999) The dimensions of the triangle of Koch in children. Am J Cardiol 83:117–120, A119

39. Gouin S, Ali S (2003) A patient with chaotic atrial tachycardia. Pediatr Emerg Care 19:95–98

40. Gross GJ, Epstein MR, Walsh EP, Saul JP (1998) Characteristics, management, and midterm outcome in infants with atrioventricular nodal reentry tachycardia. Am J Cardiol 82:956–960

41. Haissaguerre M, Cauchemez B, Marcus F, Le Metayer P, Lauribe P, Poquet F, Gencel L, Clementy J (1995) Characteristics of the ventricular insertion sites of accessory pathways with anterograde decremental conduction properties. Circulation 91:1077–1085

42. Haissaguerre M, Extramiana F, Hocini M, Cauchemez B, Jais P, Cabrera JA, Farre J, Leenhardt A, Sanders P, Scavee C, Hsu LF, Weerasooriya R, Shah DC, Frank R, Maury P, Delay M, Garrigue S, Clementy J (2003) Mapping and ablation of ventricular fibrillation associated with long-QT and Brugada syndromes. Circulation 108: 925–928

43. Hamdan M, Van Hare GF, Fisher W, Gonzalez R, Dorostkar P, Lee R, Lesh M, Saxon L, Kalman J, Scheinman M (1996) Selective catheter ablation of the tachycardia focus in patients with nonreentrant junctional tachycardia. Am J Cardiol 78:1292–1297

44. Harrison DA, Connelly M, Harris L, Luk C, Webb GD, McLaughlin PR (1996) Sudden cardiac death in the adult with congenital heart disease. Can J Cardiol 12:1161–1163

45. Huang SK, Bharati S, Graham AR, Lev M, Marcus FI, Odell RC (1987) Closed chest catheter desiccation of the atrioventricular junction

using radiofrequency energy – a new method of catheter ablation. J Am Coll Cardiol 9:349–358

46. Inoue K, Igarashi H, Fukushige J, Ohno T, Joh K, Hara T (2000) Long-term prospective study on the natural history of Wolff-Parkinson-White syndrome detected during a heart screening program at school. Acta Paediatr 89:542–545

47. Kampmann C, Wiethoff CM, Wenzel A, Stolz G, Betancor M, Wippermann C-F, Huth R-G, Habermehl P, Knuf M, Emschermann T, Stopfkuchen H (2000) Normal values of M mode echocardiographic measurements of more than 2000 healthy infants and children in central Europe. Heart 83:667–672

48. Khanal S, Ribeiro PA, Platt M, Kuhn MA (1999) Right coronary artery occlusion as a complication of accessory pathway ablation in a 12-year-old treated with stenting. Catheter Cardiovasc Interv 46:59–61

49. Kirsh JA, Walsh EP, Triedman JK (2002) Prevalence of and risk factors for atrial fibrillation and intra-atrial reentrant tachycardia among patients with congenital heart disease. Am J Cardiol 90:338–340

50. Klein GJ, Guiraudon GM, Kerr CR, Sharma AD, Yee R, Szabo T, Wah JA (1988) "Nodoventricular" accessory pathway: evidence for a distinct accessory atrioventricular pathway with atrioventricular node-like properties. J Am Coll Cardiol 11:1035–1040

51. Ko JK, Deal BJ, Strasburger JF, Benson DW Jr (1992) Supraventricular tachycardia mechanisms and their age distribution in pediatric patients. Am J Cardiol 69:1028–1032

52. Kugler JD, Danford DA, Houston KA, Felix G (2002) Pediatric radiofrequency catheter ablation registry success, fluoroscopy time, and complication rate for supraventricular tachycardia: comparison of early and recent eras. J Cardiovasc Electrophysiol 13:336–341

53. Lashus AG, Case CL, Gillette PC (1997) Catheter ablation treatment of supraventricular tachycardia-induced cardiomyopathy. Arch Pediatr Adolesc Med 151:264–266

54. Lavergne T, Guize L, Le Heuzey JY, Carcone P, Geslin J, Cousin MT (1986) Closed-chest atrioventricular junction ablation by high-frequency energy transcatheter desiccation. Lancet 2:858–859

55. Lesh MD, Van Hare GF, Schamp DJ, Chien W, Lee MA, Griffin JC, Langberg JJ, Cohen TJ, Lurie KG, Scheinman MM (1992) Curative percutaneous catheter ablation using radiofrequency energy for accessory pathways in all locations: results in 100 consecutive patients. J Am Coll Cardiol 19:1303–1309

56. Linker NJ, Fitzpatrick AP (1998) The transseptal approach for ablation of cardiac arrhythmias: experience of 104 procedures. Heart 79:379–382

57. Lisowski LA, Verheijen PM, Benatar AA, Soyeur DJ, Stoutenbeek P, Brenner JI, Kleinman CS, Meijboom EJ (2000) Atrial flutter in the perinatal age group: diagnosis, management and outcome. J Am Coll Cardiol 35:771–777

58. McClelland JH, Wang X, Beckman KJ, Hazlitt HA, Prior MI, Nakagawa H, Lazzara R, Jackman WM (1994) Radiofrequency catheter ablation of right atriofascicular (Mahaim) accessory pathways guided by accessory pathway activation potentials. Circulation 89:2655–2666

59. Mehta AV, Sanchez GR, Sacks EJ, Casta A, Dunn JM, Donner RM (1988) Ectopic automatic atrial tachycardia in children: clinical characteristics, management and follow-up. J Am Coll Cardiol 11:379–385

60. Miyazaki A, Blaufox AD, Fairbrother DL, Saul JP (2005) Cryo-ablation for septal tachycardia substrates in pediatric patients: mid-term results. J Am Coll Cardiol 45:581–588

61. Morwood JG, Triedman JK, Berul CI, Khairy P, Alexander ME, Cecchin F, Walsh EP (2004) Radiofrequency catheter ablation of ventricular tachycardia in children and young adults with congenital heart disease. Heart Rhythm 1:301–308

62. Munger TM, Packer DL, Hammill SC, Feldman BJ, Bailey KR, Ballard DJ, Holmes DR Jr, Gersh BJ (1993) A population study of the natural history of Wolff-Parkinson-White syndrome in Olmsted County, Minnesota, 1953–1989. Circulation 87:866–873

63. Ouali S, Anselme F, Savoure A, Cribier A (2002) Acute coronary occlusion during radiofrequency catheter ablation of typical atrial flutter. J Cardiovasc Electrophysiol 13:1047–1049

64. Packer DL, Bardy GH, Worley SJ, Smith MS, Cobb FR, Coleman RE, Gallagher JJ, German LD (1986) Tachycardia-induced cardiomyopathy: a reversible form of left ventricular dysfunction. Am J Cardiol 57:563–570

65. Pappone C, Manguso F, Santinelli R, Vicedomini G, Sala S, Paglino G, Mazzone P, Lang CC, Gulletta S, Augello G, Santinelli O, Santinelli V (2004) Radiofrequency ablation in children with asymptomatic Wolff-Parkinson-White syndrome. N Engl J Med 351:1197–1205

66. Perry JC, Garson A Jr (1990) Supraventricular tachycardia due to Wolff-Parkinson-White syndrome in children: early disappearance and late recurrence. J Am Coll Cardiol 16:1215–1220

67. Prager NA, Cox JL, Lindsay BD, Ferguson TB Jr, Osborn JL, Cain ME (1993) Long-term effectiveness of surgical treatment of ectopic atrial tachycardia. J Am Coll Cardiol 22:85–92

68. Salerno JC, Kertesz NJ, Friedman RA, Fenrich AL Jr (2004) Clinical course of atrial ectopic tachycardia is age-dependent: results and treatment in children <3 or >or =3 years of age. J Am Coll Cardiol 43:438–444

69. Sanchez C, Benito F, Moreno F (1995) Reversibility of tachycardia-induced cardiomyopathy after radiofrequency ablation of incessant supraventricular tachycardia in infants. Br Heart J 74:332–333

70. Sassone B, Leone O, Martinelli GN, Di Pasquale G (2004) Acute myocardial infarction after radiofrequency catheter ablation of typical atrial flutter: histopathological findings and etiopathogenetic hypothesis. Ital Heart J 5:403–407

71. Saul JP, Hulse JE, Papagiannis J, Van Praagh R, Walsh EP (1994) Late enlargement of radiofrequency lesions in infant lambs. Implications for ablation procedures in small children. Circulation 90:492–499

72. Scheinman M, Calkins H, Gillette P, Klein R, Lerman BB, Morady F, Saksena S, Waldo A (2003) NASPE policy statement on catheter ablation: personnel, policy, procedures, and therapeutic recommendations. Pacing Clin Electrophysiol 26:789–799

73. Schneider C (2004) Das EPU-Labor. Steinkopff, Darmstadt

74. Shih HT, Miles WM, Klein LS, Hubbard JE, Zipes DP (1994) Multiple accessory pathways in the permanent form of junctional reciprocating tachycardia. Am J Cardiol 73:361–367

75. Sternick EB, Timmermans C, Sosa E, Cruz FE, Rodriguez LM, Fagundes MA, Gerken LM, Wellens HJ (2004) The electrocardiogram during sinus rhythm and tachycardia in patients with Mahaim fibers: the importance of an "rS" pattern in lead III. J Am Coll Cardiol 44:1626–1635

76. Strobel GG, Trehan S, Compton S, Judd VE, Day RW, Etheridge SP (2001) Successful pediatric stenting of a nonthrombotic coronary occlusion as a complication of radiofrequency catheter ablation. Pacing Clin Electrophysiol 24:1026–1028

77. Sturm M, Hausmann D, Bokenkamp R, Bertram H, Wibbelt G, Paul T (2004) Incidence and time course of intimal plaque formation in the right coronary artery after radiofrequency current application detected by intracoronary ultrasound. Z Kardiol 93:884–889

78. Tanel RE, Walsh EP, Triedman JK (1998) Minimizing maximum radiofrequency lesion size: effects of catheter tip size in vivo animal preparations. Pacing Clin Electrophysiol 21:833

79. Tang CW, Scheinman MM, Van Hare GF, Epstein LM, Fitzpatrick AP, Lee RJ, Lesh MD (1995) Use of P wave configuration during atrial tachycardia to predict site of origin. J Am Coll Cardiol 26:1315–1324

80. Tchou P, Lehmann MH, Jazayeri M, Akhtar M (1988) Atriofascicular connection or a nodoventricular Mahaim fiber? Electrophysiologic elucidation of the pathway and associated reentrant circuit. Circulation 77:837–848

81. Teixeira OH, Balaji S, Case CL, Gillette PC (1994) Radiofrequency catheter ablation of atrioventricular nodal reentrant tachycardia in children. Pacing Clin Electrophysiol 17:1621–1626

82. Ticho BS, Saul JP, Hulse JE, De W, Lulu J, Walsh EP (1992) Variable location of accessory pathways associated with the permanent form of junctional reciprocating tachycardia and confirmation with radiofrequency ablation. Am J Cardiol 70:1559–1564

83. Triedman JK, Alexander ME, Berul CI, Bevilacqua LM, Walsh EP (2000) Estimation of atrial response to entrainment pacing using electrograms recorded from remote sites. J Cardiovasc Electrophysiol 11:1215–1222

84. Vaksmann G, D'Hoinne C, Lucet V, Guillaumont S, Lupoglazoff JM, Chantepie A, Denjoy I, Villain E, Marcon F (2005) Permanent junctional reciprocating tachycardia in children: a multicenter study on clinical profile and outcome. Heart

85. Van Hare GF, Javitz H, Carmelli D, Saul JP, Tanel RE, Fischbach PS, Kanter RJ, Schaffer M, Dunnigan A, Colan S, Serwer G (2004) Prospective assessment after pediatric cardiac ablation: demographics, medical profiles, and initial outcomes. J Cardiovasc Electrophysiol 15:759–770

86. Van Hare GF, Velvis H, Langberg JJ (1990) Successful transcatheter ablation of congenital junctional ectopic tachycardia in a ten-month-old infant using radiofrequency energy. Pacing Clin Electrophysiol 13:730–735

87. Vedel J, Frank R, Fontaine G, Fournial JF, Grosgogeat Y (1979) [Permanent intra-hisian atrioventricular block induced during right intraventricular exploration]. Arch Mal Coeur Vaiss 72:107–112

88. Villain E (1993) [Disorders of supraventricular rhythm in children]. Rev Prat 43:1538–1543

89. Villain E, Attali T, Iserin L, Aggoun Y, Kachaner J (1994) [Outcome of Wolff-Parkinson-White syndrome in children. Transesophageal study of anterograde permeability of the accessory pathway and of atrial vulnerability]. Arch Mal Coeur Vaiss 87:649–652

90. Villain E, Vetter VL, Garcia JM, Herre J, Cifarelli A, Garson A Jr (1990) Evolving concepts in the management of congenital junctional ectopic tachycardia. A multicenter study. Circulation 81:1544–1549

91. Weng KP, Wolff GS, Young ML (2003) Multiple accessory pathways in pediatric patients with Wolff-Parkinson-White syndrome. Am J Cardiol 91:1178–1183

92. Wetzel U, Hindricks G, Schirdewahn P, Dorszewski A, Fleck A, Heinke F, Kottkamp H (2002) A stepwise mapping approach for localization and ablation of ectopic right, left, and septal atrial foci using electroanatomic mapping. Eur Heart J 23:1387–1393

12 Mapping and ablation in congenital heart disease

GABRIELE HESSLING, ANDREAS PFLAUMER, BERNHARD ZRENNER

▌ Introduction

Advances in the diagnosis and treatment of congenital heart disease over recent decades have led to a dramatic improvement of outcome and long-term survival in this patient population [48]. However, the incidence of cardiac arrhythmias as a sequela of palliative or corrective heart surgery has increased significantly in adolescent and adult survivors of congenital heart disease surgery [5, 16, 48, 49]. Cardiac arrhythmias are the leading cause for emergency admissions in adult congenital heart disease patients with or without surgical interventions [24].

The incidence of late arrhythmias has been associated with long-term abnormal pressure-volume load, hypoxia, surgically created scars or suture lines [22, 28, 32, 38]. Autonomic [9] as well as congenital factors [23] also seem to play a role in arrhythmia genesis. Residual hemodynamic problems as frequently encountered in these patients might be aggravated by the arrhythmia resulting in heart failure, acute collapse or cardiac arrest. The risk of sudden death in association with recurrent intraatrial tachycardia episodes is reported to be as high as 6–10% in long-term survivors of surgery for congenital heart disease [16, 48].

As patients with congenital heart disease form a heterogeneous patient population, an optimal treatment strategy for the individual patient has to be defined which includes medical therapy, catheter ablation and/or treatment with an implantable defibrillator. Medical therapy is often difficult, it may be insufficient to control the arrhythmia and exposes patients to the risk of serious side effects especially with long-term treatment [4, 39, 42]. Catheter ablation offers an alternative treatment strategy in many of these patients. New mapping and ablation techniques have improved the understanding of complex arrhythmia mechanisms which in turn has led to higher success and lower complication rates of the ablation procedure. The goal of this chapter is to show our current approach to catheter ablation of tachycardias in patients with congenital heart disease.

▌ 12.1 Approach to the ablation procedure

There are some crucial steps in approaching an ablation therapy in patients with congenital heart disease which include
1) adequate preparation of the procedure,
2) reliable identification of the tachycardia circuit and the appropriate ablation site and
3) creation of an effective tissue altering lesion.

12.1.1 Preablation workup

Indications for catheter ablation in patients with congenital heart disease are summarized in Chapter 11. Tachycardia leading to ventricular dysfunction or recurrent and frequent episodes of tachycardia are the main indications for catheter ablation in this patient population.

A complete clinical workup (including ECG, Holter and echocardiogram) and the assessment of the hemodynamic status of the patient are mandatory prior to the procedure. Previous heart catheterizations with angiography offer the opportunity to evaluate the patient's individual anatomy and to plan the ablation procedure (e.g., access to the atria and ventricles). In postoperative patients, the surgeon's operative report must be reviewed for detail, such as the location of the coronary sinus, the insertion of prosthetic material, type of intraatrial baffling or type of Fontan creation [44].

Transthoracic echocardiography is usually not sufficient to rule out intracardiac thrombi and a transesophageal echocardiogram should therefore be performed. Preprocedural anticoagulation (usually with heparin i.v.) is advisable especially in patients with low-flow hemodynamics as with the Fontan type operation. Imaging tools as CT, MRI, scintigraphy or positron emission tomography (PET) might be helpful to assess the patient's current status. Cardiac catheterization should be performed if any question remains concerning anatomy or hemodynamics [20]. Most of the patients referred to an ablation procedure are treated with antiarrhythmic medication. Prior to the ablation procedure, antiarrhythmic medication is usually discontinued (3–5 half-lives of the drug; if necessary in-hospital).

12.1.2 Arrhythmias in congenital heart disease patients

Before approaching the ablation procedure, the most frequently encountered cardiac arrhythmias in patients with congenital heart disease will be reviewed briefly as the understanding of their pathophysiology is crucial for mapping and ablation. Atrial fibrillation, focal atrial tachycardia and tachycardias due to an accessory pathway or AV nodal reentry are discussed in more detail in the corresponding chapters of this book. It is noteworthy that "accessory pathways" as muscular connections between atrium and ventricle can be acquired due to a surgical procedure [19].

■ Intraatrial reentrant tachycardia (IART)

Atrial macroreentry is the most common tachycardia mechanism in patients with congenital heart disease and may occur in up to 30% of patients after the Mustard or Senning procedure for D-transposition of the great arteries and in up to 50% following modifications of the Fontan operation (Figure 12.1) [29, 37, 48, 49]. Macroreentry can occur as 1) isthmus-dependent atrial flutter with the cavotricuspid isthmus as part of the reentrant circuit, 2) incisional tachycardia with a scar or suture line as the central obstacle or as 3) a reentrant tachycardia not related to the cavotricuspid isthmus or a suture line. The high incidence of atrial tachycardias following particular operations is not surprising as they include relatively large areas of scarring from patches or sutures and often a thickening or dilatation of the atria.

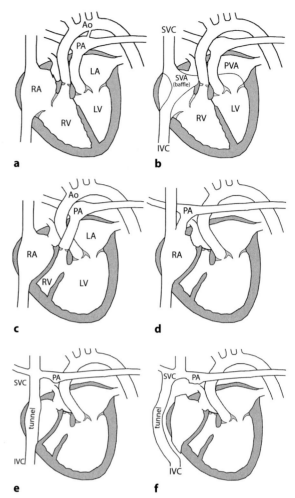

Fig. 12.1. a A Schematic representation of d-transposition of the great arteries (aorta arises from the right ventricle, pulmonary artery from the left ventricle). **b** Mustard operation with an atrial baffle created to direct blood from the superior and inferior vena cava to the mitral valve and left ventricle. **c** Tricuspid atresia with a hypoplastic right ventricle. **d** Classic Fontan type operation with direct atriopulmonary connection. **e** Intracardiac total cavopulmonary connection (TCPC). **f** Extracardiac tunnel using a Gore-tex conduit (to avoid right atrial scarring). *RA* right atrium, *RV* right ventricle, *LA* left atrium, *LV* left ventricle, *PA* pulmonary artery, *Ao* Aorta, *SVC* superior vena cava, *IVC* inferior vena cava, *SVA* systemic venous atrium, *PVA* pulmonary venous atrium

The clinical presentation of chronic intraatrial reentrant tachycardia (IART) is often unspecific or associated only with mild symptoms of heart failure [26]. Whereas typical atrial flutter involves a defined reentrant circuit around the tricuspid annulus, IART might involve different reentrant circuits around suture lines or scars and will therefore exhibit a wide spectrum of P waves on the ECG. Diagnosis from the surface ECG is therefore sometimes difficult as P waves are not easily detectable [27, 34]. Cycle length of IART is often rather long (280–450 ms) and antiarrhythmic drugs can additionally slow the atrial rate leading to 1:1 AV conduction. This makes it even more difficult to recognize the P wave as it is often superimposed on the QRS complex or T wave. A resting heart rate above the presumed level for the corresponding age group in a patient after surgery for congenital heart disease is often suggestive of IART with 2:1 or 3:1 AV conduction. Figure 12.2 shows surface and intracardiac ECG findings of a patient after the Fontan operation with IART.

▮ Ventricular tachycardia

Ventricular tachycardia (VT) is relatively rare but potentially life threatening in patients with congenital heart disease and associated with a significant risk of sudden death [48]. The largest group of congenital heart disease patients with a significant incidence of VT are patients after surgery for tetralogy of Fallot and most of the available data are derived from this popula-

tion [6, 17]. Patients often present with severe symptoms such as syncope or cardiac arrest due to the arrhythmia. Ventricular tachycardia found in these patients is usually due to a (monomorphic) macroreentrant circuit around scarred right ventricular outflow or conal septum tissue. The ECG of a typical example of a VT in a postoperative tetralogy of Fallot patient is shown in Figure 12.3.

12.1.3 General considerations of the ablation procedure

The procedure is usually performed under conscious sedation, if tolerated by the patient as this facilitates tachycardia induction and/or stability. Vascular access is often difficult due to prior procedures or underlying heart disease. We routinely use the transfemoral approach (right and/or left femoral vein and artery). A transjugular approach might be necessary in patients with complex heart disease or patients without accessible femoral vessels. There are rare instances (as with interrupted inferior caval

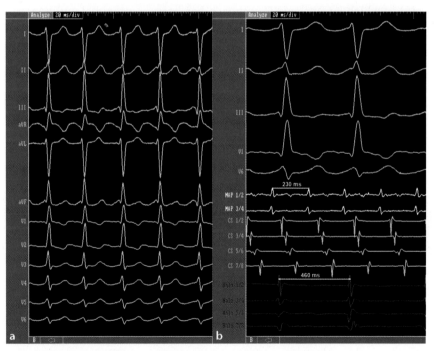

Fig. 12.2. ECG of a Fontan patient with an intraatrial reentrant tachycardia (IART). **a** 12-lead surface ECG (50 mm/s). The ventricular rhythm is regular with a rate of 130/min; distinction of P waves is difficult on the surface ECG. **b** Surface ECG and intracardiac recordings (100 mm/s) with a Map catheter positioned in the right atrium. IART with a cycle length of 230 ms (and 2:1 AV conduction to the ventricles) is detected on the Map and CS catheter (placed in the right atrium). The Halo catheter is placed in the ventricle

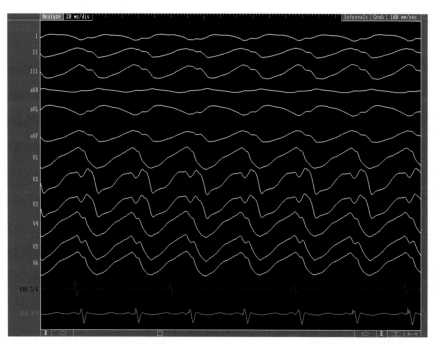

Fig. 12.3. Surface and intracardiac recordings (100 mm/s) of a patient with VT after surgical correction of tetralogy of Fallot. Tachycardia shows a LBBB morphology with inferior axis (QRS positive in II, III, avF) corresponding to an origin in the right ventricular outflow tract. A catheter is placed in the right atrium (HRA; red) and the right ventricle (RVA; pink) clearly showing VT with a dissociation of atrial and ventricular activity

vein) in which a transhepatic approach has been used for access to the atrium [15]. In patients with the Mustard or Senning operation, a catheter is usually placed in the appendage of the systemic venous atrium (which is anatomically the left atrial appendage) as an activation reference and for atrial pacing. Access to the pulmonary venous atrium in patients after the Mustard procedure or patients with a Fontan-type operation is possible by a retrograde (transaortic, transtricuspidal/transmitral) approach [50] (Figure 12.4).

If a (residual) ASD is present, antegrade access to the left atrium is sometimes achievable. Antegrade access to the pulmonary venous atrium via transseptal puncture should be guided by intracardiac echocardiography (ICE) in patients with complex anatomy or with patch material within the septum. Depending on the underlying anatomy or surgical intervention unusual locations of the sinus node, the AV node or the bundle branches should be considered [3]. If possible, placing a catheter in the coronary sinus is helpful as a guiding and reference structure and for atrial pacing. In patients with the classic type of Fontan operation, a catheter for activation mapping is often placed in the proximal pulmonary artery (PA) via the right atrial-right ventricular outflow tract or PA anastomosis. Sometimes large ventricular spikes are also recorded over this catheter which have to be distinguished from the atrial electrograms. An angiography of the reference catheter placed in the PA might be helpful as the catheter is sometimes not in a stable position. If stable placement of an intracardiac reference catheter is very difficult or time-consuming, an esophageal electrode catheter might be used as reference. In patients after the Fontan procedure, ventricular pacing must be available (by placing a catheter retrogradely in the ventricle) as the septum is often a target for ablation and unintentional damage to the AV node might result in severe bradycardia or asystole.

Monitoring of the hemodynamic status and O_2 saturation is mandatory and we often use a small arterial sheath (4-5F) for online blood pressure and blood gas analysis. Adequate anticoagulation throughout the procedure is especially important in patients with residual lesions (right-to-left or left-to-right shunts). Intravenous heparin is administered routinely throughout the procedure and anticoagulation monitored by assessing the activated clotting time

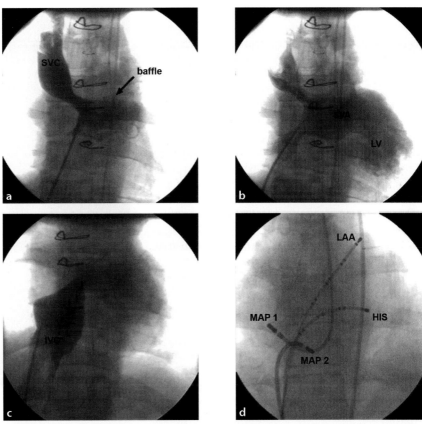

Fig. 12.4. a–c Angiographic views of the systemic venous atrium (SVA) in a patient after the Mustard operation for d-transposition of the great arteries. Superior vena cava (SVC), inferior vena cava (IVC) and atrial baffle creation form the systemic venous atrium (SVA) directing blood flow towards the mitral valve and the left ventricle (LV). **d** Catheter positions during an electrophysiological study. The reference catheter is placed in the appendage of the SVA (anatomically left atrial appendage LAA), another catheter is placed in the region of the His bundle. Two Map catheters are placed: Map 1 retrogradely over the aortic and tricuspid valve in the pulmonary venous atrium and Map 2 antegradely via the inferior vena cava in the systemic venous atrium

(ACT; aimed at 250–300). In case of an emergency, an interventional cardiac catheterization, intensive care and cardiac surgery team should be available [40]. After the procedure, an echocardiogram is performed to rule out pericardial effusion. Anticoagulation as well as ECG and hemodynamic monitoring are continued for at least 24 hours.

12.2 Mapping techniques for intraatrial reentrant tachycardia

There are two settings that are encountered when a patient with intraatrial reentrant tachycardia (IART) comes to the lab for an ablation procedure: 1) the patient is in tachycardia, he-modynamically stable and after placing the catheters mapping can be performed right away or 2) the patient is in sinus rhythm (with an ECG-documented tachycardia) and tachycardia has to be induced by programmed stimulation before mapping can be performed. In the latter case, it is often useful to perform an electroanatomical map during sinus rhythm first. Programmed atrial stimulation (including rapid atrial pacing) is used for induction of IART and sometimes aggressive burst-stimulation and/or isoprenaline are necessary for tachycardia induction. Matching the induced rhythm with a documented tachycardia is reassuring prior to mapping and ablation. Multiple tachycardia morphologies may lead to a more aggressive approach. On the other hand, induction of a previously not documented form of tachycardia after a successful ablation may represent a nonspecific finding. The two mapping techniques most helpful in patients with congenital heart disease will be discussed in more detail: electroanatomical mapping and entrainment mapping.

12.2.1 Electroanatomic mapping

Electroanatomical mapping allows a nonfluoroscopic localization of the catheter tip and generation of an activation map which shows a local activation time in reference to some spatial and/or anatomic frame of reference. The technical aspects of electroanatomical mapping are described in more detail in Chapter 3 of this book. In patients with congenital heart disease and IART we routinely use the Carto®-system (Biosense Webster, Diamond Bar, CA, USA), which has found widespread acceptance in patients with congenital heart disease [13, 28, 30, 35, 36]. A reference locator is placed on the patient's back and a 5F or 6F octapolar catheter is placed for reference as described above. A 7F deflectable, quadripolar catheter (Navi-Star® or Navistar Thermo-Cool®, Biosense Webster) is used for mapping and ablation. If the patient is in sinus rhythm at the beginning of the procedure, mapping is performed to outline the anatomy and the important landmarks of the conduction system (Figure 12.5). It should be remembered that the site of the primary pacemaker in postoperative congenital heart disease patients is often atypical.

After tachycardia is induced, a color-coded activation map is performed with local activation time on the map catheter in relation to the reference catheter. In most cases, IART is dependent on areas of surgical scarring which function as lines of conduction block. Therefore on the map, areas with absent or very low voltage (<0.03 mV) electrocardiograms are catalogued as incisional scar or patch (grey color on the maps). Two discrete electrocardiograms separated by at least 20 msec can be annotated as "double potentials". For example, a line of double potentials situated on the free wall of the right atrium might correlate with an atriotomy (line of conduction block with asynchronous activation on either side). "Fractionated" potentials show continuous low amplitude (<0.1 mV) with more than two separate positive or negative deflections also correspond to areas of slow or blocked conduction. In addition to the color-coded activation map, a voltage map

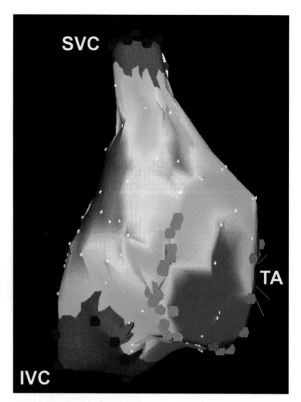

Fig. 12.5. Electroanatomical map (modified PA view) of the right atrium during sinus rhythm in a patient after an atriotomy. Activation spreads from the region of the sinus node (red) over the right atrium. The light blue dots represent "double potentials" found in this region corresponding to the atriotomy scar. Areas without electrical activity are marked in grey. *IVC* inferior vena cava, *TA* tricuspid annulus

might be displayed to show areas of scarring. An example of a color-coded activation map during tachycardia is shown in Figure 12.6.

It has recently become possible to "merge" a CT or MRT heart scan of the individual patient with the acquired electroanatomical map which allows a more precise incorporation of the underlying anatomy and facilitates mapping and ablation. An example is shown in Figure 12.7.

12.2.2 Entrainment mapping

Entrainment mapping is an electrophysiological technique that aims at differentiating bystander tissue from tissue critical to the reentrant circuit. It is discussed in more detail with examples in Chapter 1. In patients with IART, entrainment mapping is attempted at multiple sites surrounding the central barrier of an IART suggested by electroanatomical mapping [1, 11,

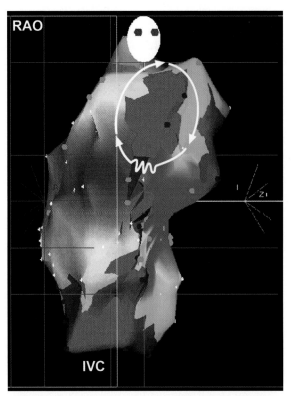

Fig. 12.6. Color-coded activation map (RAO 30° view) of a Fontan patient during intraatrial incisional reentrant tachycardia around a surgically created scar (grey) located at the right anterolateral atrial wall. The activation wavefront spreads from "early" (red) to "late" (blue) in relation to the reference catheter with a zone of slow conduction at the lower edge of the scar. *IVC* inferior vena cava

50]. A pacing cycle length 20–30 ms shorter than tachycardia cycle length is used for concealed entrainment. The postpacing interval (PPI) is measured from the pacing electrode to the beginning of the first intrinsic activation (using mostly the distal pole of the mapping catheter). Sites at which the PPI approximates tachycardia cycle length (≤20–30 ms difference) are considered to be located within the reentrant circuit. An example of positive and negative entrainment in a patient with IART is shown in Figure 1.21 in Chapter 1. It should be kept in mind that in areas of low voltage atrial capture might only be achieved by high output pacing [21]. The points of positive or negative entrainment are marked on the electroanatomical activation map to facilitate the understanding of the reentrant circuit.

12.2.3 Specific considerations in Mustard/Senning patients

One of the main findings in our patients with the Mustard procedure is that electroanatomical mapping has to be performed in both the systemic venous (SVA) and the pulmonary venous (PVA) atrium during IART to outline the reentrant circuit and to perform successful ablation [12, 50]. To map the SVA the catheter is advanced via the right femoral vein, to map the PVA via the right femoral artery across the aortic valve and across the tricuspid valve (see Figure 12.4). The His region is usually found in the SVA, the ostium of the coronary sinus in the PVA (Figure 12.4). In the great majority of patients, IART is a single-loop reentrant circuit commonly with the tricuspid annulus as a central barrier. The IART circuits are constrained inferiorly by the IVC and septally by atrial baffle. Patch, incisional scar or atriotomy can serve as additional boundaries. Peritricuspid tachycardias can rotate clockwise or counterclockwise around the tricuspid annulus (TA) and the site of ablation in these patients is most often the TA-inferior vena cava (IVC) isthmus (Figure 12.8).

The intraatrial baffle is positioned in a way that the septal TA-IVC isthmus is usually located in the PVA. The suture line at the midisthmus, however, is placed in a way that the midisthmus is confined to either PVA or to both SVA and PVA. Therefore it might be necessary not only to ablate in the PVA, but in both atria (Figure 12.9). It is important to remember that the created isthmus line must not be too septal to avoid damage of the AV node. An example of a peritricuspid IART with biatrial mapping and ablation is shown in Figures 12.8 and 12.9.

AV nodal reentrant tachycardia also occurs in patients with congenital heart disease. A retrograde (transaortic) or a transseptal access to the slow pathway region might be necessary due to anatomical or surgical reasons especially in patients after the Mustard procedure. The risk of creating AV block with RF ablation is higher and success rates are lower than in patients without heart disease [7].

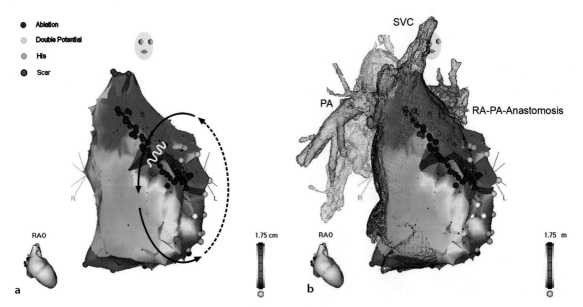

Fig. 12.7. a Electroanatomical activation map of a patient after the Fontan operation during intraatrial reentrant tachycardia. A macroreentrant circuit at the anterolateral aspect of the right atrial wall is shown. The white line represents a zone of slow conduction. The red dots show the ablation line with connection to the superior vena cava. **b** Carto-Merge: Incorporation of a CT scan from the same patient into the electroanatomical map for further detailed information about anatomic structures. The RA-PA anastomosis and peripheral PA branches are visible. *SVC* superior vena cava, *PA* pulmonary artery, *RA-PA* right atrial-pulmonary artery anastomosis

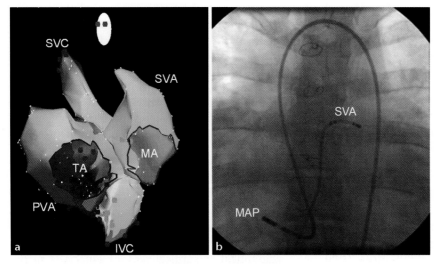

Fig. 12.8. a Activation map of peritricuspid counterclockwise IART in a patient after the Mustard procedure. Both the systemic venous and pulmonary venous atrium were mapped. Red dots refer to the ablation sites. **b** Fluoroscopic view of the successful ablation area (isthmus between tricuspid annulus and inferior vena cava). The MAP catheter was advanced retrogradely (transaortic/transtricuspid). Abbreviations see Figure 12.9. From Zrenner et al. [50] with permission

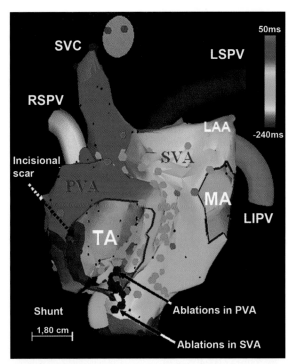

Fig. 12.9. Peritricuspid counterclockwise IART in a patient after the Mustard procedure which was mapped and ablated in the systemic venous atrium (SVA) as well as the pulmonary venous atrium (PVA). The red dots refer to the ablation sites (anatomically corresponding to the isthmus between tricuspid annulus and inferior vena cava). *SVC* superior vena cava, *RSPV* right superior pulmonary vein, *LSPV* left superior pulmonary vein, *LIPV* left inferior pulmonary vein, *LAA* left atrial appendage, *TA* tricuspid annulus, *MA* mitral annulus, *PVA* pulmonary venous atrium, *SVA* systemic venous atrium. From Dong et al. [12] with permission

12.2.4 Specific considerations in Fontan patients

In patients after a Fontan procedure, the reentrant circuit usually lies in the right atrium and involves tissue anterior to the crista terminalis. Especially in very large atria the crista terminalis is often displaced posteriorly. The site of ablation will be found to be the isthmus between the inferior vena cava and the tricuspid valve as in typical atrial flutter or more commonly it will be a region near scars on the lateral or anterior right atrial wall [1, 29, 46, 48]. Especially in patients with a Fontan operation who lack a right-sided valve annulus, successful ablation sites are more likely to be scattered around the lateral wall [29] and anterior aspect of the right atrium. In patients with an intracardiac total cavopulmonary connection (TCPC), ante-

grade access to the residual right atrium can only be accomplished through a preexistent (surgically created) opening or by puncture [10].

Identification of a reentrant tachycardia on the right atrial wall with only small, focal areas of entrainment has been reported [47]. In our experience, focal tachycardia (including a microreentrant mechanism) is not rare in patients after the Fontan procedure, accounting for up to 30% of cases. Foci are found preferentially adjacent to a scar area or the atriopulmonary conduit. Mapping and ablation techniques for FAT are described more extensively in Chapter 8.

12.3 Ablation strategies for intraatrial reentrant tachycardia

The general idea defining an ablation site in IART is to ablate the muscle tissue passing between two nonconductive boundaries. Usually linear ablation is performed to bridge the central barrier to the other barrier of the reentrant circuit. In peritricuspid IART the reentrant circuit is most often abolished by creating an ablation line connecting the tricuspid annulus to the inferior vena cava or to the incisional scar, atriotomy or patch. Ablation sites in tachycardias with the central obstacle on the right lateral wall are often treated by creating a line between the scar/suture and the SVC, IVC or the tricuspid annulus. Typical ablation lines are shown in Figures 12.7 and 12.9.

It is important to create complete conduction block by a transmural RF lesion. This can be difficult due to 1) hypertrophy of the atrial walls due to pressure and volume overload, 2) inadequate wall contact of the ablation catheter and 3) insufficient convective cooling by a low-flow circulating blood pool which limitates energy delivery to the tissue. In this setting, long sheaths often help to obtain better wall contact of the ablation catheter, and ablation with irrigated tip catheters has shown promising results [43, 47]. For mapping and ablation we either use an 8 mm distal tip catheter with a power limit of 55 W and a temperature limit of 55 °C at each site (point-by-point) for 2 minutes (Navistar, Biosense Webster) or an 4 mm irrigated tip catheter with a temperature limit of 43 °C and power limit of 40–45 W (Navistar Thermo-Cool, Biosense Webster). With the use of irrigated tip catheters, the volume load (20–30 ml/min during ablation) must be considered in hemodynamically compromised patients (and diuretics used if necessary). The His region and other structures not amenable to imaging (N. phrenicus) should be mapped or tested (by pacing) before ablation to avoid damage. Cryothermal catheters seem to be promising new tools for future developments.

Acute tachycardia termination is an indicator of acute ablation success, but a complete block line is necessary to ensure long-term success. The defined ablation lines should always be completed with the help of the electroanatomical mapping system by tagging each lesion on the map. It has been reported [36] that additional "preventive" ablation lines connecting nonconductive zones ("electrical scars") might reduce the risk of late occurring arrhythmias, but long-term clinical or EP studies addressing this issue are still lacking.

After the ablation, bidirectional block can either be verified using atrial pacing maneuvers or with creation of an electroanatomical remap during pacing. We consider ablation successful if tachycardia is no longer inducible and conduction block is established. The overall immediate success rate of ablation of IART is reported between 80 and 90%, with a recurrence rate for any type of IART of 30–50% [8, 25, 31, 36, 43, 45–47].

12.4 Mapping and ablation of postoperative ventricular tachycardia (VT)

Postoperative ventricular tachycardia (VT) occurs less frequent than IART but the techniques of electroanatomical and entrainment mapping can also be applied successfully to postoperative ventricular reentrant tachycardias [14, 18, 33, 41]. The largest group of patients with postoperative VT are patients after surgery for tetralogy of Fallot who were operated using a right ventriculotomy. Most often VT circuits use the ventriculotomy scar as the central obstacle (if they are not transannular) [14]. Mapping and ablation of scar-related VT is discussed in more detail in Chapter 9 of this book. It should be

kept in mind, however, that in patients with congenital heart disease and VT, success rates of the ablation (80% if mappable in safe location) are lower than with idiopathic VT, and the recurrence rate (40%) is higher despite using conduction block criteria to check success [33]. Therefore, the indication for an implantable defibrillator (ICD) in this population must be considered for the individual patient to prevent sudden cardiac death [2].

∎ References

1. Abrams D, Schilling R (2005) Mechanism and mapping of atrial arrhythmia in the modified Fontan circulation. Heart Rhythm 2:1138–1144
2. Alexander ME, Cecchin F, Walsh EP, Triedman JK, Bevilacqua LM, Berul CI (2004) Implications of implantable cardioverter defibrillator therapy in congenital heart disease and pediatrics. J Cardiovasc Electrophysiol 15:72–76
3. Anderson RH, Ho SY, Becker AE (1983) The surgical anatomy of the conduction tissues. Thorax 38:408–420
4. Bolens M, Friedli B, Deom A (1987) Electrophysiologic effects of intravenous verapamil in children after operations for congenital heart disease. Am J Cardiol 60:692–696
5. Brembilla-Perrot B (2000) Risk of increasing incidence of atrial flutter, the most frequent arrhythmia, after repaired congenital heart disease. Int J Cardiol 75:138–139
6. Chandar JS, Wolff GS, Garson A Jr, Bell TJ, Beder SD, Bink-Boelkens M, Byrum CJ, Campbell RM, Deal BJ, Dick M 2nd et al (1990) Ventricular arrhythmias in postoperative tetralogy of Fallot. Am J Cardiol 65:655–661
7. Chetaille P, Walsh EP, Triedman JK (2004) Outcomes of radiofrequency catheter ablation of atrioventricular reciprocating tachycardia in patients with congenital heart disease. Heart Rhythm 1:168–173
8. Collins KK, Love BA, Walsh EP, Saul JP, Epstein MR, Triedman JK (2000) Location of acutely successful radiofrequency catheter ablation of intraatrial reentrant tachycardia in patients with congenital heart disease. Am J Cardiol 86:969–974
9. Davos CH, Francis DP, Leenarts MF, Yap SC, Li W, Davlouros PA, Wensel R, Coats AJ, Piepoli M, Sreeram N, Gatzoulis MA (2003) Global impairment of cardiac autonomic nervous activity late after the Fontan operation. Circulation 108 Suppl 1:II180–185
10. Deisenhofer I, Estner H, Pflaumer A, Zrenner B (2005) Atypical access to typical atrial flutter. Heart Rhythm 2:93–96
11. Delacretaz E, Ganz LI, Soejima K, Friedman PL, Walsh EP, Triedman JK, Sloss LJ, Landzberg MJ,

Stevenson WG (2001) Multi atrial macro-re-entry circuits in adults with repaired congenital heart disease: entrainment mapping combined with three-dimensional electroanatomic mapping. J Am Coll Cardiol 37:1665–1676

12. Dong J, Zrenner B, Schreieck J, Schmitt C (2004) Necessity for biatrial ablation to achieve bidirectional cavotricuspid isthmus conduction block in a patient following senning operation. J Cardiovasc Electrophysiol 15:945–949

13. Dorostkar PC, Cheng J, Scheinman MM (1998) Electroanatomical mapping and ablation of the substrate supporting intraatrial reentrant tachycardia after palliation for complex congenital heart disease. Pacing Clin Electrophysiol 21:1810–1819

14. Downar E, Harris L, Kimber S, Mickleborough L, Williams W, Sevaptsidis E, Masse S, Chen TC, Chan A, Genga A et al (1992) Ventricular tachycardia after surgical repair of tetralogy of Fallot: results of intraoperative mapping studies. J Am Coll Cardiol 20:648–655

15. Emmel M, Brockmeier K, Sreeram N (2004) Combined transhepatic and transjugular approach for radiofrequency ablation of an accessory pathway in a child with complex congenital heart disease. Z Kardiol 93:555–557

16. Garson A Jr, Bink-Boelkens M, Hesslein PS, Hordof AJ, Keane JF, Neches WH, Porter CJ (1985) Atrial flutter in the young: a collaborative study of 380 cases. J Am Coll Cardiol 6:871–878

17. Gatzoulis MA, Till JA, Redington AN (1997) Depolarization-repolarization inhomogeneity after repair of tetralogy of Fallot. The substrate for malignant ventricular tachycardia? Circulation 95:401–404

18. Gonska BD, Cao K, Raab J, Eigster G, Kreuzer H (1996) Radiofrequency catheter ablation of right ventricular tachycardia late after repair of congenital heart defects. Circulation 94:1902–1908

19. Hager A, Zrenner B, Brodherr-Heberlein S, Steinbauer-Rosenthal I, Schreieck J, Hess J (2005) Congenital and surgically acquired Wolff-Parkinson-White syndrome in patients with tricuspid atresia. J Thorac Cardiovasc Surg 130:48–53

20. Hagler DJ (2001) Palliated congenital heart disease. Adolesc Med 12:23–34

21. Hammer PE, Brooks DH, Triedman JK (2003) Estimation of entrainment response using electrograms from remote sites: validation in animal and computer models of reentrant tachycardia. J Cardiovasc Electrophysiol 14:52–61

22. Ishii Y, Nitta T, Sakamoto S, Tanaka S, Asano G (2003) Incisional atrial reentrant tachycardia: experimental study on the conduction property through the isthmus. J Thorac Cardiovasc Surg 126:254–262

23. Jay PY, Berul CI, Tanaka M, Ishii M, Kurachi Y, Izumo S (2003) Cardiac conduction and arrhythmia: insights from Nkx2.5 mutations in mouse and humans. Novartis Found Symp 250:227–238

24. Kaemmerer H, Fratz S, Bauer U, Oechslin E, Brodherr-Heberlein S, Zrenner B, Turina J, Jenni R, Lange PE, Hess J (2003) Emergency hospital admissions and three-year survival of adults with and without cardiovascular surgery for congenital cardiac disease. J Thorac Cardiovasc Surg 126:1048–1052

25. Kannankeril PJ, Anderson ME, Rottman JN, Wathen MS, Fish FA (2003) Frequency of late recurrence of intra-atrial reentry tachycardia after radiofrequency catheter ablation in patients with congenital heart disease. Am J Cardiol 92:879–881

26. Li W, Somerville J (2000) Atrial flutter in grown-up congenital heart (GUCH) patients. Clinical characteristics of affected population. Int J Cardiol 75:129–137; discussion 138–129

27. Li W, Xiao HB, Henein MY, Somerville J, Gibson DG (2001) Progressive ECG changes before the onset of atrial flutter in adult congenital heart disease patients. Heart 85:703

28. Love BA, Collins KK, Walsh EP, Triedman JK (2001) Electroanatomic characterization of conduction barriers in sinus/atrially paced rhythm and association with intra-atrial reentrant tachycardia circuits following congenital heart disease surgery. J Cardiovasc Electrophysiol 12:17–25

29. Lukac P, Pedersen AK, Mortensen PT, Jensen HK, Hjortdal V, Hansen PS (2005) Ablation of atrial tachycardia after surgery for congenital and acquired heart disease using an electroanatomic mapping system: Which circuits to expect in which substrate? Heart Rhythm 2:64–72

30. Magnin-Poull I, De Chillou C, Miljoen H, Andronache M, Aliot E (2005) Mechanisms of right atrial tachycardia occurring late after surgical closure of atrial septal defects. J Cardiovasc Electrophysiol 16:681–687

31. Mandapati R, Walsh EP, Triedman JK (2003) Pericaval and periannular intra-atrial reentrant tachycardias in patients with congenital heart disease. J Cardiovasc Electrophysiol 14:119–125

32. McMahon CJ, Vatta M, Fraser CD Jr, Towbin JA, Chang AC (2004) Altered dystrophin expression in the right atrium of a patient after Fontan procedure with atrial flutter. Heart 90:65

33. Morwood JG, Triedman JK, Berul CI, Khairy P, Alexander ME, Cecchin F, Walsh EP (2004) Radiofrequency catheter ablation of ventricular tachycardia in children and young adults with

congenital heart disease. Heart Rhythm 1:301–308

34. Muller GI, Deal BJ, Strasburger JF, Benson DW Jr (1993) Electrocardiographic features of atrial tachycardias after operation for congenital heart disease. Am J Cardiol 71:122–124

35. Nakagawa H, Jackman WM (1998) Use of a three-dimensional, nonfluoroscopic mapping system for catheter ablation of typical atrial flutter. Pacing Clin Electrophysiol 21:1279–1286

36. Nakagawa H, Shah N, Matsudaira K, Overholt E, Chandrasekaran K, Beckman KJ, Spector P, Calame JD, Rao A, Hasdemir C, Otomo K, Wang Z, Lazzara R, Jackman WM (2001) Characterization of reentrant circuit in macroreentrant right atrial tachycardia after surgical repair of congenital heart disease: isolated channels between scars allow "focal" ablation. Circulation 103:699–709

37. Paul T, Windhagen-Mahnert B, Kriebel T, Bertram H, Kaulitz R, Korte T, Niehaus M, Tebbenjohanns J (2001) Atrial reentrant tachycardia after surgery for congenital heart disease: endocardial mapping and radiofrequency catheter ablation using a novel, noncontact mapping system. Circulation 103:2266–2271

38. Posner P, Prestwich KN, Buss DD (1985) Cardiac maturation in an hypoxic milieu: implications for arrhythmias in hypoxemic defects. Pediatr Res 19:64–66

39. Saul JP, Walsh EP, Triedman JK (1995) Mechanisms and therapy of complex arrhythmias in pediatric patients. J Cardiovasc Electrophysiol 6:1129–1148

40. Scheinman M, Calkins H, Gillette P, Klein R, Lerman BB, Morady F, Saksena S, Waldo A (2003) NASPE policy statement on catheter ablation: personnel, policy, procedures, and therapeutic recommendations. Pacing Clin Electrophysiol 26:789–799

41. Stevenson WG, Delacretaz E, Friedman PL, Ellison KE (1998) Identification and ablation of macroreentrant ventricular tachycardia with the CARTO electroanatomical mapping system. Pacing Clin Electrophysiol 21:1448–1456

42. Strasburger JF (1991) Cardiac arrhythmias in childhood. Diagnostic considerations and treatment. Drugs 42:974–983

43. Tanner H, Lukac P, Schwick N, Fuhrer J, Pedersen AK, Hansen PS, Delacretaz E (2004) Irrigated-tip catheter ablation of intraatrial reentrant tachycardia in patients late after surgery of congenital heart disease. Heart Rhythm 1:268–275

44. Triedman JK, Alexander ME, Berul CI, Bevilacqua LM, Walsh EP (2001) Electroanatomic mapping of entrained and exit zones in patients with repaired congenital heart disease and intra-atrial reentrant tachycardia. Circulation 103:2060–2065

45. Triedman JK, Alexander ME, Love BA, Collins KK, Berul CI, Bevilacqua LM, Walsh EP (2002) Influence of patient factors and ablative technologies on outcomes of radiofrequency ablation of intra-atrial re-entrant tachycardia in patients with congenital heart disease. J Am Coll Cardiol 39:1827–1835

46. Triedman JK, Bergau DM, Saul JP, Epstein MR, Walsh EP (1997) Efficacy of radiofrequency ablation for control of intraatrial reentrant tachycardia in patients with congenital heart disease. J Am Coll Cardiol 30:1032–1038

47. Triedman JK, DeLucca JM, Alexander ME, Berul CI, Cecchin F, Walsh EP (2005) Prospective trial of electroanatomically guided, irrigated catheter ablation of atrial tachycardia in patients with congenital heart disease. Heart Rhythm 2:700–705

48. Walsh EP (2002) Arrhythmias in patients with congenital heart disease. Card Electrophysiol Rev 6:422–430

49. Weipert J, Noebauer C, Schreiber C, Kostolny M, Zrenner B, Wacker A, Hess J, Lange R (2004) Occurrence and management of atrial arrhythmia after long-term Fontan circulation. J Thorac Cardiovasc Surg 127:457–464

50. Zrenner B, Dong J, Schreieck J, Ndrepepa G, Meisner H, Kaemmerer H, Schomig A, Hess J, Schmitt C (2003) Delineation of intra-atrial reentrant tachycardia circuits after mustard operation for transposition of the great arteries using biatrial electroanatomic mapping and entrainment mapping. J Cardiovasc Electrophysiol 14:1302–1310

Subject index